Neuropsychiatry
for Clinicians

Neurogenetics: A Guide for Clinicians

Edited by

Nicholas W. Wood

Galton Professor of Genetics and Head, Department of Molecular Neuroscience,
Institute of Neurology, University College London, London, UK

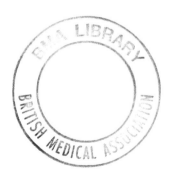

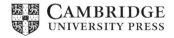

CAMBRIDGE
UNIVERSITY PRESS

CAMBRIDGE UNIVERSITY PRESS
Cambridge, New York, Melbourne, Madrid, Cape Town,
Singapore, São Paulo, Delhi, Mexico City

Cambridge University Press
The Edinburgh Building, Cambridge CB2 8RU, UK

Published in the United States of America by
Cambridge University Press, New York

www.cambridge.org
Information on this title: www.cambridge.org/9780521543729

First published 2012

Printed in the United Kingdom at the University Press, Cambridge

A catalogue record for this publication is available from the British Library

Library of Congress Cataloguing-in-Publication Data

Neurogenetics : a guide for clinicians / edited by Nicholas W. Wood.
    p. ; cm.
  Includes bibliographical references and index.
  ISBN 978-0-521-54372-9 (Paperback)
1. Nervous system–Diseases–Genetic aspects.   2. Neurogenetics.
I. Wood, N. W. (Nicholas W.)
  [DNLM: 1. Nervous System Diseases–genetics.   2. Genetic Diseases,
Inborn–etiology.   3. Genetic Testing. WL 140]
  RC346.4.N482 2012
  616.8′0442–dc23

                                                                    2011026299

ISBN 978-0-521-54372-9 Paperback

Contents

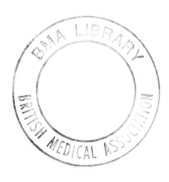

Contributors

Ammar Al-Chalabi MBChB PhD FRCP DipStat
*MRC Centre for Neurodegeneration Research,
Institute of Psychiatry, King's College London,
London, UK*

Thomas D. Bird MD
*VA Puget Sound Health Care System,
Departments of Neurology and Medical Genetics,
University of Washington,
Seattle, WA, USA*

Vincenzo Bonifati MD PhD
*Department of Clinical Genetics,
Erasmus Medical Center,
Rotterdam, the Netherlands*

Alexis Brice MD
*INSERM, UMR_S679 Neurologie and Thérapeutique
Expérimentale,
UPMC Univ Paris 06, UMR_S679 and AP-HP,
Hôpital de la Salpêtrière,
Department of Genetics and Cytogenetics,
Paris, France*

Kate Bushby MD MSc FRCP
*Institute of Human Genetics,
International Centre for Life,
Newcastle upon Tyne, UK*

John Collinge CBE MD FRCP FRS
*National Prion Clinic and MRC Prion Unit,
Department of Neurodegenerative Disease,
UCL Institute of Neurology
and the National Hospital for Neurology and
Neurosurgery, London, UK*

David Craufurd MBBS MSc FRCPsych
*Medical Genetics Research Group and Regional
Genetic Service, St Mary's Hospital,
Manchester, UK*

Odile Dubourg MD PhD
*Center of Reference for Neuromuscular Diseases,
Department of Neuropathology,
Hôpital Pitié-Salpêtrière,
Paris, France*

Rosalie E. Ferner MD MRCP
*Clinical Neuroscience,
Guy's and St Thomas' NHS Foundation Trust London
and King's College London, London, UK*

Sonia Gandhi MBBChir PhD MRCP
*Department of Molecular Neuroscience,
UCL Institute of Neurology, London, UK*

Mark Gardiner BA MD FRCP DCH
*Department of Paediatrics and Child Health,
Royal Free and University College Medical School,
London, UK*

Michael G. Hanna BSc MD FRCP
*Department of Molecular Neuroscience and
MRC Centre for Neuromuscular Disease,
UCL Institute of Neurology, London, UK*

John Hardy PhD MD(Hon) Umea FMedSci FRS
*Department of Molecular Neuroscience and
Reta Lila Weston Laboratories,
UCL Institute of Neurology, London, UK*

Peter S. Harper MA DM FRCP
*Institute of Medical Genetics,
Cardiff University, Cardiff, UK*

Dimitri M. Kullmann MA DPhil FRCP
*Department of Clinical Epilepsy,
UCL Institute of Neurology, London, UK*

Eric LeGuern MD PhD
*INSERM, UMR_S679 Neurologie and Thérapeutique
Expérimentale, UPMC Univ Paris 06,*

UMR_S679 and AP-HP, Hôpital de la Salpêtrière,
Department of Genetics and Cytogenetics,
Paris, France

Robert McFarland MA MBBS PhD MRCP MRCPCH
Mitochondrial Research Group,
Institute for Ageing and Health,
The Medical School, Newcastle University,
Newcastle upon Tyne, UK

Simon Mead PhD MRCP
National Prion Clinic and MRC Prion Unit,
Department of Neurodegenerative Disease,
UCL Institute of Neurology and the National Hospital
for Neurology and Neurosurgery, London, UK

Andrew Schaefer MBBS MRCP
Department of Neurology,
Newcastle upon Tyne Hospitals NHS Foundation
Trust, Newcastle upon Tyne, UK

**Christopher E. Shaw MBChB MD FRACP
FRCP(Hon) FMedSci**
MRC Centre for Neurodegeneration Research,
Institute of Psychiatry, King's College London,
London, UK

Una-Marie Sheerin MBBS BSc MRCP
Department of Molecular Neuroscience,
Institute of Neurology, University College London,
London, UK

Jemeen Sreedharan MBBS PhD MRCP
MRC Centre for Neurodegeneration Research,
Institute of Psychiatry, King's College London,
London, UK

S. H. Subramony MD
Department of Neurology, McKnight Brain Institute,
Gainesville, FL, USA

Sarah J. Tabrizi BSc MBChB PhD FRCP
Department of Neurodegenerative Disease,
UCL Institute of Neurology and the National
Hospital for Neurology and Neurosurgery,
London, UK

Robert Taylor PhD, FRCPath
Mitochondrial Research Group,
Institute for Ageing and Health,
The Medical School, Newcastle University,
Newcastle upon Tyne, UK

Doug Turnbull MD PhD FRCP FMedSci
Mitochondrial Research Group,
Institute for Ageing and Health,
The Medical School, Newcastle University,
Newcastle upon Tyne, UK

Caroline A. Vance MBioch MSc PhD
MRC Centre for Neurodegeneration Research,
Institute of Psychiatry, King's College London,
London, UK

Edward J. Wild MA MBBChir PhD MRCP
Department of Neurodegenerative Disease,
UCL Institute of Neurology
and the National Hospital for Neurology and
Neurosurgery, London, UK

Nicholas W. Wood PhD FRCP FMedSci
Department of Molecular Neuroscience,
UCL Institute of Neurology,
London, UK

Chapter

1

The human genome project – what it really means and where next

Sonia Gandhi and Nicholas W. Wood

Introduction

Many things in medicine and life are over-hyped and aspects of genetics and its impact are no exception. One can consider the excitement about gene therapy of a few years ago and more recently about stem cells where the public's expectations are raised so high and so quickly that nothing can survive this scrutiny. This is not the fault of the individual researchers who almost uniformly offer caution and, if anything, under-report the potential, but such is the desperation for progress in the treatment of a range of diseases that any such progress is seized upon and amplified by the press.

However, there is an area where we believe the full impact of the achievement is only just being touched on – the sequencing of the human genome. This was a huge endeavor undertaken by an international consortium and, by any measure, was a dramatic success. The United Nations Educational, Scientific, and Cultural Organization (UNESCO) universal declaration on the human genome and human rights states, "The human genome underlines the fundamental unity of all the members of the human family, as well as recognition of their inherent dignity and diversity. In a symbolic sense it is the heritage of humanity."

The 3.08 billion base pairs (bp) of *Homo sapiens*' DNA have now been sequenced and this ranks with the highest achievements of humans to date. This molecule has been reproducing itself for millions of years, and as it has mutated and under the influence of natural selection, it has resulted in the development of the myriad species on earth. To understand the significance of these mutations or variations is to start to address, at a molecular level, what makes us human and differentiates us from other species. Many more genomes have been or are being sequenced; this enables a very rapid interrogation of comparative data, what is similar and what is different between us and them. This has produced a number of really quite surprising results and we are only starting to scratch the surface of this work:

- The human genome contains somewhere between 22 000 and 25 000 genes; this is far fewer than was estimated even 10 years ago. It is also surprisingly close in number to many other vertebrates and is only about twice the number needed to produce a fruit-fly.

- Human genes show a much higher degree of alternative splicing than those of other species, so each gene can potentially make different proteins. Interestingly, it has recently been shown that sometimes these alternate transcripts can have opposing functions. There is much more work to be done here.

- Functional domains of proteins (and their DNA correlates) are frequently found in lower species. In fact, the presence of conserved sequence (DNA or amino acid) is a strong indicator of an important, even if unknown, function. This follows the idea: why would it have been so conserved across millennia of divergence if it were not important?

- More than 90% of the domains that can be identified in human proteins are also found in the fruit-fly. This indicates that the core building blocks of vertebrate biology did not need the creation of a huge number of new domains. Biology just found a new way of improving upon these core resources.

- Comparison with distant species is useful for assessing the effects and presence of evolution, but to start to better understand the function of individual genes, it will be necessary to compare closely related species – ideally, a species whose physiology, anatomy, and broad behavioral characteristics are as similar to ours as possible.

- We will also need such comparative studies not only to determine the exonic-intronic structure but also to delineate gene control mechanisms.

One of the major challenges, therefore, is how best to investigate and evaluate all these data. The field of bioinformatics is still in its infancy but one thing is certain, we are not going to be short on data. It will be the detailed and insightful organization and interrogation of the data that has the potential to deliver huge progress in the understanding of biology. The study of disease is only (albeit important) one aspect of this work. One can consider the study of the genetic aspects of disease as a way of prioritizing those variations of human DNA that should be studied in these initial stages.

Perhaps the simplest way to view disease genetics is a comparison of what we think of as simple (usually single) gene diseases and all those other traits among which are common diseases as well as the range of normal biological functions (height, intelligence, etc.). This book is concerned predominantly with the former. Of the 25 000 genes, approximately half are expressed in the nervous system (although this is a guess as one of the many other things we have to discover is the expression profiles of all the genes – both cell type and temporal). If one is to assume that mutations occur randomly, it confirms what we see in practice, namely that the nervous system has the lion's share of simple Mendelian disease. These Mendelian diseases are caused by generally rare mutation events. The changes that these mutations have produced are severe enough to produce dysfunction of the protein product, either by decreased productivity or by some novel toxic property. These mutations produce a high degree of disease risk; that is, they are the major or often the only cause of the disease. Once present on a chromosome, they carry with them a predictable recurrence risk dependent on the mode of inheritance and penetrance of the mutation.

The diseases discussed in this book are virtually all of this type, although in some cases (e.g. Parkinson's disease and Alzheimer's disease) there are familial forms caused by such mutations as well as a much greater proportion that are sporadic and where the genetic load is unknown.

Mapping the human genome
Impact of progress in sequencing

In 1980, to sequence a single 100 bp stretch in one attempt was considered a major success. Now, the large genome sequencing facilities can produce a whole human genome sequence in approximately one day. The cost of sequencing has fallen dramatically and continues to do so. Basically, the cost has halved every 22 months since 1990, and there is a stated aim to try and sequence the whole genome for $1000. This is looking increasingly achievable and it is likely that it will be a part of the medical assessment of the patient. We are entering an era where data will not be in short supply, but assigning meaning is the next great challenge.

Genetic variation and human disease

The assignment of a mutation in a gene causing a human disease is the first step in this process. In the initial phases of disease gene discovery, the defect was usually identified by the nature of its function. For example, a known enzyme deficiency was presumed and then proven to be because of a genetic defect in the gene encoding that enzyme. This only accounted for a very small proportion of disease gene discovery and most of the progress over the past 15 years has been a result of positional cloning (described in more detail in Chapter 2). As a result of this process, the gene is identified but its function is often obscure. However, the very fact that a mutation is shown to cause a phenotype quite quickly leads to testable hypotheses as to the gene's function. What is frequently forgotten, not least by the scientists themselves, is that the gene may have many functions, and labeling it as the Huntington's disease gene or the Parkinson's disease gene is just the tag line that has helped identification, and it is highly likely that its normal function is more complex than at first imagined. These major disease-causing genetic mutations are rare and yet variation throughout the genome is very common. Currently, the belief is that much of this variation is neutral and of no major genomic importance; however, such is the scale of the variation that even functionality of a tiny percentage leaves a large number of variants worthy of study. Human disease is believed by many (including these authors) to be a powerful and valuable tool for unlocking these functions. If one can identify variation that is shown to increase the risk of a disease, for example epilepsy, one can build a much more comprehensive picture of the genetic and molecular events that control seizures. Moreover, this knowledge would shed light on the normal physiology of nerve cells, how seizures start, and why they are self-limiting.

The simplest method (at least in theory) to access this, is to discover all human variants and assay them in one's case-control series of interest. However, still very few human genomes have been sequenced in their entirety and it will be some years before an attempt of this sort is feasible. Even if this were not a sufficient barrier, there is the major issue of genetic heterogeneity. One of the major lessons from Mendelian disease is that different mutations in the same gene may cause different phenotypes (allelic heterogeneity), and that mutations in different genes can cause the same phenotype (genetic heterogeneity). These facts are borne out in nearly all the subsequent disease-based chapters. Therefore, it seems fairly safe to say that genetic variation of this more subtle variety is going to be even more difficult to identify. This will require the use of large sample sizes (probably 1000s) and, more importantly, clever phenotype definition and application. It may be that relatively little progress is made using the current clinico-pathological phenotypes, and now there is much attention toward defining other phenotypes such as intermediate or endophenotypes. The basic principle here is that a component of the disease (e.g. some cognitive measure in schizophrenia) is genetically simpler, more heritable, and ultimately tractable and, therefore, will be easier to identify.

Pharmacogenetics

One human disease area for which there is rising hope of early success is the field of pharmacogenetics. The principle is that the trait (drug responsiveness or side-effect profile) is molecularly and genetically simpler. Additionally, the candidate gene list is more modest and chiefly comprises the metabolizer, transporter, or target of the drug. There is also the hope that were we to discover the variants that determine one's likelihood of responding and not developing side-effects, this would have a tremendous benefit to drug trial design and would likely impact on healthcare sooner than the discovery of disease-associated causal variants of otherwise unknown function. This field is moving rapidly, and it is highly likely that genetic testing before prescribing will become routine within a few years. Finally, if one considers a field such as epilepsy, most of the known drug targets for anti-epileptic drugs (e.g. ion channels, transporters, etc.) have also been shown to be mutated in some, usually rare forms of familial epilepsies. It is, therefore,

reasonable to expect, if one turns this around, to say that the finding of new genetic variants responsible for epilepsy provides new drug targets.

BioBank

One of the major difficulties with association study design of the sort needed to find disease susceptibility genes is the danger of biases in controls or the cases, which lead to false-positive association (discussed in more detail in Chapter 2). One way around this is to access incident cases. The United Kingdom has established a BioBank of 500 000 individuals who will provide lifestyles, environmental factors, and a DNA sample. As these individuals succumb to disease, the frequencies of DNA variations between those in the cohort who have a certain disease trait and those who do not will provide a great potential for disentangling putative gene–environment interactions. This resource has only just begun to be collected and it will be many years before its full benefits are felt.

An important initial step in creating the capacity for exploiting such a resource has come from the large case-control consortia, which recently have started to report on large-scale, systematic, genome-wide association studies in common diseases.

Other tools to help improve understanding

The encyclopaedia of DNA elements project

The ENCODE project was begun in 2003 and is endeavoring to identify the functional elements in the genome. The human genome sequence is basically a list of ingredients; we have virtually no idea how this recipe is acted upon to produce a functioning human (or any other life form, for that matter). A key element of this process is the regulatory control of switching genes on or off, and what determines the expression level and splicing variation. This project seeks to characterize enhancers, promoters, protein binding sites, and other regulatory elements. It is starting with a selected 1%, and it is hoped that what is learnt form this initial study will have lessons for the rest of the genome.

The knockout mouse project

When a disease-associated gene is found, one of the first questions is: what does it do? The usual answer is that we do not know. We gain some insights into the question by asking what it looks like, especially if it encodes domains that look very like something else about which we do know something, such as a kinase domain. However, these musings only take us so far; of major importance is what it does in a living system; better still, if it is closely related to us; for example, a mammal. Inevitably, the laboratory concerned or, more usually, one sets up experiments that manipulate the gene, knocking out or in, or doing so only when conditions are appropriate (conditional knockouts). Now there is an international project to provide publicly available knockouts of every mouse gene. It is sometimes the case that knocking out a gene, which is needed early in development, produces embryonic lethality in the homozygous state. Therefore, a system of conditional knockouts is also being generated – dependent on external triggers, the mouse gene can be knocked out at any stage, so one can let the mouse develop and then switch the gene off, as required. These resources will be hugely valuable to genomic science and understanding disease-causing mutations.

Comparative genomics

Advanced draft or complete sequences are now available for five mammals – human, mouse, rat, chimpanzee, and dog. Many other vertebrates are close behind these. The ability to compare the basic coded differences between the species is now within sight and the potential gains, as detailed above, are enormous.

Summary

The future for genetic medicine is bright. Soon we will know much more about human genetic variation, genomic control, and even how we got to the top of the evolutionary tree (at least for the time being). For those interested in the nervous system and neurobiology, the impact this field will make will be huge. It will become unimaginable to future generations that we could hope to understand the nervous system without discovering and studying the building blocks; however, that is for the future. This book attempts to synthesize what we know now and a little of how we got here. It is divided into the major disease areas and, as can be seen from scanning the contents page, the impacts have already been felt in virtually all branches of neurology. Fortunately, genetics is simple and if one can get past the jargon, one is left with a couple of rules

(formulated by Mendel) and a huge improvement in our technical ability to investigate the processes.

Neurogenetics is still in its infancy but it is now part of the core curriculum of most residency training schemes. This book hopes to provide both the neurologist in training as well as some of the neurologists who trained before these developments with the core discoveries and excitement of the field. Of course, it is a rapidly moving field and there will be some genes that will be discovered between finishing the writing and the book appearing on the shelves. However, we hope that these new discoveries can be tagged on to the basics discussed here.

Box 1 Decoding the jargon

- Allele – we all have two sets of chromosomes and hence two copies of a gene. If these vary (which they often do), these different forms are called alleles.
- BAC (bacterial artificial chromosome) – a useful packing tool used to engineer and handle quite large pieces of DNA.
- Cloning – a process of generating as many copies of a given piece of DNA as required. It has been the bedrock of the major developments.
- cDNA (complementary DNA) – a copy of a transcribed gene as it uses mRNA as its template. DNA is more stable and therefore easier to handle.
- Conservation – genes or fragments of genes can be compared across species; those present in more than one organism are said to be conserved. Generally, the greater the conservation (i.e. the more species in which any given gene is basically the same), the more fundamental and important this DNA structure is.
- EST (expressed sequence tag) – short segments of DNA corresponding to a piece of cDNA and, therefore, representing a tag for a gene as opposed to a non-transcribed part of the DNA.
- Genome – a complete description of the DNA sequence of an organism.
- Genotype – usually means the combination of two alleles that an individual carries at any given gene locus.
- Haplotype – a combination of alleles found tightly associated with one another. It forms the basis of much of the current hunt for genes underlying common forms of disease (see Chapter 2).
- Introns and exons – genes are not coded in solid blocks of sequence; the coding segments are called exons and the stretches (intervening

---

Box 1 (*cont.*)

segments) are introns. The function of introns is unknown, but it is emerging that there is some conservation in some stretches implying an as yet unknown function (see conservation). This biunitary arrangement allows for the selection of parts or all of the coding components of the gene (i.e. alternative splicing).

- mRNA – this is the message created from the DNA template. The RNA copies across the whole gene (introns and exons), and then molecular machinery (the splicesome) cuts out the intronic segments, leaving the messenger RNA to move out to the ribosome to undergo translation.
- Mutation – a change in the DNA sequence to a reference state (usually some ancestral sequence). Although used most frequently to imply a pathological state, this is most often not the case (see polymorphism).
- Phenotype – the physical characteristics of a cell or organism. From a medical point of view, it is used as the description of a disease state.
- Polymorphism – a mutation that is above a certain frequency in the population (usually >1%). Generally used to denote a variation that is not implicated in disease causation, but even this will change as more functional characteristics are applied to these polymorphisms (see Chapter 2).
- Proteome – the complete set of proteins encode by the genome.
- Recombination – along with mutation, this is the engine behind diversity and evolution. It is also the point of gender as it allows crossing-over of DNA from one ancestral chromosome to the other. It is used by geneticists to help map disease genes.

- SNP (single nucleotide polymorphism) – hugely common polymorphisms (about one every 1000 bp). These are receiving a lot of attention to inform on our evolutionary past and help map the risk of common diseases (see Chapter 2).
- Splicing – the process of intron removal and also of excluding certain exons at certain times (alternate splicing).
- Transcription – the process of copying from the DNA code into RNA.
- Transcriptome – the complete set of mRNAs transcribed from a gene.
- Translation – the process of building a specific sequence of DNA based upon the mRNA message. This is performed by ribosomes.

Useful websites

OMIM: http://www.ncbi.nlm.nih.gov/sites/entrez?db=omim

GeneClinics and Gene Tests: http://www.geneclinics.org/

UKGTN: http://www.ukgtn.nhs.uk/gtn/

Rare diseases: http://www.orpha.net/consor/cgi-bin/home.php?Lng=GB

GENDIA (Genetic diagnostics): http://www.gendia.net/index.html

Web pages with useful documents related to genetic counseling and testing:

http://www.hdfoundation.org/resources/testing.php

http://www.genome.gov/19516567

http://www.eurogentest.org/

http://www.gig.org.uk/index.html

Chapter 2

Genetic counseling and genetic testing for neurogenetic disorders

David Craufurd and Peter S. Harper

Introduction

Advances in genetics have probably had more practical applications in the field of the inherited neurological disorders than in any other area of medicine. It is thus essential that all clinicians involved with these conditions, whether as a specialist in the field or as part of more general neurological practice, are fully informed about what the applications of genetics can offer patients and their families. Being fully informed does not mean that they need to be directly involved in all these applications, although increasingly, some areas are forming part of regular clinical practice; even more important is to know one's own limitations and what can be offered by other services, including clinical and laboratory genetics for inherited disorders.

The complex and extensive field that has evolved (and is still evolving), known as neurogenetics, contains not only a very wide range of different types of disorder, but also workers with very different backgrounds and skills, a factor that greatly influences how genetic advances are applied.

Among neurologists, some will have a strong research and academic orientation, while others will have a more service oriented approach. There is a major difference in most countries between pediatric and adult neurology, while among neurologists specializing in the latter, there is often a strong distinction between those involved primarily in neuromuscular diseases and those whose focus is on central nervous system (CNS) disorders. The types of neurogenetic disorder seen will vary greatly according to these groups (see Table 2.1).

Among clinical geneticists, likewise, there is considerable variety. Some will have a strong research and clinical interest in specific areas of inherited neurological disease and, especially in the United Kingdom, may be integrally involved in long-term management, often jointly with relevant neurologists. Others may be more laboratory oriented.

Table 2.1. Principal groups of neurogenetic disorders

Childhood
Neurodevelopmental defects
Progressive childhood neurodegenerations
Non-progressive neurometabolic disorders
Neuromuscular disorders
More common childhood neurological disorders with a complex genetic basis
Mainly adult
Progressive late-onset central nervous system degenerations
Progressive neuromuscular disorders
More common adult disorders with a complex genetic basis

It follows from this diversity of both disorders and professionals that it is neither possible nor wise to lay down strict rules for how and by whom genetic services should be applied in practice, but some useful guidelines are possible, and we hope that some of the key points will emerge from this chapter.

Patterns of inheritance

Most professionals involved with neurogenetic disorders will have at least a simple knowledge of genetics and transmission within families, but it is worth pointing out here how this influences the various practical applications now possible for families. Some of the pitfalls are also important to note. For those requiring more detail, there are several simple books available.

A remarkably high number of serious neurological disorders follow single-gene Mendelian inheritance, in both childhood and adult life; it is in this group where genetic risks are often high and where applications are possible. Therefore, it is vital that clinicians are aware of and alert for Mendelian conditions among the much larger numbers of disorders showing a more complex inheritance that they see.

Autosomal recessive inheritance

This type of inheritance underlies numerous childhood neurogenetic disorders, many developmental in origin, others more progressive and with a defined metabolic or biochemical basis. Increasingly, these two groups are merging and the concept of inborn errors of development is becoming established alongside inborn errors of metabolism, as the molecular pathways of development are becoming clearer.

At a practical level, the only high genetic risk in families where an autosomal recessive disorder has occurred is for siblings (one in four); because almost all are extremely rare outside unusual populations, the chance of a homozygous affected individual occurring among offspring, offspring of healthy siblings, or cousins is extremely rare. Heterozygous carriers of such genes are almost invariably entirely healthy, an important factor in genetic counseling as increasing numbers found to be heterozygous after a genetic test are worried by their status and convinced that they have or will develop a mild form of the disorder in question. In fact, it should rarely be necessary to undertake carrier testing unless there are particular circumstances; if it is done, it is essential to emphasize the lack of clinical (and usually genetic) significance of being a carrier.

Consanguinity, frequent in many populations across the world, may raise special issues when a recessively inherited genetic disorder is diagnosed in the family. Here it is important that any genetic risk can be balanced against the social benefits involved; an accurate estimate of risk, based on the degree of relationship of partners to the affected individual, is essential in allowing individuals to make informed decisions.

Autosomal dominant inheritance

Such inheritance is seen in a series of important, progressive neuromuscular and CNS disorders of later life, and may present particular challenges owing to late onset, variability, and the existence of extended family at significant risk. For all these reasons, the clinical geneticist is likely to be involved in genetic applications to a much greater extent than is the case

Table 2.2. Genetic counseling issues in Huntington's disease and other late-onset autosomal dominant disorders

Stigma of disorder – family and wider attitudes
Variability – in severity and age at onset
Uncertainty – arising from variability
Numerous relatives often at risk – issues of extended family
Serious implications for unaffected heterozygotes
Possibility of unusual genetic mechanisms (see Table 2.3)

for many childhood autosomal recessive disorders, where the pediatrician or pediatric neurologist often will have the principal role. Despite the deceptively simple inheritance pattern – a 50% risk for offspring of an affected patient and no significant risk for offspring of an unaffected relative – the practical situation is often complex and full of pitfalls. A paradigm of the problems is provided by Huntington's disease (HD), a disorder with which we, the authors, have been extensively involved over many years.

Leaving aside the issues of predictive testing, which will be discussed later in the chapter, HD shows, in clear-cut form, many of the problems that are present, although to a lesser degree, in other neurogenetic disorders; Table 2.2 summarizes some of these. Stigma associated with the disorder remains a very real factor, despite the development of active support groups; the combination of psychiatric and physical problems creates a special burden for families and may make people reluctant to seek advice or help. Variability in age at onset (and in clinical features) has the consequence of uncertainty, which many people at risk find very hard to live with and which has major personal consequences for relationships and life decisions generally. This is one of the main reasons for people seeking predictive testing.

Extended families

Such families may indeed be extended and extensive, creating real issues as to how far a professional should go in contacting those at risk who may be unaware of it. The skills and facilities needed to handle these often difficult family situations are very different from those required for the clinically affected individual, and it is largely for such reasons that the clinical geneticist takes the main role in such cases. Indeed,

Table 2.3. Unusual genetic mechanisms in dominantly inherited neurogenetic disease that may affect genetic risks and genetic counseling

Mechanism	Examples
Gonadal mosaicism	Tuberous sclerosis, Charcot–Marie–Tooth disease
Anticipation from genetic instability	Myotonic dystrophy, Huntington's disease, spinocerebellar ataxias
Parent-of-origin effects	Juvenile Huntington's disease, congenital myotonic dystrophy
Genetic imprinting	Angelman syndrome

it is a general finding that many clinicians are not fully aware of the fact that most individuals requesting and requiring genetic services are not patients at all but are healthy individuals. Most neurologists (like other clinicians) wish to spend their time with those actually affected with a particular disorder, rather than with healthy family members, so it is here (as discussed in relation to general principles of genetic counseling) that establishing the appropriate balance and relationships between neurologist and clinical geneticist is important.

Implications for gene carriers

For gene carriers, the implications are completely different in dominant from recessive inheritance, a point obvious to professionals but often less so to families. Thus, a healthy carrier for the mutation almost inevitably will develop the condition at some future point, in contrast to carriers for autosomal recessive disorders, who will remain healthy. Not all dominant disorders are similar to HD in this respect, however. For myotonic dystrophy, the detection of a mutation in a healthy adult may well mean a milder (possibly minimal) disorder in later life in comparison to those showing early onset disease.

Unusual genetic mechanisms

Unusual genetic mechanisms are a particular pitfall for autosomal dominant disorders and some of these are summarized in Table 2.3. Inherited neurological disorders have proved to involve a remarkable number of these and their elucidation has led to major discoveries in our understanding of genetic mechanisms and pathogenesis, having implications for medicine more widely. At the practical level of

genetic counseling, these may considerably modify risks given to those seeking advice. Thus, gonadal mosaicism means that the recurrence risk for the siblings of an apparently isolated case is not zero but about 1%–3% according to the disorder, on account of the possibility of a parent carrying the mutation in the germline even though appearing to be entirely normal clinically. Such affected sibships with normal parents may mimic recessive inheritance (as in Charcot–Marie–Tooth disease). Anticipation resulting from genetic instability, seen notably in myotonic dystrophy but also in other trinucleotide repeat disorders, means that not only may the severity be greater and onset earlier for offspring, but that parent-of-origin effects may be seen, as in the greater likelihood of juvenile HD with paternal transmission, and the predominant paternal origin of kindreds from healthy individuals with an intermediate allele. Genetic imprinting, owing to differences in gene activation during male and female transmission, may also underlie parent-of-origin effects.

An important cause of variability in dominantly inherited disorders, in particular tumors, is the necessity for a somatic mutation, often a result of chromosomal loss, to occur on the opposite chromosome in order for a dominantly inherited condition to express itself. This two-hit hypothesis is seen in such tumor syndromes as von Hippel–Lindau disease and in other (mainly non-neurological) cancers determined by tumor suppressor genes. As a result, while the transmission pattern for susceptibility is dominant, there may be considerable variability according to whether or where the necessary second somatic event takes place.

In summary, genetic counseling for autosomal dominant disorders may be straightforward, but frequently is not, as the space devoted to the topic in this chapter has tried to indicate.

X-linked inheritance

Although the number of neurogenetic disorders inherited on the X chromosome is relatively limited, they produce practical issues out of all proportion to their frequency, with potential difficulties not seen in autosomal inheritance. Table 2.4 lists some of the more frequent and important conditions in this group.

The first point to be noted is that X-linked disorders usually cannot be classified strictly as recessive or

Table 2.4. Important neurogenetic disorders following X-linked inheritance

Neurodevelopmental

    Hydrocephalus (specific type)

    Incontinentia pigmenti (lethal in males)

    Pelizaeus Merzbacher disease

Metabolic

    Adrenoleukodystrophy

    Lesch–Nyhan syndrome (hypoxanthine-guanine phosphoribosyltransferase deficiency)

    Menkes syndrome

    Mucopolysaccharidosis type 2 (Hunter syndrome)

Neuromuscular

    Charcot–Marie–Tooth disease (one type)

    Muscular dystrophy (Duchenne and Becker types)

    Muscular dystrophy (Emery–Dreifuss type)

    Myotubular myopathy (one type)

Central nervous system

    Kallmann syndrome

    Spinobulbar muscular atrophy (Kennedy's disease)

dominant. Heterozygous females commonly show some degree of clinical involvement, and the frequency and extent of this varies greatly according to the disorder. Thus, for some disorders (e.g. type 2 mucopolysaccharidosis and Lesch–Nyhan disease) significant clinical involvement in heterozygotes is exceptional, while in others (e.g. adrenoleukodystrophy and X-linked Charcot–Marie–Tooth disease) it is relatively frequent. A manifesting female may present with an apparently different phenotype and, in the absence of an affected male in the family, be misdiagnosed (e.g. Duchenne muscular dystrophy, adrenoleukodystrophy). In some disorders (e.g. X-linked hyperammonemia), clinical problems may occur only under conditions of metabolic stress.

In the past, this clinical variability of heterozygotes, reflecting variation in X-chromosome inactivation, was also seen in tests of carrier detection, making it impossible to reassure women at risk completely, on the basis of a normal result (e.g. creatine kinase in Duchenne dystrophy). This problem has largely been removed by DNA-based tests, where the heterozygous state can be seen unambiguously.

A surprising number of clinicians are still confused by the basic pattern of X-linked transmission for the offspring of affected males (e.g. Becker muscular dystrophy, X-linked Charcot–Marie–Tooth disease). Because a man cannot transmit his only X chromosome to a son, all such sons (and their descendants) have no genetic risk; however, as all his daughters will receive his X chromosome, they will all (not 50%!) be heterozygous carriers. This is one of the few genetic situations (barring issues of paternity) where one comes close to certainty.

Mitochondrial inheritance

A small but important group of neurogenetic disorders are determined not by nuclear genes but by genes forming part of the mitochondrial genome. Included in this group are progressive disorders of childhood and adult life, which may affect either the CNS, muscle, or both, as well as other systems. From the viewpoint of genetic counseling, the key factor is whether the germline is involved. Some disorders (e.g. most cases of myoclonic epilepsy with ragged red fibers [MERRF] and mitochondrial myopathy, encephalopathy, lactic acidosis, and stroke [MELAS]) are associated often with large somatic deletions of mitochondrial DNA and are usually sporadic. Others (notably Leber's hereditary optic neuropathy) are the result of germline mitochondrial point mutations and may be maternally inherited; there is virtually no risk of transmission through the male line – a helpful point for genetic counseling.

For female transmissions, this situation is made more complicated by the frequent occurrence of heteroplasmy, the presence of both a normal and abnormal mitochondrial cell line, which gives a variable risk for offspring of affected women. Unfortunately, molecular testing is often unable to give greater precision, as the degree of heteroplasmy varies from tissue to tissue, and can only be an approximate guide to the likelihood of clinical problems occurring.

General principles of genetic counseling

No attempt is made here to cover the psychological or even the more generic counseling aspects of genetic counseling, although these are of great importance and need to be considered by all those intending to be involved. It is important, however, to consider

Table 2.5. General aims of genetic counseling

Information on genetic risks
Information on wider aspects of the disorder
Clarification of genetic and diagnostic uncertainties
Information on further genetic options (including genetic testing)
Information on possibilities for management, therapy, prenatal diagnosis
Supportive but nondirective framework for all the above

some of the main general factors, and the first of these is: what are the aims of genetic counseling? Table 2.5 summarizes some of these, and also some of the aspects that are not (at least in our opinion) valid aims, but which may be considered as such (and have been, in the distant past), at times with disastrous consequences.

The main reason why people request genetic counseling is to obtain accurate information on the risks of a possibly genetic disease occurring in themselves, their children, existing or future, or in other relatives. Alongside this numerical risk, accurate information is needed on the disease itself, its range of severity, age at onset, and system involvement, as well as present and likely future possibilities for therapy. Such information is often more important, although also often less certain, than the actual risk of recurrence, and assessing it may require considerable clinical as well as genetic expertise.

Particularly for those where the genetic risk is high and the disorder serious, genetic testing may be required, as covered more fully later in the chapter. Such testing may be a necessary part of making a specific genetic diagnosis in an affected individual; it may be needed for establishing or excluding the heterozygous carrier state; it may be used for predictive (presymptomatic) testing, or prenatal or (at a very early stage) preimplantation genetic diagnosis.

All these important options need to be considered in the light of the more general aspects of genetic counseling. The interpretation of and need for genetic tests may depend critically on the risk situation of the individual and on his/her wishes; indiscriminate use of tests on those not at significant risk or not wishing for them is not good clinical practice. In this respect, it should be noted that people often may request testing when what they really wish for (and need) is

a more general provision of information, which may (or may not) involve an actual laboratory test. Unfortunately, often it is easier to fill in a form and send a sample to the laboratory than to undertake the more time-consuming course of exploring what a person's wishes and worries actually are.

An essential component of genetic counseling is a nondirective approach, allowing the individual (or couple) to make their own informed decision, rather than being told what is best for them. This approach differs considerably from most in diagnostic or therapeutic medicine, where patients generally will wish to be guided regarding the best course. As clinicians ourselves, involved in both genetic counseling and management of particular disorders, we have found it a considerable challenge at times to separate the different roles. It is important, however, not to confuse nondirectiveness with lack of support – providing a supportive framework is essential if people are to be able to reach often difficult and traumatic decisions, as with presymptomatic or prenatal testing – while continuing support, regardless of what decision has been made, is equally important.

An essential component of genetic counseling is adequate time, and this actually is the most difficult and most expensive factor to preserve in most healthcare systems. It is simply not possible to deal with the complex issues, genetic and personal, that arise in genetic counseling without having adequate time, generally one hour for a new consultation. If one does not have this time available, it is better not even to try to be involved in genetic counseling, as it is likely to do more harm than good. A hurried consultation may leave people confused, with vital questions unanswered and the real issues never surfacing. Most patients and their families remain remarkably considerate of doctors and, when faced with an obviously busy or hurried clinician, often will decide not to raise questions that they know are going to be difficult to answer.

It goes without saying that anyone involved with genetic counseling needs to be a good communicator. We all consider ourselves to be able at this (although an objective opinion from others is likely to be a better guide!). Important elements include a sympathetic as well as knowledgeable approach; enjoying relating to people and their problems; willingness to listen, not just to talk; an ability to use simple language and to avoid technical details; and projecting a feeling of supportiveness. Even those who are good communicators can become much better by learning some of the underlying principles from someone already expert in counseling and psychotherapeutic skills. Of course, these communication aspects are no substitute for detailed genetic and neurological expertise, but they are equally necessary.

In the same way as time is the main general prerequisite for genetic counseling, so the setting is the most important facility. Here again, the busy management or diagnostic setting is not appropriate, especially as most people seen are healthy individuals. A less medical and more reassuring environment is required, even though examination and other medical facilities need to be at hand. Similarly, while most children's clinics now go out of their way to be informal and child-friendly, the general noise and distraction makes them an unsatisfactory environment for genetic counseling.

The previous comments may make more general clinicians feel excluded from undertaking genetic counseling, but this is not what we intend, both of us being practicing clinicians ourselves. Rather, it is essential for any clinician to recognize that genetic counseling requires approaches, skills, and settings different from those of most conventional medical clinics; increasingly in neurogenetics, neurologists and geneticists need to and are working in partnership to provide optimal services to families with inherited neurological disorders.

Genetic testing for inherited neurological disorders

Genetic testing now forms an important and integral part of both neurological and clinical genetics practice and has greatly enhanced both diagnostic precision and the options associated with genetic counseling. This situation has been the result almost entirely of the development of molecular tests for specific genes, initially based on linked genetic markers, but now mainly on techniques that directly detect the mutations responsible for neurogenetic disorders. Chromosome analysis and molecular cytogenetic *in situ* hybridization techniques and fluorescence *in situ* hybridization (FISH) are also relevant, especially for childhood neurodevelopmental disorders. The technological aspects are not covered in this chapter, and the focus will be on the use and implications of testing, especially in relation to genetic counseling.

Genetic tests can be used in several different contexts for inherited neurological disorders: primary diagnosis, carrier detection, presymptomatic (predictive) testing, and prenatal (including preimplantation) diagnosis. While the laboratory aspects of these three categories are often similar, or even identical, the implications and appropriate use differ widely, and it is essential that all those using these tests appreciate this.

Primary diagnostic genetic testing

Molecular analysis of a blood sample can replace more invasive neurological procedures, such as muscle biopsy or electrophysiology, in making a primary diagnosis; the specificity and sensitivity of the test will vary greatly according to the number of mutations or presence of multiple loci, as well as technical factors. These are discussed in some of the following chapters. For some disorders, notably trinucleotide repeat disorders such as myotonic dystrophy and HD, both specificity and sensitivity of molecular testing are remarkable.

Such diagnostic molecular genetic testing now is increasingly integrated with other aspects of diagnosis and used by relevant clinicians when a particular neurogenetic disorder is suspected. This is entirely acceptable provided that those involved have used them appropriately; in particular, it is essential that clinicians inform the patient of the nature of the test and any genetic implications that an abnormal result might have. Equally, a test is only diagnostic when carried out on a symptomatic patient, where symptoms or clinical features are consistent with the disorder being tested for. Use of tests in a random or blanket manner is inappropriate, while use in a relative whose symptoms are nonspecific or unrelated may end in a predictive test for which the individual is unprepared and which may be unwanted.

Carrier detection

The distinction between autosomal (and most X-linked) recessive disorders where carriers are likely to remain healthy and those late-onset disorders where a healthy mutation carrier is likely to develop the condition at a later date has already been emphasized; testing of this latter group should be regarded as presymptomatic and is discussed later in the chapter. Most carrier testing needs to be undertaken in the wider context of genetic counseling so that the overall genetic risk situation for offspring can be given, taking into account the specific family situation. A laboratory result in isolation is often meaningless. In addition, it needs to be remembered that in a family with a rare autosomal recessive disorder, the risk for offspring will be affected much more by the carrier status of the unrelated partner than by that of the relative, something that will depend on the population frequency of the disorder. Risk estimations in relation to carrier testing for both autosomal and X-linked recessive disorders may, in fact, be quite complex and may need the overall family structure to be considered.

Presymptomatic (predictive) testing

For the relatively small but often serious group of late-onset autosomal dominant disorders, presymptomatic testing is a complex process that can tax the counseling skills of the most experienced person. Our greatest experience has come from HD, for which such testing has been possible for nearly 20 years. In the United Kingdom during this time, about 5000 individuals have received a presymptomatic test result, and the existence of a consortium of all centers involved has allowed a large amount of anonymous information to be pooled and valuable lessons to be learnt about problems and how to achieve best practice. The issues for other late-onset neurological disorders, such as familial Alzheimer's disease (AD), prion dementias, spinocerebellar ataxias, and cerebral autosomal dominant arteriopathy with subcortical infarcts and leukoencephalopathy (CADASIL), are essentially similar, while outside the neurological field, presymptomatic testing for the familial cancers has developed along comparable lines.

Table 2.6 summarizes some of the numerous issues that need to be considered in relation to presymptomatic testing; it can be seen immediately that their complexity makes it completely inappropriate for such testing to be undertaken as a laboratory-only activity, without an appropriate framework for preparation and support. As a result of the time needed and family-based nature of many of the principal issues, this is a field best handled by those trained in clinical genetics, although there are important occasions when a neurologist or psychiatrist will need to be involved, particularly when an individual requesting testing shows suspicious neurological or psychiatric features raising the possibility that they may be clinically affected already.

Table 2.6. Presymptomatic testing for Huntington's disease and related disorders: the main issues

Does the individual really wish for testing?

Can the person give full consent?

Do the individual and family understand all the implications (and limitations)?

Issues involving family

Issues involving work, insurance, wider life

Disclosure and confidentiality issues

Support following test result

Among the issues listed in Table 2.6, some deserve particular mention. Given that only about 20% of those at high risk actually decide to be tested [1–3], it is essential to be sure that the person requesting testing really wishes for it and has not made a request under pressure from family or professionals, and that he/she understands the serious implications that an abnormal result may have for numerous aspects of his/her life. Because fully informed consent for such a serious step is clearly essential, there is general agreement that the testing of young children unable to consent is unethical [4], even if the parents are requesting this. Requests for predictive testing from individuals at 25% risk (i.e. with an affected grandparent) also give rise to significant ethical concerns where there is an intervening at-risk parent who would prefer not to know his/her carrier status. Family dynamics and wishes in relation to the presymptomatic testing are frequently complex and conflicting at times; clearly such issues need to be resolved before testing is done. Given the complexity and gravity of these and other issues, it is not surprising that some people change their minds, or decide to postpone testing until they feel clearer about their wishes.

The large amount of experience with presymptomatic testing has resulted in internationally agreed protocols suitable for application in practice [5]. Table 2.7 summarizes the main features. Generally, two specific interviews are required before the result is given; not only is there too much information to be fitted into a single interview, but an interval is necessary to allow the individual to reassess whether testing is indeed the right course for him/her.

Given the problematic nature of HD presymptomatic testing, it may well be asked whether it has

Table 2.7. Presymptomatic testing for Huntington's disease: internationally agreed framework (also appropriate for other late-onset neurogenetic disorders)

Interview one

    Sociodemographic details

    Confirmation of family and clinical data

    Assessment of impact of Huntington's disease and test results

    Assessment of knowledge of Huntington's disease and presymptomatic testing

    Reasons for requesting prediction

    Neurological examination

Interview two

    Assessment of psychological, personality, and social characteristics using standardized instruments

    Further counseling and discussion of disclosure session

    Nomination of professional supporter

    Signing and consent form

    Final blood sample

Interview three (held 4 weeks later)

    Disclosure of results

Formal followup

    1 week (telephone)

    3 months

    12 months

resulted in major adverse events in those tested. Fortunately, UK and international data show that this is not the case. Very few instances of suicide, attempted suicide, or major psychiatric episodes have occurred [6]; most of these have been in individuals close to the onset of the disorder but, importantly, some have been in people proving to have a normal test result. There is some evidence that individuals who choose to proceed with testing may be a self-selected group who are more confident of their ability to cope with the emotions associated with an unfavorable test result than are those who decide against testing [7]. Even so, it seems likely, though is not proven, that the thorough preparation and supportive framework used universally in the United Kingdom and most other countries has allowed for this difficult process to be undertaken with as few problems as can be expected. Where there are adjustment problems after unfavorable test results, it is as likely to be the spouse/partner of the at-risk person who experiences difficulty, especially when the partner would not have chosen to be tested [8,9].

Prenatal diagnosis

In contrast to presymptomatic testing, which is used mainly in the context of late-onset neurogenetic disorders, prenatal diagnosis has its main role with serious childhood conditions, especially those following autosomal recessive inheritance, where the one-in-four recurrence risk may deter couples from having further children unless prenatal diagnosis is available. In this group, biochemical prenatal diagnosis has been available for many years, and now is used often in conjunction with molecular analysis.

Development of molecular and, in some cases, molecular cytogenetic techniques has widened the scope of prenatal diagnosis for serious childhood neurogenetic disease to include many developmental disorders involving the brain. Many of the tests involved are for exceptionally rare disorders and may only be possible in a small number of laboratories worldwide. Fortunately, the development of effective networks among genetics laboratories is increasingly allowing the service delivery of tests for these rare disorders to families, as well as ensuring satisfactory experience and quality for the laboratories involved.

While it is the pediatric neurologist who will be involved with the care of most families requiring neurological prenatal diagnosis, it is also an issue that clinical geneticists and adult neurologists may encounter in relation to late-onset disorders. However, even for such serious conditions as HD, prenatal diagnosis is requested relatively rarely, in about one tenth of the frequency of presymptomatic tests shown by a collaborative European study [10].

Most prenatal diagnosis using molecular techniques uses samples of chorionic villi obtained at approximately 10 weeks of pregnancy. It should be remembered that the risk to the pregnancy of this procedure is not negligible (1%–2%), and that plans for the analysis, with identification of the appropriate molecular defect in an affected individual, need to be made before pregnancy whenever possible.

Preimplantation genetic diagnosis may prove to be a preferable alternative to the use of prenatal diagnosis and avoid the necessity for termination of pregnancy; for the foreseeable future, however, there are likely to remain considerable limitations to its use. The technology of using a single cell from an early embryo for molecular analysis is now well established in a small number of specialist centers, and experience has been reported for HD [11] and myotonic dystrophy. The success rate of in vitro fertilization (IVF), in terms of established pregnancies, remains low (about 20% per cycle), and the combination of uncertainty of outcome, complex technological procedures, and limited availability mean that most couples still prefer to utilize early prenatal diagnosis.

Population screening and neurogenetic disorders

Most genetic counseling, and indeed most medical practice, takes place in the context of help being actively sought by individuals because of the disorder in themselves or in a family member. In this situation, it is not surprising that even limited degrees of therapeutic help or information on genetic risks are welcomed and that most people receiving genetic counseling are less worried as a result of it. By comparison, with population screening, those detected as being at high risk will generally not have been aware of the problem beforehand and are likely to be poorly informed, although extremely concerned, if a problem is indeed found.

Currently, there are few situations in neurogenetics where such an active approach is justified; the most widespread is prenatal screening for neural tube defects, initially developed using biochemical serum markers but now largely dependent on sensitive ultrasound imaging. It is of interest that the techniques involved are not themselves genetic, and that while there is an undoubted genetic susceptibility, the dramatic recent decline in incidence of neural tube defects has been associated mainly with folic acid dietary supplementation – an environmental measure.

Common neurological disorders

Almost everything written in this chapter about genetic counseling and genetic testing has related to the numerous but individually rare neurogenetic disorders following single-gene inheritance. However,

Table 2.8. General factors affecting risks for relatives in common multifactorial disorders

Population frequency of the disorder (recurrence risk is higher when the disorder is more common)
Gender ratio (risk is greater for the more frequently affected gender, but also greater when the proband is of the more rarely affected gender)
Severity (risk is greater when the disorder is more severe or bilateral)
Number of affected individuals in the kindred (risk is greater when multiple individuals are involved)
Closeness to the affected individual (risks diminish steeply with increasing genetic distance)

most common neurological disorders, despite having a significant genetic component, do not follow a clear Mendelian inheritance pattern. Attempts to identify the specific genes involved are proving to be complex and it seems increasingly likely that for most disorders in this group, numerous genes, interacting with each other and with external factors, will prove to be responsible. Details of such research are given in the following chapters of this book.

From the practical viewpoint of genetic counseling, recurrence risks in this multifactorial or polygenic group are generally low by comparison with those for Mendelian disorders, except when multiple family members are affected (in this case, one should always be alert to the possibility of a Mendelian subset within a broader group). In contrast to the well-established and fixed genetic risks for different types of Mendelian inheritance, recurrence risks for multifactorial disorders are influenced by a range of particular factors (Table 2.8). These include frequency of the disorder, severity (where this can be clearly defined), gender of the parent and of the affected individual (where frequency differs according to gender), and the number and genetic distance of affected individuals in the family.

Empirical risks based on large family studies are available for some disorders, but are mostly not recent, so that reclassification as a result of new molecular knowledge or changes in frequency from environmental measures (e.g. neural tube defects) are not taken into account. Likewise, it is often unclear how far risk estimates based on one population can be applied to another. All these factors result in risk estimates being approximate.

Fortunately, these limitations generally do not affect genetic counseling seriously, particularly as the relative commonness of some of these conditions means that risk cannot be eliminated, merely reduced to close to the population frequency. Risks of 1%–5% are commonly encountered, often less for relatives more distant than first degree (offspring and siblings), so that most families seen are reassured when realizing that the risks are not of the order of 25% or 50%, as often encountered with Mendelian conditions.

The possibility of widespread genetic testing based on susceptibility genes related to neurological disorders has been suggested as a scenario resulting from the human genome project but, at least at present, this seems most unlikely, apart from a very small number of situations. Not only are proven associations with DNA polymorphisms currently very few, but they are relatively weak; even the clearest, such as the HLA locus or the association of ApoE variants with AD, are too weak to be of significant predictive or diagnostic use. It will be important for clinicians to maintain a critical attitude toward claims of association in this field and their applications.

Thus, genetic counseling for common Mendelian neurological disorders currently rests on approximate but well-established principles and risk estimates, with genetic tests not playing a significant role. The strong contrast between this situation and that for Mendelian disorders makes it especially important that clinicians correctly identify Mendelian subsets in situations where family history may be inconspicuous and clinical features not distinctive.

Conclusion

The practical applications of genetics to neurological disease are numerous and of the greatest importance to families, especially for the uncommon but numerous conditions following Mendelian inheritance. All those involved with patients and families need to be aware of these issues and familiar with the basic principles.

Assessing genetic risks and the overall practice of genetic counseling can, at times, be complex and requires a very different approach to that generally used in diagnostic and therapeutic practice, but this should not deter interested and concerned clinicians who are prepared to adapt their approach and who have adequate time and facilities. A close partnership with clinical geneticists forms a vital part of genetic counseling and wider genetic services for inherited neurological disorders.

Genetic tests, especially and increasingly those based on the direct analysis of gene mutations, have already had a major impact on the detection and prevention of neurogenetic disorders and are now an integral part of much primary neurological diagnosis. Tests of genetic prediction, especially presymptomatic tests for late-onset disorders, involve complex and often difficult issues, as does prenatal diagnosis.

For common, multifactorial neurological disorders, genetic advances remain at a very early stage and genetic tests are, at present, rarely helpful in predicting genetic susceptibility or in genetic counseling. However, because the field of neurological disease contains a particularly large number of Mendelian single-gene disorders where important applications are possible, there is ample scope for all clinicians, whether involved in childhood or adult neurological disorders, to identify important genetic issues and to ensure that, through their own practice and their links with colleagues, the highest possible standard of genetic services is provided for all families affected by neurogenetic disorders.

References

1. Harper PS, Lim C, Craufurd D. Ten years of presymptomatic testing for Huntington's disease: the experience of the UK Huntington's Disease Prediction Consortium. *J Med Genet* 2000; **37**: 567–571.

2. Maat-Kievit A, Vegter-van der Vlis M, Zoeteweij M, *et al.* Paradox of a better test for Huntington's disease. *J Neurol Neurosurg Psychiatry* 2000; **69**: 579–583.

3. Creighton S, Almqvist EW, MacGregor D, *et al.* Predictive, pre-natal and diagnostic genetic testing for Huntington's disease: the experience in Canada from 1987 to 2000. *Clin Genet* 2003; **63**: 462–475.

4. Clarke A. The genetic testing of children: report of a working party of the Clinical Genetics Society. *J Med Genet* 1994; **31**: 785–797.

5. International Huntington Association and World Federation of Neurology Research Group on Huntington's Chorea. Guidelines for the molecular genetics predictive test

in Huntington's disease. *Neurology* 1994; **44**: 1533–1536.

6. Almqvist EW, Bloch M, Brinkman R, Craufurd D, Hayden MR, on behalf of an international HD collaborative group. A world-wide assessment of the frequency of suicide, suicide attempts, or psychiatric hospitalisation after predictive testing for Huntington disease. *Am J Hum Genet* 1999; **64**: 1293–1304.

7. van der Steenstraten IM, Tibben A, Roos RA, van de Kamp JJ, Niermeijer MF.

Predictive testing for Huntington disease: nonparticipants compared with participants in the Dutch program. *Am J Hum Genet* 1994; **55**: 618–625.

8. Quaid KA, Wesson MK. Exploration of the effects of predictive testing for Huntington disease on intimate relationships. *Am J Med Genet* 1995; **57**: 46–51.

9. Decruyenaere M, Evers-Kiebooms G, Boogaerts A, *et al.* Partners of mutation-carriers for Huntington's

disease: forgotten persons? *Eur J Hum Genet* 2005; **13**: 1077–1085.

10. Simpson SA, Zoeteweij MW, Nys K, *et al.* Prenatal testing for Huntington's disease: a European collaborative study. *Eur J Hum Genet* 2002; **10**: 689–693.

11. Lashwood A, Flinter F. Clinical and counselling implications of preimplantation genetic diagnosis for Huntington's disease in the UK. *Hum Fertil (Camb)* 2001; **4**: 235–238.

Alzheimer's disease and related dementias

John Hardy

Introduction

In our aging societies, dementias, especially Alzheimer's disease (AD) but also frontal temporal dementias (FTD) and Lewy body (LB) disease, are increasing societal problems afflicting perhaps 5% of those over 65 and 20% of those over 80 years of age. These latter diseases, while sharing the main symptoms of AD, are usually clinically distinguishable from AD: in FTD, personality changes are an early feature of the disease and in LB disease, parkinsonism can be a feature. Treatment for all these diseases, as in all neurodegenerative diseases, remains palliative. However, based largely on genetic analysis, we now have an outline of the pathogenic mechanisms involved and also a clearer view of the progression of the disease. This increased understanding has led to the identification of several plausible drug targets for these diseases and a general sense of optimism that mechanistic therapy may soon be available. The purpose of this chapter is to discuss this progress. I will focus on AD and discuss other dementias to the extent to which they contribute to our understanding of AD.

Alzheimer's disease

Alzheimer's disease is the major cause of dementia in the elderly and afflicts about four million Americans (US population ~300 million: http://www.frost.com/prod/servlet/dsd-fact-file.pag?docid=38565311). It is defined as a dementing illness characterized *post mortem* by the presence of extracellular plaques largely made of the Aβ peptide and intracellular tangles consisting mainly of the tau (MAPT) protein. While most cases of AD are late onset and show familial clustering, a small proportion has onset ages below 60 years and shows autosomal dominant inheritance. All reported cases with early onset, autosomal dominant AD have mutations in either the amyloid β precursor protein gene (*APP*) or in the presenilin 1 (*PSEN1*) or

presenilin 2 (*PSEN2*) genes [1]. The only currently accepted genetic risk factor for late-onset AD is the apolipoprotein E gene (*APOE*), in which the ε4 allele is a risk factor and the ε2 allele is protective [2]. While it is widely believed that there must be other genetic risk factors for late-onset disease, a recent genome screen suggested that there were unlikely to be any other alleles that had as large an effect as APOE [3].

Amyloid precursor protein and Alzheimer's disease

The occurrence of Alzheimer pathology in Down syndrome (DS) (trisomy 21) has long been recognized, and when Glenner and Wong identified the Aβ peptide in the meninges of, first, typical Alzheimer cases [4] and then the same peptide sequence in DS [5], they commented that it was likely that the gene was on chromosome 21 and mutated in AD. These remarkable predictions were shown to be correct with the cloning of APP and the identification of APP mutations in a few AD cases [6]. Examination of cases of DS with translocations distal to the *APP* gene showed that these individuals, although they had the obvious features of DS, did not develop AD [7]: this made it clear that the relationship between AD and DS specifically relates to overexpression of the *APP* gene rather than a nonspecific relationship with the full trisomy.

In general, families with APP missense mutations have typical AD with onset ages in the 50s with little variance. However, some cases, particularly those with mutations within the Aβ sequence, have a phenotype that resembles hereditary cerebral hemorrhage with amyloidosis (Dutch type) (HCHWA-D) [8]. The reason for the variability in the phenotype is not clear. More recently, several families with duplications of the *APP* gene have been identified. Individuals with these duplications also have a variable phenotype, with approximately half the duplication carriers developing hemorrhagic strokes and half developing typical AD [9]. These data, of course, fit very well with the observations in DS, yet hemorrhagic stroke is rare in DS. The reason for this slight discrepancy is unclear.

Apolipoprotein E genotype affects the age of onset in families with APP mutations and dementia, but does not affect the age of onset of hemorrhagic stroke. In dementia, essentially single copies of the ε4 allele reduce the age of onset by five years relative to ε3 homozygotes, and ε4 homozygotes have an onset age 10 years earlier. Single copies of the ε2 allele increase the age of onset by five years and ε2 homozygotes have an onset age 10 years later [10]. These general rules of thumb also appear to be true for AD in DS [11].

One large gap in our current knowledge is that we have little idea about the function of APP. When it was first cloned, it was suggested to be a receptor [12], and that seems likely to be the case; but its ligand and downstream targets are not known. This means we do not know whether, in some way, Alzheimer pathogenesis relates to the normal function of APP (see following discussion).

The presenilins

A minority of families (~10%) had mutations in the *APP* gene. Genetic linkage analysis demonstrated that the majority of families showed linkage to chromosome 14 [13], while a minority, largely of Russo-German origin, showed linkage to chromosome 1 [14]. Position cloning identified the genes for the former, which are the majority (~80%), as mutations in the *PSEN1* gene [15], while the others (~10%), including the Russo-German families, had mutations in its homolog, *PSEN2* [16,17]. Most of the mutations are simple missense variants, but some in-frame deletions, most notably PSEN1 Δex9, have also been described. No nonsense or frameshift mutations have been identified, suggesting that the mutations are not simple loss of function variants but not eliminating the possibility that the mutations lead to a partial loss of function.

A very large number of families with PSEN1 and PSEN2 mutations have now been described (http://www.molgen.ua.ac.be/ADMutations/) (see Figure 3.1). In general, families with PSEN1 mutations have typical AD with ages of onset from 35 to 50 years, with some of the variability in onset age being

accounted for by the APOE genotype as with APP families [18]. Families with PSEN2 mutations have a very variable onset age, and while a proportion of the variance is accounted for by the APOE genotype, much of the variance remains unexplained [19]. Some families with PSEN1 mutations have an unusual phenotype of initial spastic paraparesis, and these families are generally characterized by having large "cotton wool" plaques rather than neuritic plaques [20]. While the reason for the difference in pathogenesis is not clear, it seems that the mutations involved are those which have the largest effect on APP processing [21].

In contrast to APP, the function of the presenilins is now well understood in outline. They are the central subunit of intramembranous proteases, which are responsible for the regulated cleavage of Notch, APP, and many other type 1 membrane proteins [22] (see Figure 3.1).

The effects of pathogenic mutations: the amyloid hypothesis of Alzheimer's disease

In general terms, we have a clear understanding of the effects of the APP and presenilin mutations: most APP mutations and all presenilin mutations alter APP processing such that Aβ deposition is a more likely event [23] (see Figure 3.2). Slightly less certain and less well studied is the possibility that some of the intra-Aβ mutations' primary effect is on reducing the solubility of Aβ without altering the position of cleavage [24]. These findings are the central intellectual basis for the amyloid hypothesis of AD (Figure 3.2).

Although the general framework of the effects of the pathogenic mutations is clear, the details are not, and the precise mechanisms of the effects of the mutations on APP cleavage are not understood (see Figure 3.2). There are three cleavage processes that occur: α-secretase, which is a cleavage within the Aβ part of the molecule and is an alternative to β-secretase cleavage, which occurs at the N terminus of the Aβ fragment; and γ-secretase, which occurs at the C terminus of the Aβ stub (see Figure 3.2). In fact, γ-secretase's action is complex and seems to involve multiple cleavages [25] (named γ at around codons 711 to 713, ζ at around codon 717 [Aβ46] [26], and ε at around codons 721 and 722 [Aβ49 and Aβ50] [27]). It is not clear whether these multiple cleavages are independent events occurring in different APP molecules, or sequential events on single

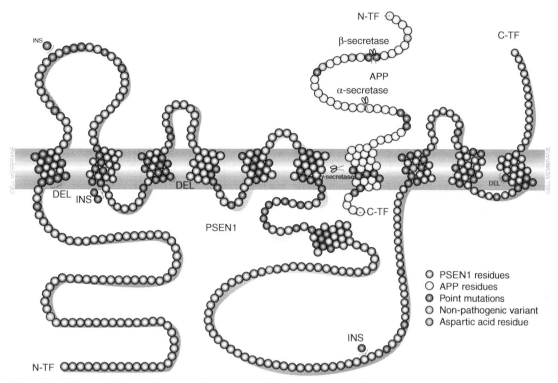

Figure 3.1. A diagram of the central structure of γ-secretase with APP in the active site of presenilin 1. The central role of presenilins in γ-secretase action was shown by the creation of *presenilin* knockout mice, which fail to metabolize the C-terminal stub of APP [121]. The critical aspartate residues at the active site were identified by mutagenesis experiments [122]. The whole active γ-secretase complex containing presenilin and other accessory proteins has been reconstituted in yeast [123]. The structure of presenilin 1 is derived from Laudon *et al.* (2005) [124].

molecules [25]. γ-Secretase liberates Aβ from the stub of APP, but this liberated Aβ has a marginal but important variability: the majority of Aβ has 40 amino acids (Aβ40), but a minor species has 42 amino acids (Aβ42).

Despite this uncertainty over the molecular detail of the effects of the mutations, most researchers have reached a consensus that, in general, the effects of the mutations are related directly to their effects on APP processing, and this has been the basis for the amyloid hypothesis of the disorder [28]. Recently, two groups have independently suggested an alternative: the crucial effect is that all the mutations cause a partial inhibition of presenilin function [29, 30]. They point out that γ-secretase has many vital functions and is involved in the processing of many type 1 membrane proteins beyond APP including Notch cleavage [22], but that APP is the major substrate in terms of expression. They argue that all the pathogenic mutations may act to inhibit γ-secretase, either directly in the case of presenilin mutations, or indirectly through the effects of mutations in or increased dose of its major substrate. This argument fits equally well with the genetic data as the amyloid hypothesis, but it seems less likely when one considers the admittedly inconclusive evidence suggesting neurotoxicity of Aβ and also the analogy with the other plaque and tangle diseases, Worster drought syndrome, and some prion dementias. In these latter diseases, there are amyloid deposits, tangles, and cell death, and in these the pathogenic mutations are, as in AD, in the extracellular deposited amyloid protein. This analogy suggests that the route to cell death directly involves the deposited protein. Neither of these arguments against the presenilin inhibition hypothesis of AD is conclusive and this hypothesis remains a credible alternative.

Recent data in transgenic animals [31] support earlier in vitro data [32] showing that Aβ42 is the primary molecule in terms of the deposition process. However, it is not clear exactly what the toxic species

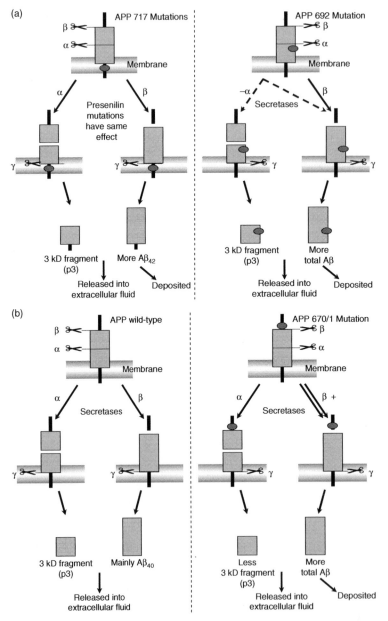

Figure 3.2. A simplistic diagram showing APP processing, which occurs through two alternative pathways [125]. In the first pathway (a), APP is cleaved at codon 671 by the enzyme β-secretase (BACE) [126] and then by γ-secretase. This pathway releases Aβ. In the second pathway (b), α-secretase cleavage occurs within the Aβ sequence, predominantly at residue 682, by a mixture of ADAM10 and ADAM17 [127], followed by γ-secretase cleavage. This yields a fragment designated p3 [125]. The APP670/1 mutation potentiates BACE cleavage yielding more total Aβ [129–131]. Some of the mutations in the APP sequence, particularly the APP692 mutation, inhibit the α-secretase cleavage, indirectly causing more flux through a β-cleavage pathway [130]. APP mutations close to the C-terminus of the Aβ sequence marginally alter the final length of a proportion of Aβ, causing an increase in the proportion of Aβ42 [131]. Presenilin mutations have the same effect essentially [132]. The approximate positions of mutations are illustrated by black circles, and the strength and number of the arrows illustrated convey the amount of flux through the pathway. The γ-secretase cleavage is a more complex event than conveyed in the diagram (see text and [25]).

of Aβ may be. The original formulations of the amyloid hypothesis [33] envisaged the plaques as the toxic elements, but more recent formulations [25,28] have acknowledged the increasing data supporting the suggestion that smaller Aβ oligomers may have a role. This, however, is an extremely difficult issue to resolve precisely because there are several oligomeric forms that may be dissociable in terms of their involvement in the Alzheimer phenotype. These are the intermediates in the deposition process: the intermediates in the neuronal toxicity and the species responsible for the well-established acute effects on memory and long-term potentiation. In addition, in all cases, it may be that the plaques act as reservoirs for the toxic species because we now know that these are dynamic structures rather than the static structure we used to envisage [34].

With regard to the deposition process, recent remarkable studies in transgenic mice [35] confirmed and extended earlier work in marmosets [36] showing that intracortical injections of human Alzheimer brain or APP transgenic mouse-derived Aβ, but not synthetic Aβ, seeded plaque deposition. This work clearly showed that some structural ("prion-like") form of the Aβ oligomer was responsible for this seeding, but the precise stoichometry (and whether other molecular components were also involved) is not clear. The fact that aggregated Aβ can be toxic in neuronal culture has long been recognized [37], but the precise structure(s) of the toxic species, although probably consisting of low subunit oligomers (reviewed in [25]), remains unclear. It is also unclear whether the toxicity seen in cell systems is directly relevant to the loss of neurons in the Alzheimer's brain, as one presumes these species would be present in the transgenic APP models in which neuronal loss is subtle at best [38]. Unfortunately, this area is further complicated by different groups using different nomenclatures (e.g. ADDLS, protofibrils) for oligomeric species that probably describe overlapping although not identical distributions of structures and which, regrettably, are hazy in their cross attributions.

With regard to the acute synaptic effects of Aβ: while APP transgenic mice had rather modest cell loss [38], they did have quite severe behavioral impairments [39]. Remarkably, passive Aβ immunization, which clearly can prevent plaque deposition over a period of weeks [40], causes some improvements in memory performance almost immediately [41], strongly suggesting that some pool of Aβ that was accessible to Aβ antibodies was responsible for some of the synaptic and behavioral effects. This oligomer, designated Aβ*, appears to be a duodecamer in large part [42].

Late-onset Alzheimer's disease

As detailed previously, most but not all researchers would acknowledge that the most likely mechanism leading to AD in the early onset kindreds and in DS is the amyloid hypothesis. However, the applicability of the amyloid hypothesis to late-onset AD (which is more than 95% of cases) is much more widely debated (see following discussion).

Apolipoprotein E

The only established risk factor for late-onset disease is the *APOE 4* gene [2] and the only protective factor is the *APOE 2* gene [43]. However, the increase in familial clustering encoded at the APOE locus is widely believed not to be sufficient to account for more than a modest proportion of the total familial clustering [44], leading to the belief that there are likely to be about five other genetic risk loci [45].

Are there other Alzheimer risk genes?

Extensive research using both linkage approaches and candidate gene association studies has failed so far to give consistent proof that any of the other candidates are involved in the etiology of the disease. The Alzgene website (http://www.alzforum.org/res/com/gen/alzgene/default.asp) keeps a continually updated meta-analysis of genes that have been tested extensively for involvement [46]. Only two genes, *ACE* and *IL1B*, pass (in July 2007) the criteria of 95% confidence intervals not including unity when the initial report is excluded, and the analysis is confined to a single ethnic group (the standard practice in meta-analysis of genetic effects). Both of these have reported odds ratios of between 1.1 and 1.2: far lower than the odds ratios of >3.5 reported for the APOE 4 locus [44].

This finding is consistent with the first reports of a whole genome study in AD, which clearly identified the APOE 4 locus [3], but found nothing else before the sample was fractionated by the APOE genotype [47]. There are many possible explanations for this: the coverage of the whole genome chip arrays is not complete and this methodology would not pick up genes that had many different risk alleles; but the simplest explanation is that there are no other alleles of major effect. This would suggest that the rest of the risk of disease is predisposed to by common alleles with low risk ratios (>1.5), or by rare variants with large effect size but low population attributable risk, as well, of course, by environmental influences and chance. The recent success of the dissection of type II diabetes by whole genome association studies suggests that the best initial approach to this problem is through the pooling of the data from several large studies to achieve very large sample sizes.

One particularly plausible risk gene is *APP*, because we know from the example of DS and the APP duplication families that increases of expression of 50% (three copies of the gene) give disease with ages of onset in the 50s. This means that if there are alleles in the general population with a relative expression level increased by 25% when homozygote, these would also be associated with disease onset at the same age, and presumably, slightly lower expression alleles would be associated with a higher onset age. In addition, in the other protein deposition disorders where autosomal dominant genes have been found, genetic variability in the expression of the same protein has shown a robust association with the sporadic disease [48]. Recently, two studies have reported such an association [49, 50], and genetic linkage analysis has also suggested that chromosome 21 may be involved [51]. However, a recent and thorough analysis failed to confirm this association [52], so even with this plausible candidate, strict genetic evidence for involvement is lacking.

Does the amyloid hypothesis apply to late-onset Alzheimer's disease?

Parsimony would suggest that the overall mechanism in late-onset disease would be generally similar to the mechanism in the autosomal dominant kindreds. However, this point has, rightly, been much more extensively debated than the mechanism of pathogenesis of the autosomal dominant kindreds. A major gap in our knowledge is a precise understanding of the functions of APP. From the perspective of the amyloid hypothesis, one worrying suggestion is that amyloid deposition is a damage response mechanism. One known function of APP is in the blood clotting cascade [53], and one intriguing suggestion is that amyloid deposition is a physiological response to microhemorrhaging [54]; certainly, there is extensive although not incontrovertible evidence that plaque formation occurs centered on blood vessel walls [55,56]. In such a scheme, the amyloid deposition may have a damage response role [57], initially at least, although such an idea is difficult to reconcile with the development of the disease in the autosomal dominant kindreds. Some have suggested that this damage response role underlies the side-effect profile of the amyloid vaccine [58] (see following discussion).

This debate will be helped as we develop an understanding of the role of APP and identify and understand more risk factor genes. Most importantly, however, it will be resolved when/if we develop treatments for the disorder.

Insights from other dementing diseases

While AD is easily the most prevalent dementing disease, other rarer dementias offer useful comparators. These include dementia with Lewy bodies (DLB), prion disease, Worster drought syndrome (British dementia), and FTD with tangles (FTDP-17T).

Dementia with Lewy bodies

The nosological separations of DLB from AD and from Parkinson's disease (PD) has proved extremely difficult [59]. In some cases of AD, including those with APP mutations [60], DS [61], and presenilin [62] mutations, there are a variable number of LB, the presence of which has become much clearer with the advent first of ubiquitin and later α-synuclein staining. This observation suggests that LB formation, like tangle formation, can be a downstream pathology to APP mismetabolism [63]. Individuals with large numbers of cortical LB have a dementing phenotype which, on a group although not an individual level, is distinguishable from typical AD in having a fluctuating course and some parkinsonian features. This latter phenotype, unsurprisingly, overlaps with that in individuals who present with PD and later develop dementia [64]. Parkinson's disease and Parkinson's dementia can occasionally be caused by α-synuclein mutations [65], including gene duplications [66], and the sporadic diseases show a genetic association with the α-synuclein haplotype [67].

Insights into Alzheimer's disease

The nosological confusion between AD and DLB is likely to obscure a rather simple and revealing underlying biology. As is true for prion (see following discussion), tau (see following discussion), and APP (discussed previously), α-synuclein deposition is influenced by the α-synuclein haplotype [67]. In addition, as is true for tau, α-synuclein deposition is increased by APP mismetabolism [68,69]. These data suggest that α-synuclein can be downstream of APP mismetabolism in an analogous way to tau (see Figure 3.3 and following discussion). From a treatment perspective, the implication of overlap between AD and DLB is that one may expect both syndromes to respond to anti-Aβ therapies but differently to anti-tau and anti-synuclein therapies.

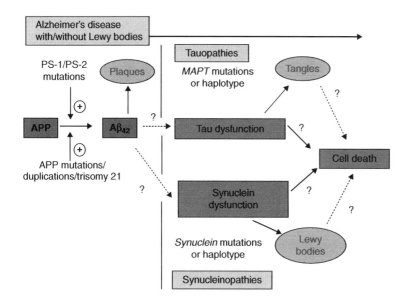

Figure 3.3. The proposed relationship between Aβ and tau and α-synuclein, between Alzheimer's disease and dementia with Lewy bodies [63,94]. The genetic data on British dementia and the prion diseases suggest that the cognate proteins (ABri and prion) can behave in a similar way to Aβ42. While this diagram is consistent with the Mendelian forms of the disease, it is difficult to understand precisely how apolipoprotein E fits into this schema, although there are data implicating apolipoprotein E in amyloid deposition [133]. In addition, the number of "?"s is notable.

Prion disease

A full description of prion diseases is beyond the scope of this chapter (see [70]). Prion diseases fall into three classes: hereditary, acquired (infectious, iatrogenic, cannibalistic), and sporadic. At the center of these etiologies is the prion protein: mutations in the prion gene causing the hereditary disorder [71]; a pathological conformation of the protein is the infectious agent in the human and animal acquired forms of the disease, and genetic variability in the prion gene contributes to the risk of the sporadic disease [72].

Insights into Alzheimer's disease

There are a number of interesting parallels between prion diseases and AD. First, the obvious similarity is that both disorders involve abnormal aggregates of the cognate protein. Some forms of prion diseases involve extracellular depositions of the prion protein as plaques, which have a superficial resemblance to the amyloid plaques of AD. However, there are other perhaps deeper parallels. Some of the hereditary prion diseases have secondary tangle and LB pathology [71], indicating that these pathologies can also be secondary to a prion etiology as they are to an Aβ etiology. In addition, genetic variability in prion expression contributes to the risk of the sporadic disease, with high expressors being at higher risk for disease in a broadly analogous way to that in which APP expression can cause AD [72]. Perhaps most interesting

has been the recent demonstration that extracts of Alzheimer brain amyloid (but not synthetic Aβ) can precipitate plaque pathology in APP transgenic mice [35], suggesting that the difference between the prion diseases' infectivity and the spread of Alzheimer pathology in AD, at its basis, is quantitative and not qualitative. Perhaps all these diseases of β-sheet protein deposition are diseases of pathological templating [73].

Worster drought syndrome (British dementia)

Worster drought syndrome [74] (now, unfortunately, redesignated as British dementia) refers to a large English family that has a plaque and tangle disease which, before immunostaining, was considered to be a form of either early onset AD or hereditary prion disease. The disease is caused by a stop codon mutation at the C terminus of a type 2 membrane protein (ABri). This frameshift mutation adds 23 nonsense amino acids to the protein [75]. Furin cleavage of the 34 terminal amino acids yields an amyloidogenic peptide, which is deposited as both congophilic angiopathy and neuritic plaques [76].

Insights into Alzheimer's disease

Tangles are the secondary pathology in this disease as in AD. The importance of this disease for AD is that it shows that the deposition of a completely unphysiological amyloidogenic peptide can lead to plaque and tangle disease. Through the manipulation of the ABri sequence in mouse transgenic models and a replacement of the pathological ABri sequence with either Aβ42 or Aβ40, McGowan and colleagues [31] showed that Aβ42 was essential for deposition to occur.

Frontal temporal dementia with parkinsonism linked to chromosome 17 with tangles (FTDP-17T: Pick's disease) and other tangle-only diseases

Hereditary FTD has long been recognized as a comparatively rare cause of morbidity and mortality, but its nosology has been extremely difficult. In the last 10 years, genetic analysis has considerably clarified this difficult issue. To date, three genes have been found, although it is likely that there are others. A nonsense mutation in CHMP2b probably explains the disease in a single Danish family [77], but the majority of families showed genetic linkage to chromosome 17 markers [78]. About half of these families had tau pathology [79]: either tangles, Pick bodies, or wispy tau filaments, and about half of them had ubiquitin-positive inclusions [80]. Initially, these were grouped together as a single entity, FTDP-17 [78], but we now know they are unrelated diseases despite their clinical and genetic linkage similarities. Those with tau pathology have mutations in the tau gene (*MAPT*) [81,82], whereas those with ubiquitin inclusions have mutations in the progranulin gene (*PGRN*) [83,84], and have the RNA binding protein TDP-43 [85] as the central protein in their inclusions. In this chapter, only the pathogenesis of those dementias with MAPT mutations will be discussed, as these offer insight into AD.

Two types of MAPT mutations have been discovered: missense changes, which decrease the binding of tau to microtubules and increase tau's propensity to aggregate [86], and splicing mutations, which increase the inclusion of exon 10 in the protein [81]. Exon 10 encodes one of the four microtubule binding domains, so this form of the protein is commonly described as 4-repeat tau.

Interestingly, the sporadic tangle diseases (including progressive supranuclear palsy (PSP) [87], corticobasal degeneration (CBD) [88], and Parkinson's dementia complex of Guam [89], show a genetic association with the *MAPT* gene. The MAPT haplotype, which shows association with PSP and CBD (designated H1c in Europeans [90]), is that which shows greatest expression of 4-repeat tau [91]. The simplest way of thinking of this is to consider these diseases as the same disorder as FTDP-17T, but separated from it by an accident of nosology, as both their pathological and clinical features also overlap with this latter disorder.

Mice with MAPT transgenes containing FTDP-17T mutations develop both tangles and cell loss, clearly implicating tau dysfunction in neuronal cell death [92].

Insights into Alzheimer's disease

The importance of FTDP-17 in our understanding of the pathogenesis of cell death in AD is clear. The fact that tau mutations cause tangles and cell death suggests that this is likely to be the same cell death pathway as the predominant pathway in AD. This suggestion is strengthened by the observation that crossing mutant APP transgenic mice with such MAPT mice leads to an augmentation of the tangle pathology without altering the amyloid pathology [93]. This observation is consistent with the view that Aβ is upstream of MAPT in AD (Figure 3.3) and is thus also consistent with the amyloid hypothesis of the disorder [33,94]. Also consistent with this view are observations that reducing tau levels reduces Aβ toxicity on cells [95] and decreases the behavioral decrements induced by Aβ overexpression in transgenic mice [96].

In addition, some [97] although not all studies [98] have reported that the same H1c MAPT haplotype that shows an association with PSP and CBD shows a weaker association with AD, suggesting that increased expression of 4-repeat tau increases the likelihood of developing AD [97].

Genetics-based clinical progress in Alzheimer's disease

If we are to develop mechanism-based therapies for AD, we will want to be able to diagnose the disease both accurately and early, and to monitor whether therapies are having beneficial effects. In both of these areas, use of the families with autosomal dominant disease has proven extremely useful because of the predictable nature of the disease. Such families have been used extensively to determine the earliest clinical symptoms of the disease [99]. However, possibly the most promising techniques for assessing both preclinical change and the rate of progression of disease are imaging techniques – two different and complementary approaches are being used: magnetic resonance (MR) image registration [100] and positron emission tomography (PET) amyloid imaging [101].

MR image registration is a technique for measuring atrophy as a change in volume in a single person over time [100], and its use has shown that detectable hippocampal atrophy begins about six years before clinical symptoms of disease are apparent, and that a more generalized atrophy is detectable about three years before the onset of clinical symptoms [102]. The analysis also showed that the global rate was relatively similar between persons at the same stage of the development of disease, but that the rate of atrophy increased as the disease spread to affect different brain regions [103]. The clinical utility of the approach was demonstrated when it was used to assess the effects of Aβ immunization when it showed the unexpected outcome that brain volume was decreased by the immunization [104], although it remains unclear as to whether this reflected a reduction in brain mass or was caused by loss of amyloid or a change in brain water balance [105].

PET amyloid imaging has recently been developed, using radiolabeled, Pittsburgh Compound B (PIB), an analogue of thioflavin S [101]. This compound allows imaging of amyloid deposition in vivo, and has shown that this deposition process begins many years (~10 years) before clinical symptoms appear in presenilin mutation carriers [106] and, when combined with MR registration, the rate of atrophy correlates with the amyloid load [107].

Animal models and experimental therapeutics

The genetic findings outlined previously have enabled the creation of transgenic mice that model parts of the disease process. Mice with mutant APP transgenes develop plaques [108], but no tangles, little cell loss [39], and only subtle behavioral changes [38]; crossing in presenilin mice increased this pathology, but did not change its basic pattern [109,110]. These mice, therefore, have been extremely useful in developing anti-amyloid therapies [111]. As one example among many, the amyloid immunization therapy came directly from such mouse experiments

[40,112]. Mice with mutant *MAPT* genes develop tangles and extensive cell loss [92], and have been useful in developing anti-tangle therapies [113]. Mice with both mutant *APP* and mutant *MAPT* genes have increased tangle formation, and such mice could be used to explore the relationship between the pathologies [94,114], although this important relationship has not yet been extensively investigated.

These mice and the mechanistic understanding we have developed offer a plethora of molecular targets for intervention (see [115]). The amyloid therapeutic approach that has attracted the most attention has been the amyloid vaccine approach. This was borne out by the surprising observation that immunization of APP transgenic mice led to the partial clearance of plaque deposits and almost immediate improvement of the APP transgenic mice on behavioral testing [41,116,117]. Clinical trials of amyloid immunization were stopped after a small proportion of patients, who received the test but not the control immunization, developed meningioencephalitis for reasons that are unclear [118]. While this trial could be seen as hopeful in that it showed that amyloid plaques could be cleared [118,119] from the Alzheimer brain, because the trial was aborted, it has remained unclear whether there were beneficial behavioral consequences [120]. It is also unclear whether the meningioencephalitis was merely an unfortunate side-effect or whether it reflected an unanticipated role for Aβ in the pathological brain [57]. Thus, this trial has been seen by amyloid optimists as a useful proof of principle [119] and by amyloid pessimists as a harbinger of other likely unsuccessful trials [58]. Many potential therapies have passed the test of working in the transgenic mice; in most cases, human trials are either underway or in the planning stage. These trials include statins and non-steroidal anti-inflammatory drugs, both of which showed reductions in Aβ42 production in transgenic mice and cell lines [111,115]. Little information concerning clinical trials is currently in the public domain, but several studies are expected to report results in 2012 or 2013. If they work, they will be a powerful validation of the use of the pathological gene, through transgenic animals, to test therapies as a route to treat all neurological diseases. If none of them work, then it should cause us to re-evaluate all of our assumptions, not just about the amyloid hypothesis, but also about this whole genetics-based approach to disease treatment.

Conclusion

Genetic analysis of AD has led to a widespread belief that we have a basic understanding of the pathogenesis of the disease. It has also led to the development of animal models, which appear to replicate aspects of this pathogenesis, as well as to the identification of credible molecular targets for therapy. Finally, it has helped in the accurate characterization of the prodrome and clinical course of the disease. However, while there have been many successful therapies in the mouse models of the disease, none has yet shown utility in clinical trials. While Alzheimer patients are undoubtedly better treated than they were 15 years ago, the only direct benefit to patients from this gene-based approach to research, to date, has been the availability of genetic testing in the kindreds with APP and presenilin mutations.

Acknowledgments

The author's laboratory is supported by the MRC. Thanks to Richard Crook for Figure 3.1.

References

1. Rogaeva E. The solved and unsolved mysteries of the genetics of early-onset Alzheimer's disease. *Neuromolecular Med* 2002; **2**: 1–10.

2. Corder EH, Saunders AM, Strittmatter WJ, *et al.* Gene dose of apolipoprotein E type 4 allele and the risk of Alzheimer's disease in late onset families. *Science* 1993; **261**: 921–923.

3. Coon KD, Myers AJ, Craig DW, *et al.* A high-density whole-genome association study reveals that APOE is the major susceptibility gene for sporadic late-onset Alzheimer's disease. *J Clin Psychiatry* 2007; **68**: 613–618.

4. Glenner GG, Wong CW. Alzheimer's disease: initial report of the purification and characterization of a novel cerebrovascular amyloid protein. *Biochem Biophys Res Commun* 1984; **120**: 885–890.

5. Glenner GG, Wong CW. Alzheimer's disease and Down's syndrome: sharing of a unique cerebrovascular amyloid fibril protein. *Biochem Biophys Res Commun* 1984; **122**: 1131–1135.

6. Goate A, Chartier-Harlin MC, Mullan M, *et al.* Segregation of a missense mutation in the amyloid precursor protein gene with familial Alzheimer's disease. *Nature* 1991; **349**: 704–706.

7. Prasher VP, Farrer MJ, Kessling AM, *et al.* Molecular mapping of Alzheimer-type dementia in Down's syndrome. *Ann Neurol* 1998; **43**: 380–383.

8. Levy E, Carman MD, Fernandez-Madrid IJ, *et al.* Mutation of the Alzheimer's disease amyloid gene in hereditary cerebral hemorrhage, Dutch type. *Science* 1990; **248**: 1124–1126.

9. Rovelet-Lecrux A, Hannequin D, Raux G, *et al.* APP locus duplication causes autosomal dominant early-onset Alzheimer disease with cerebral amyloid angiopathy. *Nat Genet* 2006; **38**: 24–26.

10. Houlden H, Collinge J, Kennedy A, *et al.* Apolipoprotein E genotype and Alzheimer's disease. Alzheimer's Disease Collaborative Group. *Lancet* 1993; **342**: 737–738.

11. Royston MC, Mann D, Pickering-Brown S, *et al.* Apolipoprotein E epsilon 2 allele promotes longevity and protects patients with Down's syndrome from dementia. *Neuroreport* 1994; **5**: 2583–2585.

12. Kang J, Lemaire HG, Unterbeck A, *et al.* The precursor of Alzheimer's disease amyloid A4 protein resembles a cell-surface receptor. *Nature* 1987; **325**: 733–736.

13. Schellenberg GD, Bird TD, Wijsman EM, *et al.* Genetic linkage evidence for a familial Alzheimer's disease locus on chromosome 14. *Science* 1992; **258**: 668–671.

14. Levy-Lahad E, Wijsman EM, Nemens E, *et al.* A familial Alzheimer's disease locus on chromosome 1. *Science* 1995; **269**: 970–973.

15. Sherrington R, Rogaev EI, Liang Y, *et al.* Cloning of a gene bearing missense mutations in early-onset familial Alzheimer's disease. *Nature* 1995; **375**: 754–760.

16. Rogaev EI, Sherrington R, Rogaeva EA, *et al.* Familial Alzheimer's disease in kindreds with missense mutations in a gene on chromosome 1 related to the Alzheimer's disease type 3 gene. *Nature* 1995; **376**: 775–778.

17. Levy-Lahad E, Wasco W, Poorkaj P, *et al.* Candidate gene for the chromosome 1 familial Alzheimer's disease locus. *Science* 1995; **269**: 973–977.

18. Pastor P, Roe CM, Villegas A, *et al.* Apolipoprotein Eepsilon4 modifies Alzheimer's disease onset in an E280A PS1 kindred. *Ann Neurol* 2003; **54**: 163–169.

19. Wijsman EM, Daw EW, Yu X, *et al.* APOE and other loci affect age-at-onset in Alzheimer's disease families with PS2 mutation. *Am J Med Genet B Neuropsychiatr Genet* 2005; **132**: 14–20.

20. Crook R, Verkkoniemi A, Perez-Tur J, *et al.* A variant of Alzheimer's disease with spastic paraparesis and unusual plaques due to deletion of exon 9 of presenilin 1. *Nat Med* 1998; **4**: 452–455.

21. Houlden H, Baker M, McGowan E, et al. Variant Alzheimer's disease with spastic paraparesis and cotton wool plaques is caused by PS-1 mutations that lead to exceptionally high amyloid-beta concentrations. Ann Neurol 2000; 48: 806–808.

22. Parks AL, Curtis D. Presenilin diversifies its portfolio. Trends Genet 2007; 23: 140–150.

23. Scheuner D, Eckman C, Jensen M, et al. Secreted amyloid beta-protein similar to that in the senile plaques of Alzheimer's disease is increased in vivo by the presenilin 1 and 2 and APP mutations linked to familial Alzheimer's disease. Nat Med 1996; 2: 864–870.

24. Wisniewski T, Ghiso J, Frangione B. Peptides homologous to the amyloid protein of Alzheimer's disease containing a glutamine for glutamic acid substitution have accelerated amyloid fibril formation. Biochem Biophys Res Commun 1991; 180: 1528.

25. Walsh DM, Selkoe DJ. A beta oligomers – a decade of discovery. J Neurochem 2007; 101: 1172–1184.

26. Kakuda N, Funamoto S, Yagishita S, et al. Equimolar production of amyloid beta-protein and amyloid precursor protein intracellular domain from beta-carboxyl-terminal fragment by gamma-secretase. J Biol Chem 2006; 281: 14776–14786.

27. Weidemann A, Eggert S, Reinhard FBM, et al. A novel ε-cleavage within the transmembrane domain of the Alzheimer amyloid precursor protein demonstrates homology with Notch processing. Biochemistry 2002; 41: 2825–2835.

28. Hardy J, Selkoe DJ. The amyloid hypothesis of Alzheimer's disease: progress and problems on the road to therapeutics. Science 2002; 297: 353–356.

29. Shen J, Kelleher RJ 3rd. The presenilin hypothesis of Alzheimer's disease: evidence for a loss-of-function pathogenic

mechanism. Proc Natl Acad Sci USA 2007; 104: 403–409.

30. Sambamurti K, Suram A, Venugopal C, et al. A partial failure of membrane protein turnover may cause Alzheimer's disease: a new hypothesis. Curr Alzheimer Res 2006; 3: 81–90.

31. McGowan E, Pickford F, Kim J, et al. Abeta42 is essential for parenchymal and vascular amyloid deposition in mice. Neuron 2005; 47: 191–199.

32. Jarrett JT, Berger EP, Lansbury PT Jr. The carboxy terminus of the beta amyloid protein is critical for the seeding of amyloid formation: implications for the pathogenesis of Alzheimer's disease. Biochemistry 1993; 32: 4693–4697.

33. Hardy J, Allsop D. Amyloid deposition as the central event in the aetiology of Alzheimer's disease. Trends Pharmacol Sci 1991; 12: 383–388.

34. Lazarov O, Lee M, Peterson DA, Sisodia SS. Evidence that synaptically released beta-amyloid accumulates as extracellular deposits in the hippocampus of transgenic mice. J Neurosci 2002; 22: 9785–9793.

35. Meyer-Luehmann M, Coomaraswamy J, Bolmont T, et al. Exogenous induction of cerebral beta-amyloidogenesis is governed by agent and host. Science 2006; 313: 1781–1784.

36. Ridley RM, Baker HF, Windle CP, Cummings RM. Very long term studies of the seeding of beta-amyloidosis in primates. J Neural Transm 2006; 113: 1243–1251.

37. Pike CJ, Burdick D, Walencewicz AJ, Glabe CG, Cotman CW. Neurodegeneration induced by beta-amyloid peptides in vitro: the role of peptide assembly state. J Neurosci 1993; 13: 1676–1687.

38. Takeuchi A, Irizarry MC, Duff K, et al. Age-related amyloid beta deposition in transgenic mice overexpressing both Alzheimer

mutant presenilin 1 and amyloid beta precursor protein Swedish mutant is not associated with global neuronal loss. Am J Pathol 2000; 157: 331–339.

39. Hsiao KK, Borchelt DR, Olson K, et al. Age-related CNS disorder and early death in transgenic FVB/N mice overexpressing Alzheimer amyloid precursor proteins. Neuron 1995; 15: 1203–1218.

40. Bard F, Cannon C, Barbour R, et al. Peripherally administered antibodies against amyloid beta-peptide enter the central nervous system and reduce pathology in a mouse model of Alzheimer disease. Nat Med 2000; 6: 916–919.

41. Dodart JC, Bales KR, Gannon KS, et al. Immunization reverses memory deficits without reducing brain Abeta burden in Alzheimer's disease model. Nat Neurosci 2002; 5: 452–457.

42. Lesne S, Koh MT, Kotilinek L, et al. A specific amyloid-beta protein assembly in the brain impairs memory. Nature 2006; 440: 352–357.

43. Chartier-Harlin MC, Parfitt M, Legrain S, et al. Apolipoprotein E, epsilon 4 allele as a major risk factor for sporadic early and late-onset forms of Alzheimer's disease: analysis of the 19q13.2 chromosomal region. Hum Mol Genet 1994; 3: 569–574.

44. Farrer LA, Cupples LA, Haines JL, et al. Effects of age, sex, and ethnicity on the association between apolipoprotein E genotype and Alzheimer disease. A meta-analysis. APOE and Alzheimer Disease Meta Analysis Consortium. JAMA 1997; 278: 1349–1356.

45. Daw EW, Payami H, Nemens EJ, et al. The number of trait loci in late-onset Alzheimer disease. Am J Hum Genet 2000; 66: 196–204.

46. Bertram L, McQueen MB, Mullin K, Blacker D, Tanzi RE. Systematic meta-analyses of

Alzheimer disease genetic association studies: the AlzGene database. *Nat Genet* 2007; **39**: 17–23.

47. Reiman EM, Webster JA, Myers AJ, *et al.* GAB2 alleles modify Alzheimer's risk in APOE epsilon4 carriers. *Neuron* 2007; **54**: 713–720.

48. Singleton A, Myers A, Hardy J. The law of mass action applied to neurodegenerative disease: a hypothesis concerning the etiology and pathogenesis of complex diseases. *Hum Mol Genet* 2004; 13 Spec No 1: R123–R126.

49. Guyant-Maréchal L, Rovelet-Lecrux A, Goumidi L, *et al.* Variations in the APP gene promoter region and risk of Alzheimer disease. *Neurology* 2007; **68**: 684–687.

50. Brouwers N, Sleegers K, Engelborghs S, *et al.* Genetic risk and transcriptional variability of amyloid precursor protein in Alzheimer's disease. *Brain* 2006; **129**: 2984–2991.

51. Wavrant-De Vrieze F, Crook R, Holmans P, *et al.* Genetic variability at the amyloid-beta precursor protein locus may contribute to the risk of late-onset Alzheimer's disease. *Neurosci Lett* 1999; **269**: 67–70.

52. Nowotny P, Simcock X, Bertelsen S, *et al.* Association studies testing for risk for late-onset Alzheimer's disease with common variants in the beta-amyloid precursor protein (APP). *Am J Med Genet B Neuropsychiatr Genet* 2007; **144**: 469–474.

53. Smith RP, Higuchi DA, Broze GJ Jr. Platelet coagulation factor XIa-inhibitor, a form of Alzheimer amyloid precursor protein. *Science* 1990; **248**: 1126–1128.

54. Cullen KM, Kocsi Z, Stone J. Microvascular pathology in the aging human brain: evidence that senile plaques are sites of microhaemorrhages. *Neurobiol Aging* 2006; **27**: 1786–1796.

55. Kumar-Singh S, Pirici D, McGowan E, *et al.* Dense-core plaques in Tg2576 and PSAPP mouse models of Alzheimer's disease are centered on vessel walls. *Am J Pathol* 2005; **167**: 527–543.

56. Miyakawa T, Shimoji A, Kuramoto R, Higuchi Y. The relationship between senile plaques and cerebral blood vessels in Alzheimer's disease and senile dementia. Morphological mechanism of senile plaque production. *Virchows Arch B Cell Pathol Incl Mol Pathol* 1982; **40**: 121–129.

57. Atwood CS, Bishop GM, Perry G, Smith MA. Amyloid-beta: a vascular sealant that protects against hemorrhage? *J Neurosci Res* 2002; **70**: 356.

58. Atwood CS, Perry G, Smith MA. Cerebral hemorrhage and amyloid-beta. *Science* 2003; **299**: 1014.

59. McKeith IG, Galasko D, Kosaka K, *et al.* Consensus guidelines for the clinical and pathologic diagnosis of dementia with Lewy bodies (DLB): report of the consortium on DLB International Workshop. *Neurology* 1996; **47**: 1113–1124.

60. Lantos PL, Ovenstone IM, Johnson J, *et al.* Lewy bodies in the brain of two members of a family with the 717 (Val to Ile) mutation of the amyloid precursor protein gene. *Neurosci Lett* 1994; **172**: 77–79.

61. Lippa CF, Schmidt ML, Lee VM, Trojanowski JQ. Antibodies to alpha-synuclein detect Lewy bodies in many Down's syndrome brains with Alzheimer's disease. *Ann Neurol* 1999; **45**: 353–357.

62. Lippa CF, Fujiwara H, Mann DM, *et al.* Lewy bodies contain altered alpha-synuclein in brains of many familial Alzheimer's disease patients with mutations in presenilin and amyloid precursor protein genes. *Am J Pathol* 1998; **153**: 1365–1370.

63. Hardy J. The relationship between Lewy body disease, Parkinson's disease, and Alzheimer's disease. *Ann NY Acad Sci* 2003; **991**: 167–170.

64. Lippa CF, Duda JE, Grossman M, *et al.* DLB and PDD boundary issues: diagnosis, treatment, molecular pathology, and biomarkers. *Neurology* 2007; **68**: 812–819.

65. Polymeropoulos MH, Lavedan C, Leroy E, *et al.* Mutation in the alpha-synuclein gene identified in families with Parkinson's disease. *Science* 1997; **276**: 2045–2047.

66. Singleton AB, Farrer M, Johnson J, *et al.* alpha-Synuclein locus triplication causes Parkinson's disease. *Science* 2003; **302**: 841.

67. Farrer M, Maraganore DM, Lockhart P, *et al.* alpha-Synuclein gene haplotypes are associated with Parkinson's disease. *Hum Mol Genet* 2001; **10**: 1847–1851.

68. Masliah E, Rockenstein E, Veinbergs I, *et al.* Dopaminergic loss and inclusion body formation in alpha-synuclein mice: implications for neurodegenerative disorders. *Science* 2000; **287**: 1265–1269.

69. Masliah E, Rockenstein E, Veinbergs I, *et al.* Beta-amyloid peptides enhance alpha-synuclein accumulation and neuronal deficits in a transgenic mouse model linking Alzheimer's disease and Parkinson's disease. *Proc Natl Acad Sci USA* 2001; **98**: 12245–12250.

70. Prusiner SB. Shattuck lecture – neurodegenerative diseases and prions. *N Engl J Med* 2001; **344**: 1516–1526.

71. Hsiao K, Dlouhy SR, Farlow MR, *et al.* Mutant prion proteins in Gerstmann–Sträussler–Scheinker

disease with neurofibrillary tangles. *Nat Genet* 1992; **1**: 68–71.

72. Mead S, Mahal SP, Beck J, *et al.* Sporadic – but not variant – Creutzfeldt–Jakob disease is associated with polymorphisms upstream of PRNP exon 1. *Am J Hum Genet* 2001; **69**: 1225–1235.

73. Hardy J. Expression of normal sequence pathogenic proteins for neurodegenerative disease contributes to disease risk: 'permissive templating' as a general mechanism underlying neurodegeneration. *Biochem Soc Trans* 2005; **33**: 578–581.

74. Worster-Drought C, Hill TR, McMenemey WH. Familial presenile dementia with spastic paralysis. *J Neurol Psychopath* 1933; **14**: 27–34.

75. Vidal R, Frangione B, Rostagno A, *et al.* A stop-codon mutation in the BRI gene associated with familial British dementia. *Nature* 1999; **399**: 776–781.

76. Kim SH, Wang R, Gordon DJ, *et al.* Furin mediates enhanced production of fibrillogenic ABri peptides in familial British dementia. *Nat Neurosci* 1999; **2**: 984–988.

77. Skibinski G, Parkinson NJ, Brown JM, *et al.* Mutations in the endosomal ESCRTIII-complex subunit CHMP2B in frontotemporal dementia. *Nat Genet* 2005; **37**: 806–808.

78. Foster NL, Wilhelmsen K, Sima AA, *et al.* Frontotemporal dementia and parkinsonism linked to chromosome 17: a consensus conference. Conference Participants. *Ann Neurol* 1997; **41**: 706–715.

79. Spillantini MG, Bird TD, Ghetti B. Frontotemporal dementia and Parkinsonism linked to chromosome 17: a new group of tauopathies. *Brain Pathol* 1998; **8**: 387–402.

80. Mackenzie IR, Feldman HH. Ubiquitin immunohistochemistry suggests classic motor neuron disease, motor neuron disease with dementia, and frontotemporal dementia of the motor neuron disease type represent a clinicopathologic spectrum. *J Neuropathol Exp Neurol* 2005; **64**: 730–739.

81. Hutton M, Lendon CL, Rizzu P, *et al.* Association of missense and 5′-splice-site mutations in tau with the inherited dementia FTDP-17. *Nature* 1998; **393**: 702–705.

82. Poorkaj P, Bird TD, Wijsman E, *et al.* Tau is a candidate gene for chromosome 17 frontotemporal dementia. *Ann Neurol* 1998; **43**: 815–825.

83. Baker M, Mackenzie IR, Pickering-Brown SM, *et al.* Mutations in progranulin cause tau-negative frontotemporal dementia linked to chromosome 17. *Nature* 2006; **442**: 916–919.

84. Cruts M, Gijselinck I, van der Zee J, *et al.* Null mutations in progranulin cause ubiquitin-positive frontotemporal dementia linked to chromosome 17q21. *Nature* 2006; **442**: 920–924.

85. Neumann M, Sampathu DM, Kwong LK, *et al.* Ubiquitinated TDP-43 in frontotemporal lobar degeneration and amyotrophic lateral sclerosis. *Science* 2006; **314**: 130–133.

86. Hong M, Zhukareva V, Vogelsberg-Ragaglia V, *et al.* Mutation-specific functional impairments in distinct tau isoforms of hereditary FTDP-17. *Science* 1998; **282**: 1914–1917.

87. Baker M, Litvan I, Houlden H, *et al.* Association of an extended haplotype in the tau gene with progressive supranuclear palsy. *Hum Mol Genet* 1999; **8**: 711–715.

88. Houlden H, Baker M, Morris HR, *et al.* Corticobasal degeneration and progressive supranuclear palsy share a common tau haplotype. *Neurology* 2001; **56**: 1702–1706.

89. Poorkaj P, Tsuang D, Wijsman E, *et al.* TAU as a susceptibility gene for amyotropic lateral sclerosis-parkinsonism dementia complex of Guam. *Arch Neurol* 2001; **58**: 1871–1878.

90. Pittman AM, Myers AJ, Abou-Sleiman P, *et al.* Linkage disequilibrium fine mapping and haplotype association analysis of the tau gene in progressive supranuclear palsy and corticobasal degeneration. *J Med Genet* 2005; **42**: 837–846.

91. Myers AJ, Pittman AM, Zhao AS, *et al.* The MAPT H1c risk haplotype is associated with increased expression of tau and especially of 4 repeat containing transcripts. *Neurobiol Dis* 2007; **25**: 561–570.

92. Lewis J, McGowan E, Rockwood J, *et al.* Neurofibrillary tangles, amyotrophy and progressive motor disturbance in mice expressing mutant (P301L) tau protein. *Nat Genet* 2000; **25**: 402–405.

93. Lewis J, Dickson DW, Lin WL, *et al.* Enhanced neurofibrillary degeneration in transgenic mice expressing mutant tau and APP. *Science* 2001; **293**: 1487–1491.

94. Hardy J, Duff K, Hardy KG, Perez-Tur J, Hutton M. Genetic dissection of Alzheimer's disease and related dementias: amyloid and its relationship to tau. *Nat Neurosci* 1998; **1**: 355–358.

95. Rapoport M, Dawson HN, Binder LI, Vitek MP, Ferreira A. Tau is essential to beta-amyloid-induced neurotoxicity. *Proc Natl Acad Sci USA* 2002; **99**: 6364–6369.

96. Roberson ED, Scearce-Levie K, Palop JJ, *et al.* Reducing endogenous tau ameliorates amyloid beta-induced deficits in an Alzheimer's disease mouse model. *Science* 2007; **316**: 750–754.

97. Myers AJ, Kaleem M, Marlowe L, *et al.* The H1c haplotype at the MAPT locus is associated with

Alzheimer's disease. *Hum Mol Genet* 2005; **14**: 2399–2404.

98. Mukherjee O, Kauwe JS, Mayo K, Morris JC, Goate AM. Haplotype-based association analysis of the MAPT locus in late onset Alzheimer's disease. *BMC Genet* 2007; **8**: 3.

99. Fox NC, Warrington EK, Seiffer AL, Agnew SK, Rossor MN. Presymptomatic cognitive deficits in individuals at risk of familial Alzheimer's disease. A longitudinal prospective study. *Brain* 1998; **121**: 1631–1639.

100. Freeborough PA, Woods RP, Fox NC. Accurate registration of serial 3D MR brain images and its application to visualizing change in neurodegenerative disorders. *J Comput Assist Tomogr* 1996; **20**: 1012–1022.

101. Klunk WE, Engler H, Nordberg A, *et al.* Imaging brain amyloid in Alzheimer's disease with Pittsburgh Compound-B. *Ann Neurol* 2004; **55**: 306–319.

102. Ridha BH, Barnes J, Bartlett JW, *et al.* Tracking atrophy progression in familial Alzheimer's disease: a serial MRI study. *Lancet Neurol* 2006; **5**: 828–834.

103. Chan D, Janssen JC, Whitwell JL, *et al.* Change in rates of cerebral atrophy over time in early-onset Alzheimer's disease: longitudinal MRI study. *Lancet* 2003; **362**: 1121–1122.

104. Fox NC, Black RS, Gilman S, *et al.* Effects of Abeta immunization (AN1792) on MRI measures of cerebral volume in Alzheimer disease. *Neurology* 2005; **64**: 1563–1572.

105. Gilman S, Koller M, Black RS, *et al.* Clinical effects of Abeta immunization (AN1792) in patients with AD in an interrupted trial. *Neurology* 2005; **64**: 1553–1562.

106. Klunk WE, Price JC, Mathis CA, *et al.* Amyloid deposition begins in the striatum of presenilin-1 mutation carriers from two unrelated pedigrees. *J Neurosci* 2007; **27**: 6174–6184.

107. Edison P, Archer HA, Hinz R, *et al.* Amyloid, hypometabolism, and cognition in Alzheimer disease: an [11C]PIB and [18F] FDG PET study. *Neurology* 2007; **68**: 501–508.

108. Games D, Adams D, Alessandrini R, *et al.* Alzheimer-type neuropathology in transgenic mice overexpressing V717F beta-amyloid precursor protein. *Nature* 1995; **373**: 523–527.

109. Duff K, Eckman C, Zehr C, *et al.* Increased amyloid-beta42(43) in brains of mice expressing mutant presenilin 1. *Nature* 1996; **383**: 710–713.

110. Borchelt DR, Ratovitski T, van Lare J, *et al.* Accelerated amyloid deposition in the brains of transgenic mice coexpressing mutant presenilin 1 and amyloid precursor proteins. *Neuron* 1997; **19**: 939–945.

111. Duff K, Suleman F. Transgenic mouse models of Alzheimer's disease: how useful have they been for therapeutic development? *Brief Funct Genomic Proteomic* 2004; **3**: 47–55.

112. Schenk D, Barbour R, Dunn W, *et al.* Immunization with amyloid-beta attenuates Alzheimer-disease-like pathology in the PDAPP mouse. *Nature* 1999; **400**: 173–177.

113. Noble W, Planel E, Zehr C, *et al.* Inhibition of glycogen synthase kinase-3 by lithium correlates with reduced tauopathy and degeneration in vivo. *Proc Natl Acad Sci USA* 2005; **102**: 6990–6995.

114. Oddo S, Caccamo A, Shepherd JD, *et al.* Triple-transgenic model of Alzheimer's disease with plaques and tangles: intracellular Abeta and synaptic dysfunction. *Neuron* 2003; **39**: 409–421.

115. Golde TE. Disease modifying therapy for AD? *J Neurochem* 2006; **99**: 689–707.

116. Morgan D, Diamond DM, Gottschall PE, *et al.* A beta peptide vaccination prevents memory loss in an animal model of Alzheimer's disease. *Nature* 2000; **408**: 982–985.

117. Janus C, Pearson J, McLaurin J, *et al.* A beta peptide immunization reduces behavioural impairment and plaques in a model of Alzheimer's disease. *Nature* 2000; **408**: 979–982.

118. Nicoll JA, Wilkinson D, Holmes C, *et al.* Neuropathology of human Alzheimer disease after immunization with amyloid-beta peptide: a case report. *Nat Med* 2003; **9**: 448–455.

119. Schenk D. Hopes remain for an Alzheimer's vaccine. *Nature* 2004; **431**: 398.

120. Hock C, Konietzko U, Streffer JR, *et al.* Antibodies against beta-amyloid slow cognitive decline in Alzheimer's disease. *Neuron* 2003; **38**: 547–554.

121. De Strooper B, Saftig P, Craessaerts K, *et al.* Deficiency of presenilin-1 inhibits the normal cleavage of amyloid precursor protein. *Nature* 1998; **391**: 387–390.

122. Wolfe MS, Xia W, Ostaszewski BL, *et al.* Two transmembrane aspartates in presenilin-1 required for presenilin endoproteolysis and gamma-secretase activity. *Nature* 1999; **398**: 513–517.

123. Edbauer D, Winkler E, Regula JT, *et al.* Reconstitution of gamma-secretase activity. *Nat Cell Biol* 2003; 5: 486–488.

124. Laudon H, Hansson EM, Melen K, *et al.* A nine-transmembrane domain topology for presenilin 1. *J Biol Chem* 2005; **280**: 35352–35360.

125. Haass C, Schlossmacher MG, Hung AY, *et al.* Amyloid beta-peptide is produced by cultured cells during

normal metabolism. *Nature* 1992; **359**: 322–324.

126. Vassar R, Bennett BD, Babu-Khan S, *et al.* Beta-secretase cleavage of Alzheimer's amyloid precursor protein by the transmembrane aspartic protease BACE. *Science* 1999; **286**: 735–741.

127. Asai M, Hattori C, Szabo B, *et al.* Putative function of ADAM9, ADAM10, and ADAM17 as APP alpha-secretase. *Biochem Biophys Res Commun* 2003; **301**: 231–235.

128. Cai XD, Golde TE, Younkin SG. Release of excess amyloid beta protein from a mutant amyloid beta protein precursor. *Science* 1993; **259**: 514–516.

129. Citron M, Teplow DB, Selkoe DJ. Generation of amyloid beta protein from its precursor is sequence specific. *Neuron* 1995; **14**: 661–670.

130. De Jonghe C, Zehr C, Yager D, *et al.* Flemish and Dutch mutations in amyloid beta precursor protein have different effects on amyloid beta secretion. *Neurobiol Dis* 1998; **5**: 281–286.

131. Suzuki N, Cheung TT, Cai XD, *et al.* An increased percentage of long amyloid beta protein secreted by familial amyloid beta protein precursor (beta APP717) mutants. *Science* 1994; **264**: 1336–1340.

132. Scheuner D, Eckman C, Jensen M, *et al.* Secreted amyloid beta-protein similar to that in the senile plaques of Alzheimer's disease is increased in vivo by the presenilin 1 and 2 and APP mutations linked to familial Alzheimer's disease. *Nat Med* 1996; **2**: 864–867.

133. Bales KR, Verina T, Cummins DJ, *et al.* Apolipoprotein E is essential for amyloid deposition in the APP(V717F) transgenic mouse model of Alzheimer's disease. *Proc Natl Acad Sci USA* 1999; **96**: 15233–15238.

The epilepsies

Mark Gardiner

Introduction

Epilepsy is a chronic brain disorder affecting up to 60 million people worldwide. The human epilepsies are a heterogeneous group of disorders with many causes, but it is generally accepted that a genetic etiology may be present in up to 40% of patients.

The current classification of epileptic seizures, epilepsies, and epilepsy syndromes is considered first. The literature (and clinical practice) remains confused by outdated terminology and a clear comprehension of current terminology is essential for understanding the genetics of this group of disorders. Moreover, recent advances in the understanding of the molecular basis of several epilepsy syndromes have revealed a level of genetic and phenotypic heterogeneity that adds a new dimension of complexity to classification and terminology.

The last decade has seen spectacular advances in the understanding of the molecular genetic basis of a number of rare Mendelian epilepsies. Autosomal dominant idiopathic epilepsies have emerged as ion channelopathies, arising from mutations in a host of voltage-gated and ligand-gated ion channel genes [1–4]. Genes underlying malformations of cortical development [5] and several of the progressive myoclonic epilepsies [6] have been identified. The next decade should see similar advances with respect to common, familial human genetic epilepsies, and a translation of the new molecular information into clinical practice with new diagnostic and treatment modalities.

Definitions, classification, and etiology

The definitions of seizures and epilepsy are considered, followed by an account of the current International League Against Epilepsy (ILAE) classifications of each [7,8]. These have recently been updated [9].

Epileptic seizure

An epileptic seizure is a transient episode of abnormal cortical neuronal activity apparent either to the patient or to an observer. The abnormal cortical activity may be manifest as a motor, sensory, autonomic, cognitive, or psychic disturbance. An epileptic seizure is, therefore, a transient event. It is neither a disease nor a syndrome. Epileptic seizure is a clinical diagnosis, although electrophysiological data may be used in determining the precise variety of seizure.

Epilepsy

Epilepsy is a disorder of the brain, characterized by recurrent, unprovoked epileptic seizures. Epilepsy may occur as a feature of a disease in which there is a common etiology, or a syndrome in which there is a particular pattern of seizures, and physical and investigative findings that occur together in a nonfortuitous manner. Epilepsy does not, therefore, include single epileptic seizures, occasional provoked epileptic seizures, or seizures that occur during an acute illness (e.g. encephalitis). Epileptic seizures and the epilepsies are classified separately, although the classification and terminology for each have features in common.

Classification of epileptic seizures

The first major division is into partial and generalized seizures.

Partial (focal, local) seizures

A partial seizure is an epileptic seizure in which the first clinical and electroencephalographic (EEG) changes indicate initial activation of a pool of neurons limited to part of one cerebral hemisphere. Partial seizures are divided further into simple and complex, according to whether consciousness is impaired. Simple seizures are those in which consciousness is retained, and complex seizures those in which it is impaired.

Generalized seizures

A generalized seizure is an epileptic seizure in which the first clinical changes indicate initial involvement of both cerebral hemispheres. In generalized seizures, consciousness may or may not be impaired. Any motor manifestations are bilateral. The two main varieties include absence and tonic-clonic seizures.

Absence seizure

Sudden onset of a brief impairment of consciousness, which may be mild or incomplete, characterizes absence seizures. Ongoing activities, such as speaking or walking, are interrupted.

Tonic-clonic seizures

In tonic-clonic seizures, there is a sudden loss of consciousness with sharp, tonic bilateral or axial muscular contraction, which may be asymmetric. This is followed by clonic jerking – rhythmic alternation of tonic phases with briefer relaxed phases – which builds up in amplitude and frequency and then subsides in frequency.

Classification of epilepsies and epileptic syndromes

The initial division follows that for seizures. A generalized epilepsy is one in which generalized seizures occur; a partial epilepsy is one in which partial seizures occur. Subsequent categorization is quite different, according to whether the etiology is idiopathic or symptomatic.

Idiopathic denotes a disorder that is "not preceded or occasioned by another". There is no underlying cause other than a possible hereditary predisposition. Symptomatic epilepsies are those that are "considered the consequence of a known or suspected disorder of the CNS". The disorder may originate in or outside the central nervous system (CNS).

Partial epilepsies

Idiopathic partial epilepsies include benign childhood epilepsy with centrotemporal spikes, autosomal dominant nocturnal frontal lobe epilepsy, and familial partial epilepsy with variable foci. Symptomatic partial epilepsies include chronic progressive epilepsia partialis continua of childhood (Kojewnikow syndrome) and a number of syndromes characterized by anatomical origin: temporal lobe epilepsy, frontal lobe epilepsy, parietal lobe epilepsy, and occipital lobe epilepsy.

Generalized epilepsies

The idiopathic generalized epilepsies include syndromes such as benign neonatal familial convulsions, childhood absence epilepsy (CAE), juvenile absence epilepsy (JAE), juvenile myoclonic epilepsy (JME), and epilepsy with generalized tonic-clonic seizures on awakening.

The symptomatic generalized epilepsies can be divided into those of nonspecific etiology (syndromes) and those of specific etiology (diseases). The former include entities such as West syndrome, Lennox–Gastaut syndrome, epilepsy with myoclonic absences, early myoclonic encephalopathy, and early infantile epileptic encephalopathy with suppression burst (Ohtahara syndrome). Symptomatic generalized epilepsies of specific etiology include a very large number of conditions, mostly genetic in etiology, in which seizures are the prominent or presenting feature. They include those with recognizable anatomical abnormalities in the CNS such as the neurocutaneous disorders and lissencephaly, inborn errors of metabolism such as phenylketonuria and nonketotic hyperglycinemia, storage disorders such as Tay–Sachs disease and the neuronal ceroid lipofuscinoses, disorders of mitochondrial function such as myoclonic epilepsy with ragged red fibers (MERRF) and mitochondrial encephalopathy with lactic acidosis and stroke-like episodes (MELAS), and a miscellaneous group of neurodegenerative conditions such as early onset Huntington's disease (HD), Unverricht–Lundborg disease, and Lafora disease.

Clinical diagnosis
History

When a patient presents with seizures, a crucial first step is to establish whether the attacks described are epileptic in nature. A number of paroxysmal episodes may mimic seizures [10,11]. Breath-holding spells in young children can, if of sufficient length, lead to unconsciousness, a fall to the ground, and myoclonic jerking. Syncope, from a variety of causes, may be mistaken for epileptic seizures. The possibility that the attacks have a psychological basis must also be considered. Other aspects of the history will be important in enabling the clinician to classify the epilepsy as idiopathic or symptomatic. A history of an abnormal pregnancy or birth may suggest that perinatal events have contributed to the etiology. A previous history of a significant head injury or an episode of intracranial infection may be the cause of subsequent epilepsy. The presence of developmental delay, intellectual deterioration, or evolving neurological symptoms suggests that the epilepsy is symptomatic, caused by either a progressive disorder or another of the Mendelian conditions described later. A detailed family pedigree may reveal a clear Mendelian pattern of inheritance or maternal inheritance, and suggest possible diagnoses.

Clinical examination

Dysmorphic features and cutaneous stigmata should be sought. Particular dysmorphic features in an individual with epilepsy may indicate a diagnosis. For example, patients with Angelman syndrome or fragile-X syndrome exhibit epilepsy. The neurocutaneous syndromes that may present with epilepsy include tuberous sclerosis complex (TSC), neurofibromatosis type 1 (NF 1), hypomelanosis of Ito, incontinentia pigmenti, linear sebaceous nevus syndrome, Sturge–Weber syndrome, and Klippel–Trenaunay–Weber syndrome.

Patients who give a history of partial seizures and who display localizing neurological signs should be considered to have a focal lesion requiring cranial imaging. The presence of progressive neurological signs is a cause for concern and suggests a degenerative disorder. Fundal examination should be included; it may reveal a retinal phakoma and lead to a diagnosis of tuberous sclerosis or the optic glioma of NF 1. The presence of choroidoretinitis would suggest congenital infection as a cause. Pigmentary retinopathy is a feature of many conditions, including the mitochondrial disorders and the neuronal ceroid lipofucinoses.

Investigations

Investigations may include biochemical investigation, EEG, videotelemetry, cranial imaging, and DNA diagnostics.

The electroencephalograph

Electroencephalographic criteria form part of the ILAE classification of many epileptic syndromes. Routine EEG examination usually consists of a standard 12-lead EEG performed in the waking state, but this may be followed by prolonged monitoring in individuals who have infrequent episodes or in whom seizures occur at night or in the early morning. A sleep-deprived EEG or sleep EEG may reveal abnormalities not seen on the standard recording. In addition, provocation by hyperventilation and intermittent photic stimulation may enhance features that are present already or may elicit abnormalities in otherwise normal EEGs. It is important to recognize that a normal EEG does not exclude epilepsy.

The EEG may be recorded during a seizure (the ictal EEG) or between seizures (interictal). Ictal changes seen on the EEG consist of typical epileptiform activity such as spikes, sharp waves, or spike wave discharges. The interictal EEG is more likely to be abnormal in children than in adults with epilepsy. The only features that are directly supportive of a diagnosis of epilepsy are epileptiform discharges.

Photosensitive epilepsy is a term that probably encompasses a heterogeneous group of conditions that include seizures in response to photic stimulation. Photosensitivity is defined by the occurrence of spikes or spike waves in response to intermittent photic stimulation (IPS), known as the photoparoxysmal response (PPR).

Investigations in which twins have been studied at different stages of life have shown a remarkably high concordance in the EEGs of monozygotic twins, suggesting that the EEG is almost entirely genetically determined [12,13].

Imaging

Modern imaging techniques, in particular structural magnetic resonance imaging (MRI) and methods of functional imaging, are being used increasingly for the assessment of patients with epilepsy. The main application of improved imaging techniques has been in the development of epilepsy surgery, now a recognized treatment for children and adults with intractable epilepsy and focal brain lesions. In addition, increasingly subtle abnormalities of cortical development, some of which have a genetic basis, are now detectable on MRI. In order to provide accurate genetic counseling, an MRI is an essential tool in diagnosis.

The plain skull radiograph has a limited role in the investigation of an individual with epilepsy. Intracerebral calcification is apparent on a skull radiograph; when considered with other clinical features, it may point to a diagnosis of congenital infection or tuberous sclerosis. It will demonstrate the railroad calcification associated with Sturge–Weber syndrome.

Cerebral ultrasound is the imaging modality of choice for the assessment of infants in the perinatal period. Ultrasound is useful in making diagnoses in infants with hypoxic-ischemic encephalopathy, suspected developmental malformations, infarctions, microcephaly, and cerebral hemorrhage.

The place for further imaging of the brain in epilepsy largely depends on the type of epilepsy present. Computerized tomography (CT) has certain limitations; most notably, its inability to image in the multiplanar dimension, exposure to ionizing radiation, and interference with imaging of the temporal lobe because of bony artifacts from the middle fossa. For these reasons, CT has now been largely superseded by MRI in the investigation of the epileptic patient.

The main indications for an MRI scan in a patient with epilepsy include [14]: focal epilepsy or a focal abnormality on EEG, seizures in the first year of life, seizure onset after the age of 20 years, focal neurological signs, loss of seizure control or change in the pattern of seizures, and generalized seizures resistant to medication.

DNA diagnostics

DNA-based tests are available for a number of genetic epilepsies for which the gene has been identified. These include, of course, conditions such as fragile-X, HD, TSC, and NF 1. A single common mutation, in most patients, accounts for several autosomal recessive epilepsies such as Unverricht–Lundborg disease (EPM1) and juvenile-onset neuronal ceroid lipofuscinosis (NCL) (CLN3); but locus and allelic heterogeneity render DNA analysis problematic in the idiopathic autosomal dominant epilepsies caused by mutations in ion channel genes, such as autosomal dominant nocturnal frontal lobe epilepsy, benign familial neonatal convulsions, and generalized epilepsy with febrile seizures plus (GEFS+).

Mendelian epilepsies

X-linked

Fragile-X

Affected males with fragile-X have an increased frequency of epilepsy. Estimates of its prevalence vary from 28% to 45%. Seizures may be generalized tonic-clonic, partial with or without secondary generalization, or of multiple types.

Rett syndrome

Rett syndrome (RTT) [15] is a progressive neurodevelopmental disorder that affects females almost exclusively, with an incidence of 1 in 10 000–15 000 [16]. It is an X-linked dominant condition with lethality in hemizygous males. Epilepsy may occur during the stagnant or pseudostationary stage, between the ages of 2 and 10 years. Seizures are frequently preceded by EEG abnormalities including paroxysmal spikes or spike waves, and a progressive slowing and deterioration of the background activity. Mutations in the X-linked *MECP2* gene encoding methyl-CpG-binding protein 2 (MeCP2) are responsible for the primary defect in RTT [17].

West syndrome

This classical form of epilepsy with onset in early infancy is etiologically heterogeneous. The existence of an X-linked form has been observed [18,19] and was confirmed by demonstration of linkage to Xp11.4-Xpter in two families [20]. Mutations in the human ortholog of Aristaless were recently found to cause X-linked mental retardation and epilepsy [21].

X-linked lissencephaly and subcortical band heterotopia

X-linked lissencephaly (XLIS) causes classical lissencephaly in hemizygous males and a milder phenotype in affected female heterozygotes. Males have profound mental retardation, epilepsy with multiple seizure types including infantile spasms, and a shortened lifespan. Nearly all patients with sporadic subcortical band heterotopia (SBH) are female. A wide range of seizure types may occur including infantile spasms, and the disorder may underlie Lennox–Gastaut syndrome. The brains of affected females have a subpopulation of neurons that migrate abnormally and arrest in the subcortical white matter, leading to a double-cortex appearance or SBH [22]. The gene that is mutated in XLIS/SBH, *DCX*, was recently cloned. It encodes doublecortin, a novel protein of 360 amino acids [23,24].

Periventricular heterotopia

Periventricular heterotopia (PH), the existence of normal tissue in an abnormal location, occurs when neurons of the developing cerebral cortex fail to migrate from the ventricular zone and remain as nodules lining the walls of the ventricles. It is an X-linked dominant condition, usually lethal in male embryos. Affected females have normal intelligence and present with seizures and other systemic signs [25,26]. Multiple seizure types may occur.

The locus for PH was mapped to chromosome Xq28. The candidate region included the gene *FLN1*, which encodes the protein filamin 1, an actin-binding protein that binds other cytoskeletal regulators and plays an important role in migration of many cell types. Mutation analysis of the exons that encode the actin-binding domain in 25 affected females (both sporadic and familial) identified four point mutations and a frameshift mutation. The failure of neurons to migrate from their point of origin suggests a functional role at the initial stage of migration.

Autosomal dominant

Symptomatic

Miller–Dieker syndrome and isolated lissencephaly sequence

Nearly all patients who have Miller–Dieker syndrome (MDS) and approximately one third of those patients who have isolated lissencephaly sequence (ILS) have a hemizygous deletion or a mutation in the *LIS1* gene, which encodes a noncatalytic subunit of the platelet-activating factor (PAF) acetylhydrolase, a heterotrimeric enzyme that inactivates PAF [27,28]. Miller–Dieker syndrome comprises classical lissencephaly (grade 1 or 2) together with characteristic facial abnormalities, which include prominent narrow forehead, long philtrum, short nose, and flat midface. Isolated lissencephaly sequence consists of classical lissencephaly (grades 1–4) with normal facial appearance. In both, clinical features include severe mental retardation, diplegia, and mixed seizure types that often include partial seizures and infantile spasms.

Tuberous sclerosis complex

Mutations of two different genes cause TSC. *TSC1* at 9q34 encodes hamartin and *TSC2* at 16p13.3 encodes tuberin. The gene products are known to interact in vivo although the nature of this interaction remains undetermined. Early reports of what now is called TSC described it as the classical triad of epilepsy, mental retardation, and facial angiofibromas [29]. Estimates of the incidence of epilepsy in TSC vary from 60% to 100%. A number of seizure types may occur in tuberous sclerosis, including infantile spasms, which are the most common seizure type at presentation, myoclonic, and generalized tonic-clonic seizures. Up to 25% of babies presenting with infantile spasms have TSC. Tuberous sclerosis complex is the most common identifiable cause of the Lennox–Gastaut syndrome, a syndrome of multiple seizure types, interictal diffuse slow spike waves on EEG, and developmental delay.

Neurofibromatosis type 1

The incidence of epilepsy in NF 1 is low compared with TSC and is estimated to occur in 5%–10% of affected individuals [30]. A variety of seizure types are seen, including infantile spasms, absence, generalized tonic-clonic, and complex partial seizures. Complex partial seizures appear to be the most common type.

Idiopathic

Autosomal dominant nocturnal frontal lobe epilepsy: mutations in *CHRNA4* and *CHRNB2*

Autosomal dominant nocturnal frontal lobe epilepsy (ADNFLE) is a rare autosomal dominant epilepsy with high penetrance, first described in 1995 [31]. The phenotype is characterized by clusters of brief nocturnal motor seizures, including hyperkinetic activity or tonic stiffening, normally with retained consciousness.

Autosomal dominant nocturnal frontal lobe epilepsy was the first human idiopathic epilepsy for which the genetic basis was identified. Five distinct mutations have now been identified in genes encoding the α4 (*CHRNA4*) and β2 (*CHRNB2*) subunits of the neuronal nicotinic acetylcholine receptor (NNR). There is marked heterogeneity, however. One family is linked to the cluster of NNR-subunit genes on chromosome 15q [32] (although no mutations in their genes have been identified) and more families link to none of these loci.

A locus for ADNFLE was first mapped to chromosome 20q13.2 in a large Australian pedigree [33], and a missense c839C>T mutation in *CHRNA4* was identified, associated with substitution of phenylalanine for serine (Ser280Phe) in the M2 domain [34]. (Numbering is based on Antonarakis 1998 and differs from that in the original report: Ser248Phe.) This mutation has arisen independently in a Norwegian family [35], and two further mutations have been described in the M2 domain: c873–874insGCT associated with Leu301–302 [36] and c851C>T associated with Ser284Leu (Ser252Leu in old numbering) in a Japanese family [37].

Further loci were identified on 15q24 and 1q and two mutations have been identified at the *CHRNB2* gene locus on 1q. These are both missense mutations, changing the valine residue at 287 to leucine [38] or to methionine [39]. The ADNFLE loci at the three chromosomal regions are designated epilepsy, nocturnal frontal lobe (ENFL) type 1: 20q13.2, type 2: 15q24, and type 3: 1q.

It remains uncertain how mutations in genes encoding neuronal nicotinic acetylcholine receptor subunits cause an age-dependant, nocturnal frontal lobe epilepsy [40]. In the mammalian brain, most NNRs are heteromultimers more commonly consisting of three α4 and two β2 subunits, the very two subunits encoded by the genes mutated in ADNFLE.

The functional effects of the naturally occurring mutations described previously have been examined in vitro by expression in *Xenopus laevis* oocytes and other cells. Results have varied, partly because of the difficulty of replicating the in vivo situation, in which both wild type and mutant are coexpressed. The only common characteristic observed in the analysis of four mutations is an increase in acetylcholine sensitivity, indicating a gain of function [41].

Benign familial neonatal convulsions: mutations in *KCNQ2* and *KCNQ3*

Benign familial neonatal convulsions (BFNC) is a rare, autosomal dominant, idiopathic epilepsy [42]. Seizures occur in otherwise well neonates from the second or third day of life and remit by six weeks. Typical seizures are generalized and include tonic and clonic phases. However, focal components may occur, including motor automatisms and ocular manifestations. Affected neonates usually show normal neurological and intellectual development. Seizures may recur in later life in approximately 10% of individuals.

Benign familial neonatal convulsions exhibits both clinical and genetic heterogeneity. The first epilepsy locus to be identified by linkage analysis, designated EBN1, was found on chromosome 20q in a four-generation family with 19 individuals with BFNC [43]. Six other pedigrees confirmed this linkage [44]. However, clinical heterogeneity was demonstrated by another family, which showed no linkage to EBN1. This family included members with seizures persisting up to two years of age, and in one individual, into adolescence [45]. Genetic heterogeneity was subsequently demonstrated by another family, none of whose members had seizures after two months of age. EBN1 was excluded by linkage analysis, and a second locus (EBN2) was identified on chromosome 8q [46]. The genes for EBN1 and EBN2, *KCNQ2* and *KCNQ3*, were both identified as voltage-dependent potassium channels. *KCNQ2* was identified by characterization of a submicroscopic deletion on chromosome 20q13.3 and shows significant homology with a voltage-dependent potassium channel gene, *KCNQ1* [47].

At least six allelic variants of *KCNQ2* segregate with the disease in families with BFNC, including one family whose affected members subsequently developed myokymia [48]. *KCNQ3* was identified by the discovery of a cDNA sequence with significant homology to *KCNQ2*. A novel gene, *KCNQ3*, shows 69% similarity to *KCNQ2* and maps to the EBN2 critical region on chromosome 8q24. Mutations in *KCNQ3* were identified in affected members of the BFNC/EBN2 family [49].

The *KCNQ* gene family encodes voltage-dependent potassium channels mainly expressed in the heart, CNS (especially hippocampus, neocortex, and cerebellum), inner ear, and skeletal muscle. In the CNS, they are important in regulating neuronal excitability by controlling the duration of the action potential and responsiveness to synaptic inputs. Mutations in *KCNQ1* can cause the paroxysmal cardiac dysrhythmias, long QT syndrome, and Jervell–Lange–Nielson cardioauditory syndrome [50,51], and mutations in *KCNQ4* cause congenital deafness [52].

The heteromeric assembly of *KCNQ2* and *KCNQ3* encoded potassium channel subunits has been shown to form the M-channel [53,54]. This mediates the slowly activating and noninactivating M-current, which is a widespread regulator of neuronal excitability. It limits repetitive firing by tending to repolarize the neuronal membrane back toward resting membrane potential during long-lasting depolarizing inputs [55]. The coassembly of *KCNQ2* and *KCNQ3* enhances, by about 10-fold, the current size of *KCNQ3* alone [56]. Mutations in *KCNQ2* and *KCNQ3*, which cause BFNC, occur either in the critical pore-forming region or in the C-terminus, which is thought to mediate formation of the M-channel. The reduction in M-current caused by the *KCNQ2* and *KCNQ3* gene mutations seems relatively small (20%–25%), indicating that the brain may be particularly sensitive to changes in potassium conductance causing hyperexcitability [57].

Generalized epilepsy with febrile seizures plus and severe myoclonic epilepsy of infancy: mutations in *SCN1A*, *SCN2A*, *SCN1B*, and *GABRG2*

Generalized epilepsy with febrile seizures plus (GEFS+) is an autosomal dominant epilepsy first described in 1997 [58]. The commonest GEFS+ phenotype comprises a childhood onset of multiple febrile seizures persisting beyond the age of six years, together with afebrile seizures including absences, myclonic seizures, atonic seizures and, rarely, myoclonic-astatic epilepsy. A large Australian GEFS+ family was linked to chromosome 19q13.1, and a point mutation identified in the gene *SCN1B*, which encodes the β1 subunit of the voltage-gated sodium channel [59].

Two French families with GEFS+ showed linkage to chromosome 2q24, and mutations were identified in *SCN1A*, the gene encoding the sodium channel α1 subunit [60–62]. Novel *SCN1A* gene mutations were also identified in two unrelated Japanese families with febrile seizures associated with afebrile partial seizures [63].

De novo mutations in *SCN1A* have been identified in patients with severe myoclonic epilepsy of infancy (SMEI), which also involves fever-associated seizures but shows a more malignant course [64–66]. SMEI was first described in 1978 by Dravet and is characterized by early normal development before the onset of seizures in the first year of life [67]. Generalized or partial febrile seizures are followed by afebrile seizures, including myoclonic, absence, tonic-clonic, and partial seizures. Seizures are often refractory to treatment and developmental arrest and regression occur. Many patients with SMEI have a family history of seizures consistent with the spectrum of seizure phenotypes seen in GEFS+, suggesting that SMEI is the most severe phenotype in the GEFS+ spectrum [68]. A mutation in a third sodium channel gene, *SCN2A*, encoding the α2-channel subunit, has been identified in a patient with febrile seizures associated with afebrile seizures, consistent with GEFS+. Mutations in *SCN2A* have also been found in families with benign familial neonatal-infantile seizures (BFNIS), an epilepsy similar to benign familial neonatal convulsions (see previous discussion), but in which seizures begin after one month of age [69]. In fact, *SCN2A* gene mutations appear to be specific for BFNIS [70].

Mutations in sodium channel α-subunit genes also cause several paroxysmal disorders of muscle, including hyperkalemic periodic paralysis, paramyotonia congenita (*SCN4A*), and long QT syndrome (*SCN5A*) [71]. Sodium channels are modulated by anti-epileptic drugs such as phenytoin and carbamazepine [72].

The original *SCN1B* (C121W) mutation has recently been found in a second GEFS+ family [73]. It changes a conserved cysteine residue that disrupts a disulfide bridge normally maintaining an immunoglobulin-like fold in the β-subunit extracellular domain. Coexpression of C121W mutant human β1

subunit with a rat brain α subunit in *Xenopus laevis* oocytes caused slower sodium channel inactivation, which is likely to cause persistent inward neuronal sodium currents, increased membrane depolarization, and neuronal hyperexcitability [59]. This may also exaggerate the normal effects of temperature on both conductance and gating of neuronal sodium channels, explaining the apparent temperature dependence of the GEFS+ phenotype.

The initial *SCN1A* gene mutations discovered in GEFS+ altered amino acids within the voltage-sensing S4 segments [62]. The functional effects of three *SCN1A* mutations have been investigated by heterologous expression with β1 and β2 subunits in cultured mammalian cells [74]. All three mutations alter channel inactivation, resulting in persistent inward sodium current. Thus, neuronal hyperexcitability is again likely to result from increased membrane depolarization, as with the *SCN1B* gene mutation. The *SCN1A* mutations causing SMEI generally predict introduction of a stop codon and truncation of the protein with predicted complete loss of function. Thus, severe *de novo* truncation mutations of *SCN1A* underlie many cases of SMEI. Those cases occurring within GEFS+ families may suggest interaction of *SCN1A* mutations with modifier genes.

The GEFS+ phenotype is not only caused by mutations in voltage-gated sodium channels. In two GEFS+ families, mutations have been identified in the GABA$_A$ receptor γ-subunit gene, *GABRG2* [75,76]. Binding of GABA opens an integral chloride channel, with resultant inhibition of neuronal activity. The first GEFS+ mutation substitutes a serine for a methionine in the extracellular loop between transmembrane segments M2 and M3. This decreased the amplitude of GABA-activated currents when expressed in *Xenopus laevis* oocytes and HEK293 cells, but did not alter diazepam potentiation [75,77]. The second mutation introduces a premature stop codon in the mature protein [76]. This completely abolished GABA sensitivity in *Xenopus laevis* oocytes expressing the mutant γ2 subunit. Receptors containing the mutant subunit failed to reach the cell surface when expressed in HEK293 cells. Mutations in *GABRG2* also cause a phenotype of CAE and febrile seizures [78].

Autosomal dominant juvenile myoclonic epilepsy: mutation in *GABRA1*

GABA$_A$ receptors are the major sites of fast synaptic inhibition in the brain and dysfunction of this receptor has long been suspected in the development of epilepsy. Mutations were recently described (see previous discussion) in the *GABRG2* gene, which encodes the $GABA_A$ receptor γ2 subunit, in several families. The associated phenotypes encompassed GEFS[+], absence epilepsy, and SMEI.

A mutation in the *GABRA1* gene has been described in a large French Canadian kindred with autosomal dominant segregation of a phenotype consistent with JME [79]. All affected individuals had myoclonic and generalized tonic-clonic seizures with generalized polyspike and wave discharges on EEG. A genome scan provided evidence of linkage to chromosome 5q34 encompassing a cluster of $GABA_A$ receptor subunit genes: *GABRB2*, *GABRA1*, and *GABRG2*. A mutation, Ala322Asp, in *GABRA1* was found to segregate in a heterozygous state with affected individuals but none of the unaffected. $GABA_A$ receptors containing the mutant subunit showed a lesser amplitude of GABA activated current in vitro compared with wild-type receptors.

This is the first example of a mutation segregating with a Mendelian phenotype corresponding to a common idiopathic generalized epilepsy (IGE) syndrome. This mutation was not found in 83 patients with sporadic IGE (including JME and CAE), some of whom had a positive family history for various epilepsy syndromes. It will be of great interest to determine whether common sequence variants in genes encoding $GABA_A$ receptor subunits contribute to the common non-Mendelian form of JME.

Mutations in *KCNA1* and *CACNA1A* associated with episodic ataxia and epilepsy

It is noteworthy that epilepsy occurs as a component of the phenotype in some patients with the rare autosomal dominant episodic ataxias EA1 and EA2, associated with mutations in *KCNA1* and *CACNA1A*.

A Scottish EA1 family with five affected individuals, two of whom had partial epilepsy, were found to be heterozygous for a missense point mutation in *KCNA1*, predicted to cause a substitution of arginine for threonine at position 226 in the second transmembrane segment [80]. Functional studies suggested a dominant negative effect. Another family, in which the two affected individuals had muscle twitching and seizures but no episodic ataxia, had a missense mutation (G724C) predicted to cause substitution of proline for alanine at position 242 [81], and associated with a profound reduction in current amplitude

without evidence of a dominant negative effect. Mice that have had the homologous *KCNA1* gene deleted develop a lethal epilepsy phenotype in the homozygous state [82].

A mutation in *CACNA1A* was recently described in an 11-year-old boy with a complex phenotype including primary generalized epilepsy, episodic and progressive ataxia, and mild learning difficulties [83]. The heterozygous point mutation (C5733T) introduces a premature stop codon (R1820 stop) resulting in complete loss of the C-terminal region. Expression studies revealed that the mutation impairs calcium channel function and coexpression studies indicated a dominant negative effect. It is noteworthy that polymorphisms in *CACNA1A* appear to be associated with IGE [84].

Mutations in *CLCN2* associated with idiopathic generalized epilepsies

A genome-wide search in a large number of families with common IGE subtypes identified a susceptibility locus on chromosome 3q26 [85]. One of the candidate genes in this region was *CLCN2*, which encodes the voltage-gated chloride channel CLC-2.

Mutation analysis of this gene in affected individuals from 46 unrelated families led to identification of three different heterozygous mutations in three families in which affected individuals had any of the four most common IGE subtypes: CAE, JAE, JME, and epilepsy with grand-mal seizures on awakening [86]. The mutations resulted in a premature stop codon (M200fs × 231), an atypical splicing event (del 74–117), and a single amino acid substitution (G715E).

CLC-2 is expressed in the brain, especially in neurons inhibited by GABA, and is believed to play a role in maintaining the low intracellular chloride concentration that is necessary for an inhibitory GABA response. Functional analysis of mutant channels indicated a loss of function for the first two mutations, predicted to result in intracellular chloride accumulation and a reduction in the inhibitory GABA response, or even conversion to an excitatory response. In contrast, G715E mutant channels had normal current amplitudes but altered voltage-dependent gating causing them to open at less negative potentials. This gain of function may render GABAergic synapses hyperexcitable by allowing an increased outward chloride current during repolarization.

Autosomal dominant lateral temporal lobe epilepsy and mutations in *LGI1*: chromosome 10q-linked partial epilepsy

Autosomal dominant lateral temporal lobe epilepsy (ADLTE) is an epilepsy syndrome characterized by focal seizures arising from the lateral temporal lobe, usually preceded by nonspecific auditory phenomena, such as a ringing or humming noise. It is also termed autosomal dominant partial epilepsy with auditory features (ADPEAF) or lateral temporal epilepsy with acoustic aura.

Ottman and colleagues provided the first description of this disorder and identified the linkage to a 10-cM interval on chromosome 10q in a family with 11 affected individuals [87]. Additional kindreds were defined, which confirmed and refined the locus on 10q22-q24 [88,89]. Using a positional candidate approach, five disease mutations were found in *LGI1* (leucine-rich gene, glioma-inactivated) in five families with this disorder [90], and additional mutations were subsequently identified in two Spanish ADLTE families [91], one Norwegian family [92], and one Italian family [93]. The majority of the mutations are predicted to cause protein truncation, the remainder being missense mutations altering conserved amino acids.

The human *LGI1* gene (also called the *Epitempin* gene) was first discovered in a glioblastoma cell line in which it is rearranged as a result of a balanced translocation. The expression pattern of the highly conserved homologous mouse gene (*Lgi1*) is mostly neuronal. The encoded protein has several interesting features. There are three leucine-rich repeats (LRRs) in the predicted N-terminal domain, flanked by conserved cysteine-rich clusters. LRR-containing genes are involved in a variety of functions including signal transduction, regulation of cell growth, adhesion, and migration.

The LGI1/epitempin protein was also noted to contain a novel homology domain consisting of a seven-fold repeated 44-residue motif predicted to form a seven-bladed β-propellor fold [94,95]. This repeat, variously called the epilepsy associated repeat (EAR) and epitempin (EPTP) repeat, defines a subfamily of genes, some of which have also been implicated in epilepsy in mice and humans. Genes that encode proteins with this repeat include a subfamily of leucine-rich repeat proteins and are designated *LGI2* (chromosome 4p15.2), *LGI3* (chromosome 8p21.3), and *LGI4* (chromosome 19q13.13). The loci of *LGI3* and *LGI4* are confusingly also referred to as LGIL4 and LGIL3 (i.e. numbers reversed) in the literature.

In addition to proteins having the typical LGI-like domain organization, the EPTP repeat is found in the human and mouse very large G-protein coupled receptors (VLGR) and a protein called TSPEAR or TSP-EAR (gene *TNEP1*) on chromosome 21q22.3. Part of the human *VLGR1* gene (exons 5–39 form a transcript of *MASS1*) on chromosome 5q14.1 is homologous to the mouse *Mass1* gene, which is mutated in the Frings mouse, a model of audiogenic seizures [96]. A mutation in *MASS1* has recently been described in a family with febrile and afebrile seizures, although cosegregation of trait and mutant allele cannot be established unequivocally [97]. The EPTP repeat is the only sequence motif that links the three subfamilies represented by genes *LGI1*, *VLGR1*, and *TNEP1*. The functional basis of its link with epilepsy remains unknown but is of great interest.

Autosomal recessive

Symptomatic

Metabolic disorders

Epileptic seizures are a feature of many of the inborn errors of metabolism, all of which are individually rare and together are found in about 1 in 5000 live births. Seizures may be a presenting symptom or may form part of the evolving clinical picture. In general, any infant with seizures without obvious cause (e.g. hypoxic-ischemic encephalopathy, hypoglycemia, hypocalcemia, or other electrolyte disturbance, sepsis, brain infarction, or hemorrhage) should be investigated. Hypoglycemia is a common feature of many metabolic disorders, and should be investigated in any child outside the neonatal period, or in a neonate with recurrent, unexplained hypoglycemia. A metabolic disorder should be suspected in any patient found to have an unexplained neurological process. Myoclonic seizures appear to be particularly common in this group of disorders; their presence in an infant should alert the clinician to the possibility of a metabolic disease. Metabolic disorders associated with epilepsy include storage disorders such as the gangliosidoses and Gaucher disease, urea cycle defects, peroxisomal disorders (e.g. adrenoleukodystrophy), and aminoacidopathies such as phenylketonuria.

Of particular importance is the syndrome of pyridoxine dependent seizures, an autosomal recessive condition characterized by the onset of intractable seizures during the neonatal period or even prior to delivery. The seizures respond dramatically to intravenous pyridoxine coincidentally with a normalization of the EEG. Pyridoxine is required throughout life, with early treatment possibly preventing later epilepsy and mental retardation.

Nonketotic hyperglycinemia presents with early myoclonic encephalopathy with erratic myoclonus, partial seizures, and a suppression burst pattern on EEG.

Progressive myoclonus epilepsies

The progressive myoclonus epilepsies (PMEs) are a clinically and etiologically heterogeneous group of rare inherited disorders characterized by the association of epilepsy, myoclonus, and progressive neurological deterioration, in particular ataxia and dementia [98–100]. The most common forms of PME are: Unverricht–Lundborg disease, Lafora disease, the neuronal ceroid lipofuscinoses, MERRF, and sialidosis.

Unverricht–Lundborg disease (Baltic myoclonus)

Progressive myoclonic epilepsy of the Unverricht–Lundborg type (ULD, locus symbol, EPM1) is an autosomal recessive disorder, which is enriched in the Finnish population with an incidence of one in 20 000 births. Stimulus sensitive myoclonus begins between the ages of about 6 and 15 years and mild mental retardation, dysarthria, and ataxia develop with time. Nonspecific histological changes are found in the brain; Lafora bodies or autofluorescent lipopigment are not found. Evidence suggests that ULD, Baltic myoclonus [63], and so-called Mediterranean myoclonus [64] are genetically homogenous. The combination of a high degree of consanguinity and a risk rate for siblings of one in four demonstrates that inheritance is autosomal recessive [63].

Unverricht–Lundborg disease was mapped to the long arm of chromosome 21 in a group of 11 nuclear pedigrees from Finland. A genome search was undertaken and linkage found after testing 64 marker loci [65]. A maximum multipoint LOD score of 10.08 was obtained with three loci in 21q22.3. Linkage studies in non-Finnish families have demonstrated genetic (locus) homogeneity within this phenotype.

The *EPM1* gene was isolated by positional cloning and shown to be the gene encoding cystatin B [68]. Cystatin B, a small protein that is a member of a superfamily of cysteine protease inhibitors, is thought to inactivate proteases that leak out of the lysosome. Of great interest is the observation that the majority of disease-causing mutations are a result of expansion of an unstable minisatellite repeat in the $5'$ flanking region [69,71,72].

Cystatin B is ubiquitously expressed. Its role in the development of ULD is not known. Mice lacking cystatin B develop myoclonic seizures and ataxia, associated with cerebellar granule cell loss, and cellular changes characteristic of apoptotic cell death [73]. Cystatin B, therefore, may protect against cerebellar cell apoptosis.

Lafora disease

Progressive myoclonus epilepsy with polyglucosan intracellular inclusion bodies was first described in 1911 by Lafora and has become known as Lafora disease [74,75]. It is an autosomal recessive disease characterized by the presence of periodic acid–Schiff-positive cytoplasmic inclusion bodies, known as Lafora bodies, in neurons, heart, liver, and muscle. During adolescence, affected individuals develop a seizure disorder that may include generalized tonic-clonic seizures, absences, drop attacks, or focal occipital seizures. Soon after presentation, subjects develop asymmetric myoclonic jerks. The EEG shows high-voltage bilateral synchronous, spike-wave and poly-spike-wave complexes. Diagnosis is based on the presence of Lafora bodies in the eccrine sweat duct cells, most readily detected on axillary skin biopsy.

Linkage analysis performed in nine families with Lafora disease produced a maximum two-point LOD score of 10.54 at $\theta = 0$ at the marker D6S311, localizing the gene to 6q23–25 [76]. Using a positional cloning approach, the gene mutated in Lafora disease, *EPM2A*, was cloned [77]. *EPM2A* is predicted to encode an intracellular protein tyrosine phosphatase (PTP), laforin. *EPM2A* is expressed in many tissues, including brain. The PTPs act to oppose the action of tyrosine kinases in cell signaling pathways and regulate levels of phosphotyrosine in cells.

The neuronal ceroid lipofuscinoses

The neuronal ceroid lipofuscinoses (NCLs) are a group of neurodegenerative encephalopathies characterized by psychomotor deterioration, visual failure, seizures, and the accumulation of autofluorescent lipopigment in neurons and other cell types. There are five types that present as a PME: classical late infantile or CLN2 (Jansky–Bielschowsky's disease), juvenile or CLN3 (Spielmeyer–Vogt–Sjögren's or Batten's disease), adult or CLN4 (Kufs' or Parry disease), late infantile Finnish variant or CLN5, and late infantile variant or CLN6. Inheritance is autosomal recessive except for the adult form, which may present autosomal dominant inheritance. The phenotypic subtypes are classified on the basis of age of onset, clinical features, and ultrastructural content of the storage material. The main clinical features include failure of psychomotor development, impaired vision, and epilepsy. Studies of storage bodies have demonstrated that the major component in both late infantile and juvenile (but not infantile) NCL is the protein subunit c of the mitochondrial ATP synthase complex [78,79] .

Advances in human molecular genetic techniques have allowed positional cloning strategies to be applied to identification of the defective genes and their protein products. To date, six disease gene loci have been mapped and all of these genes have been isolated.

Non-Mendelian epilepsies

Complex traits

Two recent studies have clarified the genetic architecture of IGE, suggesting that CAE and JAE share a close genetic relationship and JME is a more distinct entity [101,102].

Juvenile myoclonic epilepsy

Juvenile myoclonic epilepsy is a common form of idiopathic generalized epilepsy representing 5%–10% of epilepsy as a whole. Individuals most commonly present between the ages of 8 and 26 years with early morning myoclonus, symmetrical shock-like jerks predominantly of the upper limbs, precipitated by fatigue, alcohol, and menstruation. Over 90% also have generalized tonic-clonic seizures and 30% have absence seizures. The EEG characteristically shows bilateral symmetrical 4–6 Hz polyspike and wave although it may be normal. Juvenile myoclonic epilepsy usually is readily treated with sodium valproate.

A genetic contribution to JME has long been established although the mode of inheritance is unclear. Autosomal dominant [103], autosomal recessive [104], two locus [105], and multifactorial models have been proposed.

Four studies from two groups have provided evidence for the existence of a locus predisposing to JME on chromosome 6p – designated EJM1. In 1988, Greenberg and colleagues performed linkage analysis in 24 families in which the proband had JME using the classical markers HLA and properdin factor B (BF) [106]. Asymptomatic relatives with an abnormal EEG were classified as affected. The maximum LOD score of 3.04 was obtained when HLA and BF were considered together and under the assumption of autosomal recessive inheritance with full penetrance. By increasing the family resource, the same group later obtained a maximum LOD score of 3.78 ($\theta_{m=f} = 0.01$), with HLA assuming autosomal dominant inheritance and classifying asymptomatic relatives with abnormal EEGs as affected. They suggested that EJM1 lay close to but not within the HLA region. In 1991, a study in a separately ascertained group of 33 German families, using HLA serological markers, provided further evidence for the existence of a locus on chromosome 6p [107]. A further study of a subset of 20 of these families with one additional family, using HLA-DQ RFLP markers, provided a maximum LOD score of 4.1 under the assumption of dominant inheritance with 90% penetrance [108]. More recently, a study in a single large pedigree of Belize origin, using microsatellite markers on chromosome 6p, obtained a maximum LOD score of 3.67 ($\theta_{m=f} = 0$) between the centromeric marker D6S257 and a trait defined as the presence of clinical JME or an EEG showing diffuse 3.5–6 Hz multispike and slow wave complexes [109]. Two studies from a single group have failed to find evidence for the existence of a locus on chromosome 6p [110,111]. Five missense mutations have recently been identified in EFHC1 in six of 44 families with JME. This gene maps to 6p12–p11 and encodes a protein with an EF hand motif, which may have a role in apoptosis [112].

Chromosomal regions harboring genes for subunits of the neuronal nicotinic acetylcholine receptor (nAChR) were tested for linkage to the JME trait in 35 pedigrees. A maximum multipoint LOD score of 4.18 was obtained on 15q14 under the assumption of heterogeneity at $\alpha = 0.64$. Analysis of recombinant events defined the 10-cM interval between D15S144 and D15S1012 as being the region in which the gene lies. The $\alpha 7$ subunit of the neuronal nicotinic acetylcholine receptor (CHRNA7) maps within this interval and, therefore, represents an excellent candidate gene. These results indicate that a major susceptibility locus for JME maps to this region of chromosome 15q [113]. However, it does not contribute to the broader phenotype of IGE [114]. An association with a polymorphism in the *connexin36* gene in that region has been identified [115]. More recently, linkage analysis with seven microsatellite markers encompassing the CHRNA7 region failed to replicate linkage in 11 families with at least two JME members [116].

Absence epilepsies

At least three distinct syndromes in which absence seizures dominate the clinical phenotype are recognized: CAE, JAE, and epilepsy with myoclonic absences. Unfortunately, most genetic studies of individuals with absence seizures or their electrophysiological correlates have used definitions of the trait under study that do not correspond to current terminology.

The first study using modern syndrome categorization for proband diagnosis is that of Beck–Mannagetta and Janz [117]. Among 671 first-degree relatives of 151 probands with either CAE or JAE, 33 (4.9%) had epilepsy, with a similar percentage in parents, siblings, and offspring. A variety of epilepsy syndromes were observed in these affected relatives, but approximately one third had absence epilepsy.

For obvious reasons, it is difficult to draw firm conclusions from these studies. Clearly, they do not provide strong evidence for single-gene Mendelian inheritance of any of the traits examined. Difficulties created by the age-specific penetrance of these syndromes render the recognition of a dominant pattern of inheritance difficult. The proportion of siblings either affected or displaying EEG changes on average is above the expected population risk but well below the 25% expected for an autosomal recessive disorder. This is compatible with a so-called multifactorial model of inheritance. Molecular genetic aspects of absence seizures in humans and rodents have recently been reviewed [118].

Childhood absence epilepsy

Childhood absence epilepsy is a relatively uncommon form of IGE with good evidence for a genetic predisposition [119]. The incidence is between 6 and 8 per 100 000 children at the age of birth to 15 years. Onset is at 2 to 12 years, with a peak at 6 to 7 years of age. Girls are more frequently affected than boys. Absence seizures (of any type except myoclonic absences) occur and may be very frequent. Generalized tonic-clonic seizures develop in about 40% of cases and unclassifiable seizures may also occur. The patients are usually cognitively and neurologically intact. The characteristic EEG pattern is a bilateral, symmetric, and synchronous discharge of regular 3-Hz spike and wave complexes on a normal background activity.

A recent study provided evidence of linkage of CAE with tonic-clonic seizures and EEG 3–4 Hz spike and multispike slow wave complexes to chromosome 8q24. Two-point linkage analysis assuming autosomal dominant inheritance with 50% penetrance gave a Z_{max} of 3.6 at D8S502 in a five-generation family from India [120].

Suggestive evidence of linkage to *CACNG3* and the GABA receptor gene cluster on 15q has been obtained [121], and mutations were recently identified in *CACNA1H* in Chinese patients [122].

Juvenile absence epilepsy

Juvenile absence epilepsy is an idiopathic generalized epilepsy characterized by absence seizures with onset at 12 to 26 years of age [123]. The seizure frequency is usually lower than that in CAE. Generalized tonic-clonic seizures occur frequently and may precede the absences. Myoclonic seizures may also occur, rendering the distinction from JME problematic. The interictal EEG may be normal, and the ictal EEG characteristic is a generalized symmetric spike-wave discharge with frontal accentuation and a frequency of 3.5–4 Hz.

Mitochondrial disorders

The mitochondrial genome (mtDNA) is a circular DNA molecule, 16 569 bp long, present in up to 10 copies per mitochondrion and, therefore, in up to several hundred copies per cell. Mitochondrial DNA encodes two ribosomal RNAs, 22 transfer RNAs, and 13 messenger RNAs encoding components of the inner mitochondrial membrane respiratory chain. The entire mitochondrial genotype of an individual is inherited from the mother.

Human diseases because of mutations of mtDNA include myopathies, encephalopathies, cardiomyopathies, and various multisystem disorders. Two neurological disorders manifested in part as epilepsy and which are caused by point mutations in mitochondrial transfer RNA genes have been described. These are so-called MERRF and MELAS.

Myoclonic epilepsy with ragged red fibers is characterized by epilepsy, intention myoclonus, muscle weakness, progressive ataxia, and deafness. An A to G transition mutation at nucleotide pair 8344 in the pseudouridyl loop of the *tRNA^lys* gene was first described in three unrelated MERRF families [124]. This mutation has now been described in most MERRF families. The patients are heteroplasmic – both normal and mutated mtDNA populations are found.

An A to G transition at nucleotide 3243 was reported in 26 of 31 unrelated Japanese patients with MELAS. This mutation affects a nucleotide position in the dihydrouridine loop of the transfer RNA for leucine. Heteroplasmy was present with 50%–92% of mutant mtDNA present [125].

Chromosomal disorders and epilepsy

There are 400 chromosomal imbalances associated with epilepsy, usually in the context of neurodevelopmental delay [126]. Epilepsy has been found to occur consistently in a proportion of individuals with Down syndrome (DS), and is a major feature in individuals with ring chromosome 20 and supernumerary marker chromosome 15. A variety of chromosomal deletions predispose to epilepsy, including 4p (Wolf–Hirschhorn syndrome), deletions of 15q11–13 (Angelman syndrome), and deletions of 1q [127] and 1p. Conversely, certain types of epilepsy syndrome are more likely to be associated with chromosomal abnormalities. Elia *et al.* [128] studied a group of 14 patients with myoclonic absence seizures and found that seven had chromosomal abnormalities.

Down syndrome

The prevalence of seizures in DS is estimated to be 5%–15% [129–131]. Epilepsy occurring in DS has a number of causes and the type of epilepsy present is related to the cause and age of onset. Veall [130] observed that the prevalence of epilepsy rose with increasing age – the prevalence under 20 years was 1.9% rising to 12.2% over 55 years of age in his study. A more recent study confirmed these findings, but found a much higher prevalence of 46% in those over 50 years old [132].

Infantile spasms occurring in patients with DS have been observed by others [133]. All 14 patients in this report showed hypsarrhythmia on EEG. Reflex seizures have also been reported to be common in individuals with DS [134].

Wolf–Hirschhorn syndrome

Wolf–Hirschhorn syndrome is caused by deletion involving the band 4p16.3 [135]. It is characterized by developmental delay, failure to thrive, and characteristic dysmorphic facial features. Seizures occur in about 85% of patients [136]. These are usually generalized and include generalized tonic-clonic seizures, atypical absences, and myoclonic seizures. A characteristic EEG has been reported [137].

Angelman syndrome

Angelman syndrome is a disorder characterized by mental retardation, epilepsy, ataxia, and a happy disposition. It arises by four different genetic mechanisms. In about 70% of cases a *de novo* deletion of maternal chromosome 15q11–13 is found [138]. The genes in this region of chromosome 15 show imprinting, with the result that paternal inheritance of the deletion produces a different phenotype – Prader–Willi syndrome. Two to four percent of patients have a defect of imprinting, caused either by a microdeletion involving the imprinting center (IC) or by mutation in the IC [139]. Mutations in the gene *UBE-3A*, encoding ubiquitin-protein ligase, are found in a further 5% of cases [140,141].

Epilepsy occurs in 80%–90% of patients with Angelman syndrome. Seizure onset usually occurs in childhood, and seizures are usually generalized and persist into adulthood, when the most prevalent seizure types are atypical absences and myoclonic seizures [142].

Supernumerary inverted duplication 15

Small marker chromosomes are estimated to occur in 0.05% of live births [143]. Inverted duplications of chromosome 15pter–q13 (inv dup [15]) represent about 40% of these [144] and are mainly of maternal origin [145–147]. Most reported cases have been identified because of developmental delay, but inv dup (15) have been found in clinically normal individuals, patients with Angelman syndrome, and Prader–Willi syndrome [146,148]. Wisniewski *et al.* [149] reported five cases and compared these with ten proven cases and nine suspected cases in the literature. They found the most consistent features of the phenotype to be developmental delay and hypotonia in infancy. In childhood, the majority develop seizures that may be refractory to treatment.

Ring chromosome 20

The association between ring chromosome 20 (r[20]) and epilepsy was first reported in 1972 [150–153]. Subsequent case reports have confirmed this association and delineated the ring chromosome 20 syndrome of developmental delay, epilepsy, and behavioral problems with few dysmorphic features [154–156]. Affected patients are usually mosaic for the ring chromosome 20, but the percentage of lymphocytes containing r(20) varies considerably between individuals (10%–100%) [157].

Two studies have examined the epilepsy phenotype and EEG in patients' mosaic for r(20) specifically. Inoue et al. [157] described the seizures in six patients with r(20) and provided a review of the literature. Patients experienced different seizure types. Seizures occurred frequently and most cases were refractory to treatment. Localizing features were found either on EEG or on functional imaging in their six patients, which led the authors to classify the epilepsy in this group of patients as complex partial status epilepticus. Canevini et al. [158] described three patients with r(20), including a mother and son. Some features of the seizures were similar to those described by Inoue et al. [157] and the EEG findings were also similar.

Ring chromosomes are formed by breakage in both arms of a chromosome with fusion of the points of fracture and loss of the distal fragments [159]. They usually arise de novo. A few familial cases have been reported and have been maternally inherited in over 90% of these. In all reports in the literature, the site of fusion of the ring chromosome 20 was p13q13, p13q13.3, or p13q13.33. Two epilepsy phenotypes, ADNFLE and BFNC, map to 20q13 and are caused by mutations in two different genes – CHRNA4 and KCNQ2 (see previous discussion). In addition, a locus for the normal variant low voltage EEG maps to this region [160]. One or more of these genes may be contained within the deletion or disrupted by the breakpoints of the ring chromosome, resulting in epilepsy.

Genetic counseling

Provision of genetic counseling for epilepsy is both challenging and complex. Epilepsy can occur within the context of a wide variety of genetic conditions with different modes of inheritance, making the search for associated symptoms and signs essential. When the epilepsy appears to be occurring in isolation, the possibility of an underlying structural lesion needs to be considered. If the epilepsy is thought to be truly idiopathic, the epileptic syndrome must be defined in order to give accurate advice about natural history, prognosis, and the risk to relatives.

There are predominantly three main situations in which an individual may seek genetic counseling for epilepsy [10]: (1) a couple in which one partner (or both) have epilepsy may be interested in the risk of epilepsy in their offspring, (2) a couple with one epileptic child may be concerned about the risk to subsequent children, and (3) an epileptic woman may seek advice during pregnancy particularly about the risk to the fetus of teratogenicity from anti-epileptic medication.

In the first two situations, the risk depends, of course, on the type of epilepsy present. Some family pedigrees will reveal an autosomal dominant pattern of inheritance, or at least a high genetic susceptibility to seizures. In all cases, the risk figure given must be compared with that of the general population. The cumulative incidence for developing epilepsy to the age of 20 years is 1% and to 40 years is about 1.7%, based on a study in Rochester, USA [161].

A number of studies have been performed on the incidence of epilepsy in the offspring of epileptic parents, and provide an empiric risk of 1.7%–7.3%, with a median of 4.2% for all types of seizures, including febrile convulsions and single seizures [162]. A slight increase in the risk to the children of epileptic mothers is well established [162,163].

Specific figures, albeit covering a wide range, are available for individual IGE syndromes. For a patient with CAE, the risk for offspring is 6%–7% and for a sibling 5%–10%. In JME, the risk is 5%–14% and for a sibling 4%–7%.

In the symptomatic epilepsies, counseling obviously depends on the diagnosis of one of the very wide range of potential underlying disorders described in this chapter.

References

1. Noebels J. Exploring new gene discoveries in idiopathic generalized epilepsy. *Epilepsia* 2003; **44**: 16–21.

2. Scheffer IE, Berkovic SF. The genetics of human epilepsy. *Trends Pharmacol Sci* 2003; **24**: 428–433.

3. Gourfinkel-An I, Baulac S, Nabbout R, et al. Monogenic idiopathic epilepsies. *Lancet Neurol* 2004; **3**: 209–218.

4. Steinlein OK. Genes and mutations in human idiopathic epilepsy. *Brain Dev* 2004; **26**: 213–218.

5. Mochida GH, Walsh CA. Genetic basis of developmental malformations of the cerebral cortex. *Arch Neurol* 2004; **61**: 637–640.

6. Lehesjoki A-E. Molecular background of progressive myoclonus epilepsy. *EMBO J* 2003; **22**: 3473–3478.

7. Commission on Classification and Terminology of the ILAE. Proposal for revised classification of epilepsies and epilepsy syndromes. *Epilepsia* 1989; **30**: 389–399.

8. Engel J Jr. A proposed diagnostic scheme for people with epileptic seizures and with epilepsy: report of the ILAE Task Force on Classification and Terminology. *Epilepsia* 2001; **42**: 796–803.

9. Berg AT, Scheffer IE. New concepts in classification of the epilepsies: entering the 21st century. *Epilepsia* 2011; **52**: 1058–1062.

10. Ottman R, Hirose S, Jain S, *et al.* Genetic testing in the epilepsies – report of the ILAE Genetics Commission. *Epilepsia* 2010; **51**: 655–670.

11. Stephenson JPB. Specific syncopes and anoxic seizure types. In Stephenson JPB, ed. *Fits and Faints.* Oxford, UK: MacKeith Press, 1990; 59.

12. Metrakos K, Metrakos JD. Genetics of convulsive disorders II. Genetic and electroencephalographic studies in centrencephalic epilepsy. *Neurology* 1961; **11**: 474–483.

13. Vogel F, Motulsky AG. Genetics and human behavior. In Vogel F, Motulsky AG, eds. *Human Genetics: Problems and Approaches.* Berlin, Germany: Springer-Verlag, 1986; 590.

14. Duncan JS. Imaging and epilepsy. *Brain* 1997; **120**: 339–377.

15. Rett A. On an unusual brain atrophy syndrome in hyperammonemia in childhood.

Wien Med Wochenschr 1966; **116**: 723–726.

16. Hagberg B. Rett's syndrome: prevalence and impact on progressive severe mental retardation in girls. *Acta Paediatr Scand* 1985; **74**: 405–408.

17. Amir RE, Van den Veyver IB, Wan M, *et al.* Rett syndrome is caused by mutations in X-linked MECP2, encoding methyl-CpG-binding protein 2. *Nat Genet* 1999; **23**: 185–188.

18. Feinberg AP, Leahy WR. Infantile spasms: case report of sex-linked inheritance. *Dev Med Child Neurol* 1977; **19**: 524–526.

19. Rugtveit J. X-linked mental retardation and infantile spasms in two brothers [letter]. *Dev Med Child Neurol* 1986; **28**: 544–546.

20. Claes S, Devriendt K, Lagae L, *et al.* The X-linked infantile spasms syndrome (MIM 308350) maps to Xp11.4-Xpter in two pedigrees. *Ann Neurol* 1997; **42**: 360–364.

21. Stromme P, Mangelsdorf ME, Shaw MA, *et al.* Mutations in the human ortholog of Aristaless cause X-linked mental retardation and epilepsy. *Nat Genet* 2002; **30**: 441–445.

22. Dobyns WB, Andermann E, Andermann F, *et al.* X-linked malformations of neuronal migration. *Neurology* 1996; **47**: 331–339.

23. des Portes V, Pinard JM, Billuart P, *et al.* A novel CNS gene required for neuronal migration and involved in X-linked subcortical laminar heterotopia and lissencephaly syndrome. *Cell* 1998; **92**: 51–61.

24. Gleeson JG, Allen KM, Fox JW, *et al.* Doublecortin, a brain-specific gene mutated in human X-linked lissencephaly and double cortex syndrome, encodes a putative signaling protein. *Cell* 1998; **92**: 63–72.

25. Huttenlocher PR, Taravath S, Mojtahedi S. Periventricular heterotopia and epilepsy. *Neurology* 1994; **44**: 51–55.

26. Eksioglu YZ, Scheffer IE, Cardenas P, *et al.* Periventricular heterotopia: an X-linked dominant epilepsy locus causing aberrant cerebral cortical development. *Neuron* 1996; **16**: 77–87.

27. Hattori M, Adachl H, Tsujlmoto M, *et al.* Miller-Dieker lissencephaly gene encodes a subunit of brain platelet-activating factor. *Nature* 1994; **370**: 216–218.

28. Lo Nigro C, Chong CS, Smith AC, *et al.* Point mutations and an intragenic deletion in LIS1, the lissencephaly causative gene in isolated lissencephaly sequence and Miller-Dieker syndrome. *Hum Mol Genet* 1997; **6**: 157–164.

29. Bourneville DM. Sclérose tubereuse des circonvolutions cérébrales: idiotie et épilepsie hémiplégique. *Arch Neurol* 1880; **1**: 81–91.

30. Korf BR, Carrazana R, Holmes G. Patterns of seizures found in children with neurofibromatosis type 1. *Ann Neurol* 1991; **30**: 491.

31. Scheffer IE, Bhatia KP, Lopes-Cendes I, *et al.* Autosomal dominant nocturnal frontal lobe epilepsy – a distinctive clinical disorder. *Brain* 1995; **118**: 61–73.

32. Phillips HA, Scheffer IE, Crossland KM, *et al.* Autosomal dominant nocturnal frontal-lobe epilepsy: genetic heterogeneity and evidence for a second locus at 15q24. *Am J Hum Genet* 1998; **63**: 1108–1116.

33. Phillips HA, Scheffer IE, Berkovic SF, *et al.* Localization of a gene for autosomal dominant nocturnal frontal lobe epilepsy to chromosome 20q13.2. *Nat Genet* 1995; **10**: 117–118.

34. Steinlein OK, Mulley JC, Propping P, *et al.* A missense

mutation in the neuronal nicotinic acetylcholine receptor alpha 4 subunit is associated with autosomal dominant nocturnal frontal lobe epilepsy. *Nat Genet* 1995; **11**: 201–203.

35. Steinlein OK, Stoodt J, Mulley J, *et al*. Independent occurrence of the CHRNA4 Ser248Phe mutation in a Norwegian family with nocturnal frontal lobe epilepsy. *Epilepsia* 2000; **41**: 529–535.

36. Steinlein OK, Magnusson A, Stoodt J, *et al*. An insertion mutation of the CHRNA4 gene in a family with autosomal dominant nocturnal frontal lobe epilepsy. *Hum Mol Genet* 1997; **6**: 943–947.

37. Hirose S, Iwata H, Akiyoshi H, *et al*. A novel mutation of CHRNA4 responsible for autosomal dominant nocturnal frontal lobe epilepsy. *Neurology* 1999; **53**: 1749–1753.

38. De Fusco M, Becchetti A, Patrignani A, *et al*. The nicotinic receptor beta 2 subunit is mutant in nocturnal frontal lobe epilepsy. *Nat Genet* 2000; **26**: 275–276.

39. Phillips HA, Favre I, Kirkpatrick M, *et al*. CHRNB2 is the second acetylcholine receptor subunit associated with autosomal dominant nocturnal frontal lobe epilepsy. *Am J Hum Genet* 2001; **68**: 225–231.

40. Steinlein OK. Nicotinic receptor mutations in human epilepsy. *Prog Brain Res* 2000; **145**: 275–285.

41. Bertrand D, Picard F, Le Hellard S, *et al*. How mutations in the nAChRs can cause ADNFLE epilepsy. *Epilepsia* 2002; **43**: 112–122.

42. Rett A, Teubel R. Neugeborenen Krampfe im Rahmen einer epileptisch belasteten Familie. *Wien Klin Wochenschr* 1964; **76**: 609–613.

43. Leppert M, Anderson VE, Quattlebaum T, *et al*. Benign familial neonatal convulsions linked to genetic markers on chromosome 20. *Nature* 1989; **337**: 647–648.

44. Malafosse A, Leboyer M, Dulac O, *et al*. Confirmation of linkage of benign familial neonatal convulsions to D20S19 and D20S20. *Hum Genet* 1992; **89**: 54–58.

45. Ryan SG, Wiznitzer M, Hollman C, *et al*. Benign familial neonatal convulsions: evidence for clinical and genetic heterogeneity. *Ann Neurol* 1991; **29**: 469–473.

46. Lewis TB, Leach RJ, Ward K, *et al*. Genetic heterogeneity in benign familial neonatal convulsions: identification of a new locus on chromosome 8q. *Am J Hum Genet* 1993; **53**: 670–675.

47. Singh NA, Charlier C, Stauffer D, *et al*. A novel potassium channel gene, *KCNQ2*, is mutated in an inherited epilepsy of newborns. *Nat Genet* 1998; **18**: 25–29.

48. Dedek K, Kunath B, Kananura C, *et al*. Myokymia and neonatal epilepsy caused by a mutation in the voltage sensor of the KCNQ2 K+ channel. *Proc Natl Acad Sci USA* 2001; **98**: 12272–12277.

49. Charlier C, Singh NA, Ryan SG, *et al*. A pore mutation in a novel KQT-like potassium channel gene in an idiopathic epilepsy family. *Nat Genet* 1998; **18**: 53–55.

50. Wang Q, Curran ME, Splawski I, *et al*. Positional cloning of a novel potassium channel gene: KVLQT1 mutations cause cardiac arrhythmias. *Nat Genet* 1996; **12**: 17–23.

51. Neyroud N, Tesson F, Denjoy I, *et al*. A novel mutation in the potassium channel gene KVLQT1 causes the Jervell and Lange–Nielsen cardioauditory syndrome. *Nat Genet* 1997; **15**: 186–189.

52. Kubisch C, Schroeder BC, Friedrich T, *et al*. KCNQ4, a novel potassium channel expressed in sensory outer hair cells, is mutated in dominant deafness. *Cell* 1999; **96**: 437–446.

53. Wang HS, Pan Z, Shi W, *et al*. KCNQ2 and KCNQ3 potassium channel subunits: molecular correlates of the M-channel. *Science* 1998; **282**: 1890–1893.

54. Cooper EC, Aldape KD, Abosch A, *et al*. Colocalization and coassembly of two human brain M-type potassium channel subunits that are mutated in epilepsy. *Proc Natl Acad Sci USA* 2000; **97**: 4914–4919.

55. Rogawski MA. KCNQ2/KCNQ3 K+ channels and the molecular pathogenesis of epilepsy: implications for therapy. *Trends Neurosci* 2000; **23**: 393–398.

56. Yang WP, Levesque PC, Little WA, *et al*. Functional expression of two KvLQT1-related potassium channels responsible for an inherited idiopathic epilepsy. *J Biol Chem* 1998; **273**: 19419–19423.

57. Lerche H, Jurkat-Rott K, Lehmann-Horn F. Ion channels and epilepsy. *Am J Med Genet* 2001; **106**: 146–159.

58. Scheffer IE, Berkovic SF. Generalized epilepsy with febrile seizures plus. A genetic disorder with heterogeneous clinical phenotypes. *Brain* 1997; **120**: 479–490.

59. Wallace RH, Wang D, Singh R, *et al*. Febrile seizures and generalized epilepsy associated with a mutation in the Na+-channel beta1 subunit gene SCN1B. *Nat Genet* 1998; **19**: 366–370.

60. Baulac S, Gourfinkel-An I, Picard F, *et al*. A second locus for familial generalized epilepsy with febrile seizures plus maps to chromosome 2q21-q33. *Am J Hum Genet* 1999; **65**: 1078–1085.

61. Moulard B, Guipponi M, Chaigne D, *et al*. Identification of a new locus for generalized

epilepsy with febrile seizures plus (GEFS+) on chromosome 2q24-q33. *Am J Hum Genet* 1999; **65**: 1396–1400.

62. Escayg A, MacDonald BT, Meisler MH, *et al.* Mutations of SCN1A, encoding a neuronal sodium channel, in two families with GEFS+2. *Nat Genet* 2000; **24**: 343–345.

63. Sugawara T, Mazaki-Miyazaki E, Ito M, *et al.* Nav1.1 mutations cause febrile seizures associated with afebrile partial seizures. *Neurology* 2001; **57**: 703–705

64. Claes L, Del-Favero J, Ceulemans B, *et al.* De novo mutations in the sodium-channel gene SCN1A cause severe myoclonic epilepsy of infancy. *Am J Hum Genet* 2001; **68**: 1327–1332.

65. Ohmori I, Ouchida M, Ohtsuka Y, *et al.* Significant correlation of the SCN1A mutations and severe myoclonic epilepsy in infancy. *Biochem Biophys Res Commun* 2002; **295**: 17–23.

66. Sugawara T, Mazaki-Miyazaki E, Fukushima K, *et al.* Frequent mutations of SCN1A in severe myoclonic epilepsy in infancy. *Neurology* 2002; **58**: 1122–1124.

67. Dravet C. Les épilepsies graves de l'enfant. *Vie Med* 1978; **8**: 543–548.

68. Singh R, Andermann E, Whitehouse WP, *et al.* Severe myoclonic epilepsy of infancy: extended spectrum of GEFS+? *Epilepsia* 2001; **42**: 837–844.

69. Heron SE, Crossland KM, Andermann E, *et al.* Sodium-channel defects in benign familial neonatal-infantile seizures. *Lancet* 2002; **360**: 851–852.

70. Berkovic SF, Heron SE, Giordano L, *et al.* Benign familial neonatal-infantile seizures: characterization of a new sodium channelopathy. *Ann Neurol* 2004; **55**: 550–557.

71. Bulman DE. Phenotype variation and newcomers in ion channel disorders. *Hum Mol Genet* 1997; **6**: 1679–1685.

72. Macdonald RL, Kelly KM. Mechanisms of action of currently prescribed and newly developed antiepileptic drugs. *Epilepsia* 1994; **35**: S41–S50.

73. Wallace RH, Scheffer IE, Parasivam G, *et al.* Generalized epilepsy with febrile seizures plus: mutation of the sodium channel subunit SCN1B. *Neurology* 2002; **58**: 1426–1429.

74. Lossin C, Wang DW, Rhodes TH, *et al.* Molecular basis of an inherited epilepsy. *Neuron* 2002; **34**: 877–884.

75. Baulac S, Huberfeld G, Gourfinkel-An I, *et al.* First genetic evidence of GABA(A) receptor dysfunction in epilepsy: a mutation in the gamma2-subunit gene. *Nat Genet* 2001; **28**: 46–48.

76. Harkin LA, Bowser DN, Dibbens LM, *et al.* Truncation of the GABA(A)-receptor gamma2 subunit in a family with generalized epilepsy with febrile seizures plus. *Am J Hum Genet* 2002; **70**: 530–536.

77. Bianchi MT, Song L, Zhang H, Macdonald RL. Two different mechanisms of disinhibition produced by GABA$_A$ receptor mutations linked to epilepsy in humans. *J Neurosci* 2002; **22**: 5321–5327.

78. Wallace RH, Marini C, Petrou S, *et al.* Mutant GABA$_A$ receptor gamma2-subunit in childhood absence epilepsy and febrile seizures. *Nat Genet* 2001; **28**: 49–52.

79. Cossette P, Liu L, Brisebois K, *et al.* Mutation of GABRA1 in an autosomal dominant form of juvenile myoclonic epilepsy. *Nat Genet* 2002; **31**: 184–189.

80. Zuberi SM, Eunson LH, Spauschus A, *et al.* A novel mutation in the human voltage-gated potassium channel gene (Kv1.1) associates with episodic ataxia type 1 and sometimes with partial epilepsy. *Brain* 1999; **122**: 817–825.

81. Eunson LH, Rea R, Zuberi SM, *et al.* Clinical, genetic, and expression studies of mutations in the potassium channel gene KCNA1 reveal new phenotypic variability. *Ann Neurol* 2000; **48**: 647–656.

82. Smart SL, Lopantsev V, Zhang CL, *et al.* Deletion of the K(V)1.1 potassium channel causes epilepsy in mice. *Neuron* 1998; **20**: 809–819.

83. Jouvenceau A, Eunson LH, Spauschus A, *et al.* Human epilepsy associated with dysfunction of the brain P/Q-type calcium channel. *Lancet* 2001; **358**: 801–807.

84. Chioza B, Wilkie H, Nashef L, *et al.* Association between the alpha(1a) calcium channel gene CACNA1A and idiopathic generalized epilepsy. *Neurology* 2001; **56**: 1245–1246.

85. Sander T, Schulz H, Saar K, *et al.* Genome search for susceptibility loci of common idiopathic generalised epilepsies. *Hum Mol Genet* 2000; **9**: 1465–1472.

86. Haug K, Warnstedt M, Alekov AK, *et al.* Mutations in CLCN2 encoding a voltage-gated chloride channel are associated with idiopathic generalized epilepsies. *Nat Genet* 2003; **33**: 527–532.

87. Ottman R, Risch N, Hauser WA, *et al.* Localization of a gene for partial epilepsy to chromosome 10q. *Nat Genet* 1995; **10**: 56–60.

88. Poza JJ, Saenz A, Martinez-Gil A, *et al.* Autosomal dominant lateral temporal epilepsy: clinical and genetic study of a large Basque pedigree linked to chromosome 10q. *Ann Neurol* 1999; **45**: 182–188.

89. Mautner VF, Lindenau M, Gottesleben A, *et al.* Supporting evidence of a gene for partial epilepsy on 10q. *Neurogenetics* 2000; **3**: 31–34.

90. Kalachikov S, Evgrafov O, Ross B, *et al.* Mutations in LGI1 cause

autosomal-dominant partial epilepsy with auditory features. *Nat Genet* 2002; **30**: 335–341.

91. Morante-Redolat JM, Gorostidi-Pagola A, Piquer-Sirerol S, *et al.* Mutations in the LGI1/Epitempin gene on 10q24 cause autosomal dominant lateral temporal epilepsy. *Hum Mol Genet* 2002; **11**: 1119–1128.

92. Gu W, Brodtkorb E, Steinlein OK. LGI1 is mutated in familial temporal lobe epilepsy characterized by aphasic seizures. *Ann Neurol* 2002; **52**: 364–367.

93. Pizzuti A, Flex E, Di Bonaventura C, *et al.* Epilepsy with auditory features: a LGI1 gene mutation suggests a loss-of-function mechanism. *Ann Neurol* 2003; **53**: 396–399.

94. Gu W, Wevers A, Schroder H, *et al.* The LGI1 gene involved in lateral temporal lobe epilepsy belongs to a new subfamily of leucine-rich repeat proteins. *FEBS Lett* 2002; **519**: 71–76.

95. Scheel H, Tomiuk S, Hofmann K. A common protein interaction domain links two recently identified epilepsy genes. *Hum Mol Genet* 2002; **11**: 1757–1762.

96. Skradski SL, Clark AM, Jiang H, *et al.* A novel gene causing a mendelian audiogenic mouse epilepsy. *Neuron* 2001; **31**: 537–544.

97. Nakayama J, Fu YH, Clark AM, *et al.* A nonsense mutation of the MASS1 gene in a family with febrile and afebrile seizures. *Ann Neurol* 2002; **52**: 654–657.

98. Berkovic SF, Andermann F, Carpenter S, Wolfe LS. Progressive myoclonus epilepsies: specific causes and diagnosis. *N Engl J Med* 1986; **315**: 296–305.

99. Roger J, Genton P, Bureau M, Dravet C. Progressive myoclonus epilepsies in childhood and adolescence. In Roger J, Bureau M, Dravet C, *et al.*, eds. *Epileptic Syndromes in Infancy,* *Childhood and Adolescence.* 2nd edn. London, UK: John Libbey, 1992; 381–400.

100. Serratosa JM, Gardiner RM, Lehesjoki A-E, *et al.* The molecular genetic bases of the progressive myoclonus epilepsies. *Adv Neurol* 1999; **79**: 383–398.

101. Marini C, Scheffer I, Crossland K, *et al.* Genetic architecture of idiopathic generalized epilepsy: clinical genetic analysis of 55 multiplex families. *Epilepsia* 2004; **45**: 467–478.

102. Winawer MR, Rabinowitz D, Pedley TA, *et al.* Genetic influences on myoclonic and absence seizures. *Neurology* 2003; **61**: 1576–1581.

103. Delgado-Escueta AV, Greenberg D, Weissbecker K. Gene mapping in the idiopathic generalised epilepsies. *Epilepsia* 1990; **31**: 519–529.

104. Panayiotopoulos CP, Obeid T. Juvenile myoclonic epilepsy: an autosomal recessive disease. *Ann Neurol* 1989; **25**: 440–443.

105. Greenberg DA, Delgado-Escueta AV, Widelitz H, *et al.* Strengthened evidence for linkage of juvenile myoclonic epilepsy to HLA and BF. *Cytogenet Cell Genet* 1989; **51**: 1008.

106. Greenberg DA, Delgado-Escueta AV, Widelitz H, *et al.* Juvenile myoclonic epilepsy may be linked to the BF and HLA loci on human chromosome 6. *Am J Med Genet* 1988; **31**: 185–192.

107. Weissbecker KA, Durner M, Janz D, *et al.* Confirmation of linkage between juvenile myoclonic epilepsy locus and the HLA region on chromosome 6. *Am J Med Genet* 1991; **38**: 32–36.

108. Durner M, Sander T, Greenberg DA, *et al.* Localisation of idiopathic generalised epilepsy on chromosome 6p in families of juvenile myoclonic epilepsy patients. *Neurology* 1991; **41**: 1651–1655.

109. Liu AW, Delgado-Escueta AV, Serratosa JM, *et al.* Juvenile myoclonic epilepsy locus in chromosome 6p21.2-p11:linkage to convulsions and electroencephalography trait. *Am J Hum Genet* 1995; **57**: 368–381.

110. Whitehouse W, Diebold U, Rees M, *et al.* Exclusion of linkage of genetic focal sharp waves to the HLA region on chromosome 6p in families with benign partial epilepsy with centrotemporal spikes. *Neuropediatrics* 1993; **24**: 208–210.

111. Elmslie FV, Williamson MP, Rees M, *et al.* Linkage analysis of juvenile myoclonic epilepsy and microsatellite loci spanning 61 cM of human chromosome 6p in 19 nuclear pedigrees provides no evidence for a susceptibility locus in this region. *Am J Hum Genet* 1996; **59**: 653–663.

112. Suzuki T, Delgado-Escueta AV, Aguan K, *et al.* Mutations in EFHC1 cause juvenile myoclonic epilepsy. *Nat Genet* 2004; **36**: 842–849.

113. Elmslie FV, Rees M, Williamson MP, *et al.* Genetic mapping of a major susceptibility locus for juvenile myoclonic epilepsy on chromosome 15q. *Hum Mol Genet* 1997; **6**: 1329–1334.

114. Taske NL, Williamson MP, Makoff A, *et al.* Evaluation of the positional candidate gene CHRNA7 at the juvenile myoclonic epilepsy locus (EJM2) on chromosome 15q13–14. *Epilepsy Res* 2002; **49**: 157–172.

115. Mas C, Taske N, Deutsch S, *et al.* Association of the connexin36 gene with juvenile myoclonic epilepsy. *J Med Genet* 2004; **41**: 1–7.

116. Sander T, Schulz H, Vieira-Saeker AM, *et al.* Evaluation of a putative major susceptibility locus for juvenile myoclonic epilepsy on chromosome 15q14. *Am J Med Genet* 1999; **88**: 182–187.

117. Beck-Mannagetta G, Janz D. Syndrome-related genetics in generalised epilepsy. *Epilepsy Res Suppl* 1991; **4**: 105–111.

118. Crunelli V, Leresche N. Childhood absence epilepsy: genes, channels, neurons and networks. *Nat Rev Neurosci* 2002; **3**: 371–382.

119. Loiseau P. Childhood absence epilepsy. In Roger J, Bureau M, Dravet C, *et al*. eds. *Epilepsy Syndromes in Infancy, Childhood and Adolescence*. 2nd edn. London, UK: John Libbey, 1992; 135–150.

120. Fong GC, Shah PU, Gee MN, *et al*. Childhood absence epilepsy with tonic-clonic seizures and electroencephalogram 3–4-Hz spike and multispike-slow wave complexes: linkage to chromosome 8q24. *Am J Hum Genet* 1998; **63**: 1117–1129.

121. Robinson R, Taske N, Sander T, *et al*. Linkage analysis between childhood absence epilepsy and genes encoding GABAA and GABAB receptors, voltage-dependent calcium channels, and the ECA1 region on chromosome 8q. *Epilepsy Res* 2002; **48**: 169–179.

122. Chen Y, Lu J, Pan H, *et al*. Association between genetic variation of CACNA1H and childhood absence epilepsy. *Ann Neurol* 2003; **54**: 239–243.

123. Wolf P. Juvenile absence epilepsy. In Roger J, Bureau M, Dravet C, *et al*., eds. *Epileptic Syndromes in Infancy, Childhood and Adolescence*, 2nd edn. London, UK: John Libbey, 1992; 307–312.

124. Shoffner JM, Lott MT, Lezza AMS, *et al*. Myoclonic epilepsy and ragged-red fiber disease (MERRF) is associated with a mitochondrial DNA tRNA^{Lys} mutation. *Cell* 1990; **61**: 931–937.

125. Goto Y, Nonaka I, Horai S. A mutation in the tRNA^{Leu} gene associated with the MELAS subgroup of mitochondrial encephalomyopathies. *Nature* 1990; **348**: 651–653.

126. Singh R, Gardner RJ, Crossland KM, *et al*. Chromosomal abnormalities and epilepsy: a review for clinicians and gene hunters. *Epilepsia* 2002; **43**: 127–140.

127. Vaughn BV, Greenwood RS, Aylsworth AS, Tennison MB. Similarities of EEG and seizures in del(1q) and benign rolandic epilepsy. *Pediatr Neurol* 1996; **15**: 261–264.

128. Elia M, Guerrini R, Musumeci SA, *et al*. Myoclonic absence-like seizures and chromosome abnormality syndromes. *Epilepsia* 1998; **39**: 660–663.

129. Moore BC. Some characteristics of institutionalised mongols. *J Ment Defic Res* 1973; **17**: 46–51.

130. Veall RM. The prevalance of epilepsy among mongols related to age. *J Ment Defic Res* 1974; **18**: 99–106.

131. Prasher VP. Epilepsy and associated effects on adaptive behaviour in adults with Down syndrome. *Seizure* 1995; **4**: 53–56.

132. McVicker RW, Shanks OE, McClelland RJ. Prevalence and associated features of epilepsy in adults with Down's syndrome. *Br J Psychiatry* 1994; **164**: 528–532.

133. Silva ML, Cieuta C, Guerrini R, *et al*. Early clinical and EEG features of infantile spasms in Down syndrome. *Epilepsia* 1996; **37**: 977–982.

134. Guerrini R, Genton P, Bureau M, *et al*. Reflex seizures are frequent in patients with Down syndrome and epilepsy. *Epilepsia* 1990; **31**: 406–417.

135. Fang YY, Bain S, Haan EA, *et al*. High resolution characterization of an interstitial deletion of less than 1.9 Mb at 4p16.3 associated with Wolf–Hirschhorn syndrome. *Am J Med Genet* 1997; **71**: 453–457.

136. Battaglia A, Carey JC, Cederholm P, *et al*. Natural history of Wolf–Hirschhorn syndrome: experience with 15 cases. *Pediatrics* 1999; **103**: 830–836.

137. Sgro V, Riva E, Canevini MP, *et al*. 4p(-) syndrome: a chromosomal disorder associated with a particular EEG pattern. *Epilepsia* 1995; **36**: 1206–1214.

138. Chan CT, Clayton-Smith J, Cheng XJ, *et al*. Molecular mechanisms in Angelman syndrome: a survey of 93 patients. *J Med Genet* 1993; **30**: 895–902.

139. Buiting K, Dittrich B, Gross S, *et al*. Sporadic imprinting defects in Prader–Willi syndrome and Angelman syndrome: implications for imprint-switch models, genetic counseling, and prenatal diagnosis. *Am J Hum Genet* 1998; **63**: 170–180.

140. Kishino T, Lalande M, Wagstaff J. UBE3A/E6-AP mutations cause Angelman syndrome. *Nat Genet* 1997; **15**: 70–73.

141. Matsuura T, Sutcliffe JS, Fang P, *et al*. De novo truncating mutations in E6-AP ubiquitin-protein ligase gene (UBE3A) in Angelman syndrome. *Nat Genet* 1997; **15**: 74–77.

142. Laan LA, Renier WO, Arts WF, *et al*. Evolution of epilepsy and EEG findings in Angelman syndrome. *Epilepsia* 1997; **38**: 195–199.

143. Buckton KE, O'Riordan ML, Ratcliffe S, *et al*. A G-band study of chromosomes in liveborn infants. *Ann Hum Genet* 1980; **43**: 227–239.

144. Buckton KE, Spowart G, Newton MS, Evans HJ. Forty four probands with an additional "marker" chromosome. *Hum Genet* 1985; **69**: 353–370.

145. Bundey S, Hardy C, Vickers S, *et al*. Duplication of the 15q11–13 region in a patient with autism, epilepsy and ataxia. *Dev Med Child Neurol* 1994; **36**: 736–742.

146. Cheng SD, Spinner NB, Zackai EH, Knoll JH. Cytogenetic and molecular characterization of inverted duplicated chromosomes 15 from 11 patients. *Am J Hum Genet* 1994; **55**: 753–759.

147. Guerrini R, Bonanni P, Nardocci N, *et al.* Autosomal recessive rolandic epilepsy with paroxysmal exercise-induced dystonia and writer's cramp: delineation of the syndrome and gene mapping to chromosome 16p12–11.2. *Ann Neurol* 1999; **45**: 344–352.

148. Torrisi L, Sangiorgi E, Russo L, Gurrieri F. Rearrangements of chromosome 15 in epilepsy. *Am J Med Genet* 2001; **106**: 125–128.

149. Wisniewski L, Hassold T, Heffelfinger J, Higgins JV. Cytogenetic and clinical studies in five cases of inv dup(15). *Hum Genet* 1979; **50**: 259–270.

150. Atkins L, Miller WL, Salam M. A ring-20 chromosome. *J Med Genet* 1972; **9**: 377–380.

151. De Grouchy J, Plachot M, Sebaoun M, Bouchard R. [F fing chromosome (46, XY, Fr) in a boy with multiple abnormalities]. *Ann Genet* 1972; **15**: 121–126.

152. Faed M, Morton HG, Robertson J. Ring F chromosome mosaicism (46,XY,20r-46,XY) in an epileptic child without apparent haematological disease. *J Med Genet* 1972; **9**: 470–473.

153. Uchida IA, Lin CC. Ring formation of chromosomes nos. 19 and 20. *Cytogenetics* 1972; **11**: 208–215.

154. Borgaonkar DS, Lacassie YE, Stoll C. Usefulness of chromosome catalog in delineating new syndromes. *Birth Defects* 1976; **12**: 87–95.

155. Herva R, Saarinen I, Leikkonen L. The r(20) syndrome. *J Med Genet* 1977; **14**: 281–283.

156. Stewart JM, Cavanagh N, Hughes DT. Ring 20 chromosome in a child with seizures, minor anomalies, and retardation. *Arch Dis Child* 1979; **54**: 477–479.

157. Inoue Y, Fujiwara T, Matsuda K, *et al.* Ring chromosome 20 and nonconvulsive status epilepticus. A new epileptic syndrome. *Brain* 1997; **120**: 939–953.

158. Canevini MP, Sgro V, Zuffardi O, *et al.* Chromosome 20 ring: a chromosomal disorder associated with a particular electroclinical pattern. *Epilepsia* 1998; **39**: 942–951.

159. Gardner RJM, Sutherland GR. *Autosomal Rings. Chromosome Abnormalities and Genetic Counseling.* Oxford, UK: Oxford University Press, 1996; 177.

160. Steinlein OK, Fischer C, Keil R, *et al.* D20S19, linked to low voltage EEG, benign neonatal convulsions, and Fanconi anaemia, maps to a region of enhanced recombination and is localized between CpG islands. *Hum Mol Genet* 1992; **1**: 325–329.

161. Anderson VE, Hauser WA, Rich SS. Genetic heterogeneity in the epilepsies. *Adv Neurol* 1986; **44**: 59–75.

162. Tsuboi T. Genetic risks in offspring of epileptic parents. In Beck–Mannagetta G, Anderson VE, Doose H, Janz D, eds. *Genetics of the Epilepsies.* Berlin, Germany: Springer-Verlag, 1989; 111.

163. Ottman R, Annegers K, Hauser WA, Kurland LT. Higher risk of seizures in offspring of mothers than of fathers with epilepsy. *Am J Hum Genet* 1988; **42**: 257–264.

The ataxias

S. H. Subramony

The inherited ataxias vary in their clinical and pathological features, not only between different families but also within the same family. Thus, for example, Konigsmark and Weiner (1970) [1], in their classic paper on olivopontocerebellar atrophies, ended up classifying members of the same family into different categories based on pathological findings. The studies by Anita Harding (1984) [2] led to a rational clinical-genetic classification of these diseases. Recent genetic studies have illustrated the enormous genetic heterogeneity of the inherited ataxias and paved the way to precise molecular diagnosis, allowed better genetic counseling, improved our understanding of the pathogenesis of the inherited ataxias, and raised hopes for rational treatment. In this chapter, I review the major advances in autosomal recessive and autosomal dominant ataxias, discuss the use of genetic tests in these disorders, and summarize some current ideas regarding pathogenesis. There are

websites that have more detailed descriptions of the inherited ataxias (www.ncbr.nlm.nih.gov/Omim/; www.geneclinics.org).

Autosomal recessive ataxias

Table 5.1 lists the autosomal recessive ataxias that have been genotypically characterized to date.

Friedreich's ataxia
Clinical features

This is the most common form of recessive ataxia among Indo-Caucasian populations and has a prevalence of 2×10^{-5} [3]. The classical phenotype of Friedreich's ataxia (FA) is one of progressive gait ataxia beginning before the age of 25 years, typically around puberty [4]. Rarely, the children can present with cardiomyopathy or skeletal deformity. The early

Table 5.1. Autosomal recessive ataxias with known gene loci

Disease	Gene locus/gene	Mutation
Friedreich's ataxia	9q/FA	GAA expansion (66–>1000)
AVED	8q/α TTP	Conventional mutations
Abetalipoproteinemia	4q/MTP	Conventional mutations
Ataxia telangiectasia	11q/ATM	Conventional mutations
Ataxia with oculomotor apraxia 1	9p/aprataxin	Conventional mutations
Ataxia with oculomotor apraxia 2	9q/senataxin	Conventional mutations
AT-like disorder	11q/hMRE 11	Point mutations
SCAN 1	14q/TDP-1	Point mutations
ARSACS	13q/SACS	Point mutations
IOSCA	10qc10orf2	Conventional mutations
Ataxia, deafness, optic atrophy	6p/?	Unknown
Unverricht–Lundborg disease	21q/cystatin B	Repeat expansion

AVED, ataxia with isolated vitamin E deficiency; AT, ataxia telangiectasia; SCAN 1, spinocerebellar ataxia with axonal neuropathy 1; ARSACS, autosomal recessive spastic ataxia of Charlevoix–Saguenay; IOSCA: infantile onset spinocerebellar ataxia.

features of the disease reflect the prominent pathology in dorsal root ganglion cells with evidence of proprioceptive loss in the limbs and loss of deep tendon reflexes [5–7]. The sensory nerve action potentials are typically small or absent and nerve biopsies show loss of large myelinated fibers. At this stage, some children may be misdiagnosed with pure sensory neuropathy. However, other signs reflecting cerebellar pathology develop and include abnormal eye movements (usually square wave jerks) and dysarthria. Saccades may become dysmetric and pursuit eye movements abnormal, but nystagmus is rare. Increasing imbalance and incoordination develop, with dysmetria, abnormal rapid alternating movements, and a broad-based gait; ambulation is lost 10 to 15 years after onset of the disease. Dysphagia and upper motor neuron signs such as weakness of lower limbs, extensor plantar reflexes, and flexor spasms occur in the more advanced stages. Optic atrophy and visual and hearing loss occur in a minority of individuals. Heart disease occurs in many patients, and is characterized by inverted T waves on an electrocardiograph (EKG) and by the presence of hypertrophic cardiomyopathy demonstrated by echocardiography. Symptomatic heart disease may cause arrhythmias and heart failure. Diabetes occurs in about 10% of cases. Skeletal deformities such as pes cavus and kyphoscoliosis are common. The typical imaging finding is atrophy of the cervical spinal cord [8].

Neuropathology

There is severe loss of dorsal root ganglion cells resulting in degeneration of the posterior columns and peripheral sensory axons. The Clarke's column, spinocerebellar tracts, and cerebellar dentate nuclei are also atrophic. Finally, there is predominant distal loss of the pyramidal tract.

Genetics

Friedreich's ataxia is inherited in an autosomal recessive form. Many patients are singletons, but in larger families many siblings may be affected and parental consanguinity may be found. The FA gene, on chromosome 9, codes for a 210 amino acid protein called frataxin [9]. The mutation in this gene is an unstable expansion of a trinucleotide repeat (GAA) within the first intron. Normal chromosomes have fewer than 40 GAA repeats at this locus and the pathologically expanded alleles have from 66 to more than 1000 GAA repeats. Over 95% of patients with classic FA carry an expansion in both alleles; however, about 3% of such cases are heterozygous for the expansion with the second allele carrying a point mutation [10]. In a typical case of FA, the heterozygous expansion of the GAA repeat may be enough to establish the diagnosis, but one may obtain sequencing to detect the point mutation in the unexpanded allele. If the phenotype is atypical, a heterozygous expansion may be an incidental carrier state, and clinical judgment will have to be used.

Variant phenotypes

The FA GAA expansion can be associated with phenotypes different from the classical description given previously [5–7,11]. Many patients with a typical neurological picture may have an onset of disease after 25 years of age (late-onset FA or LOFA). Alternatively, childhood-onset ataxia with preserved or even brisk deep tendon reflexes can also be associated with the FA gene mutation (FA with retained reflexes or FARR). Some patients have adult-onset as well as preserved reflexes and even old-age onset may occur [12]. Lastly, rare patients have more spasticity in their legs and minimal ataxia.

Some of the phenotypic variability is related to the unstable nature of the GAA expansion. Thus, the age at onset is inversely correlated with the size of the repeat, especially the smaller of the two alleles [5,6]. Large repeat sizes of about 700 or more are correlated with the classical phenotype and usually are associated with diabetes and cardiomyopathy as well. Late-onset cases often have fewer than 500 repeats but such correlations are not strict enough to make predictions in individual cases.

Indications for Friedreich's ataxia mutation analysis

The FA mutation study should be done in all cases of typical FA to confirm the diagnosis. However, close to 10% of patients with typical FA may not have the GAA expansion, indicating that there are unknown genotypes that can cause an identical phenotype [13]. The FA gene mutation should be considered in almost all cases of sporadic or recessive ataxia with onset at all ages to over 60 years old if the syndrome cannot be readily characterized otherwise; the yield of such testing, however, will be small. One should also consider the test in patients with uncharacterized spasticity in the legs, especially if accompanied by evidence of sensory nerve dysfunction or minor ataxia.

Pathogenesis

Frataxin is a highly conserved protein that is targeted to the mitochondrial matrix [14,15]. Friedreich's ataxia is a disease of relative frataxin deficiency because the presence of the GAA expansion reduces the transcriptional and translational efficiency of the gene proportionally to the size of the expansion. This reduced transcriptional efficiency has been shown to result from an unusual configuration of the DNA created by the expansion [16]. Complete lack of frataxin may be incompatible with life; for example, complete knockout of the frataxin gene in mice is embyonically lethal [17].

In the yeast frataxin homolog knockout model, the mitochondria accumulate iron, become sensitive to oxidative stress (which is known to occur from excessive iron), and lose their respiratory efficiency [15,18]. Human tissue from FA patients can be shown to have excess iron at autopsy or by magnetic resonance imaging (MRI) [19,20]. Frataxin deficiency may allow the ferrous form of iron to be oxidized to the ferric form, allowing the generation of toxic hydroxyl radicals (Fenton reaction) [21]. In addition, frataxin may make iron available for specific metabolic functions such as the assembly of iron–sulfur cluster enzymes [22]. Such enzymes (complex I, II, and III of the respiratory chain and mitochondrial aconitase) have been shown to be lost specifically in myocardial tissue of patients with FA. The iron–sulfur (Fe–S) enzymes are also particularly susceptible to oxidative stress. In FA patients, evidence that oxidative stress is involved has been generated by the elevation of such chemicals as 8-OH-2-deoxyguanosine and malondialdehyde [23,24]. Loss of respiratory competence has been shown by impaired ATP synthesis by exercising skeletal muscle using MR spectroscopy (MRS) [25]. Overall, loss of Fe–S cluster enzymes and excess oxidative stress may have a major role in the pathogenesis of tissue damage in FA.

Treatment

Based on the pathogenetic scenario outlined, antioxidant strategies have been tried in patients with FA. A number of studies have shown a variable effect of the coenzyme Q analogue idebenone on the cardiomyopathy and neurological status of FA patients [26,27]. Similarly, a combination of coenzyme Q and vitamin E has been shown to improve MRS findings in skeletal muscle in FA patients [28].

In addition, general supportive care is needed. The patient is monitored for cardiomyopathy and diabetes at least yearly or when symptoms occur. Skeletal deformities may need correction. Physical therapy and rehabilitative equipment are also needed.

Other well-defined autosomal recessive ataxias

Ataxia with isolated vitamin E deficiency

This disease resembles FA with onset of ataxia in childhood, areflexia, and proprioceptive loss. Cardiomyopathy and diabetes do not occur and head titubation may be more common [29]. Vitamin E levels are low, usually below 50% of the lower limit of normal. The mutation in ataxia with isolated vitamin E deficiency (AVED) involves the alpha-tocopherol transfer protein that functions in delivering vitamin E to very-low-density lipoproteins for transport to tissues [30]. Mutations in AVED are scattered throughout the gene and some of them may be associated with a mild phenotype, late onset, retinitis pigmentosa, and retained reflexes [31]. Vitamin E levels should be checked in all cases of sporadic ataxias. Vitamin E supplements can arrest progression of AVED.

Abetalipoproteinemia

Mutations in the microsomal triglyceride transfer protein cause abetalipoproteinemia [32]. Patients present with fat malabsorption, a neurological syndrome similar to AVED, retinal pigmentary degeneration, and acanthocytosis [33]. Vitamin E levels are low, serum beta lipoproteins are absent, and cholesterol and triglyceride levels are low. Vitamin E supplements can prevent neurological deterioration.

Ataxia telangiectasia

This disease typically has onset before three years of age, with truncal ataxia [34]. The children develop progressive gait problems, requiring a wheelchair by the early teen years, and other neurological deficits including hypotonia, choreoathetosis, and evidence of peripheral nerve dysfunction with areflexia. Oculomotor apraxia is a constant finding, requiring head thrusts for eye movements. Typical conjunctival telangiectasia usually develops after five years of age. Immunodeficiencies occur in about one third of cases, leading to repeated chest infections. Malignancies, especially hematologic, are common as well. Many patients with ataxia telangiectasia (AT) die in their

30s and 40s because of pulmonary infections, failure, or malignancy.

Laboratory tests that may be useful include elevated alpha-fetoprotein and abnormal chromosomal translocations on karyotyping. IgE and IgA levels are low. Brain imaging shows cerebellar atrophy. Cultured lymphoblastoid cells reveal abnormal radiosensitivity (colony survival assay). The gene mutated in AT (*ATM*) codes for a protein that functions as a protein kinase that phosphorylates many substrates involved in cell cycle control and DNA double-strand break repair [35]. The ATM protein is absent in most of the AT patients because the mutations usually lead to premature stop codons [36]. Because the gene is large and mutations found in patients diverse, there is no simple DNA strategy to confirm the diagnosis of AT, although some screening strategies that involve haplotyping or protein truncation methods may simplify the task [37]. Treatment strategies include rehabilitative measures and management of medical problems such as infections and malignancies. Radiation cannot be used to treat these malignancies.

Other DNA repair defects

Ataxia with oculomotor apraxia 1 (AOA 1) is characterized by onset of ataxia early in the first decade, ocular apraxia, and areflexia [38,39]. Hypoalbuminemia and elevated cholesterol levels may be seen many years after onset. The genetic abnormality is in a gene called *aprataxin*, which codes for a HIT (histidine triad)/Zn-finger print protein that may be involved in single-strand-DNA break repair [40,41]. There are no systemic features such as malignancy.

Spinocerebellar ataxia with axonal neuropathy (SCAN 1) is another disease related to a DNA repair defect. The mutation affects the tyrosyl-DNA phosphodiesterase 1 (TDP 1) gene [42]. This disorder can also cause hypoalbuminemia.

A disorder that can closely mimic AT (AT-like disorder or ATLD) but with a milder phenotype has been related to a mutation in still another DNA repair gene known as *hMRE 11* [43]. Other classical DNA repair defects such as Cockayne's syndrome and xeroderma pigmentosum can also affect the cerebellum.

Ataxia with oculomotor apraxia 2

Clinically, children with ataxia with oculomotor apraxia (AOA 2) resemble those with AOA 1 but often have elevated alpha-fetoprotein levels and peripheral neuropathy [44] as well. Mutations have been described in the gene coding for the protein senataxin [45].

Ataxia with blindness and deafness

A syndrome of ataxia associated with optic atrophy, visual loss, and cochlear degeneration has been mapped to chromosome 6p21–23 [45,46].

Autosomal recessive spastic ataxia of Charlevoix–Saguenay

Described primarily from a population isolated in the Canadian province of Charlevoix–Saguenay, the disorder known as autosomal recessive spastic ataxia of Charlevoix–Saguenay (ARSACS) has onset early in life (about two years of age) and is characterized by severe spasticity in the beginning and ataxia later [47]. It has a slow progression rate. The ARSACS gene codes for a protein called sacsin that may function as a protein chaperone [48]. Patients from Tunisia and Turkey have also been described [49,50].

Ataxia related to polymerase gamma 1 gene mutations

Recessive mutations of the polymerase gamma 1 gene, *POLG1*, a nuclear gene involved in the replication of mitochondrial DNA (mtDNA), can cause ataxia often associated with ophthalmoplegia, sensory neuropathy, and myoclonus [51].

Other ataxic syndromes of childhood

Other ataxias of recessive origin include Cayman ataxia, autosomal recessive cerebellar ataxia type 1 (ARCA 1), and infantile onset spinocerebellar ataxia (IOSCA) [52–54]. Other ataxic syndromes in childhood and young adult life are less well defined. Early onset ataxia with retained reflexes has phenotypic similarities to FA but for the presence of reflexes. Some of the children have the FA mutation but others do not. Another clinically defined syndrome combines ataxia and hypogonadism with or without chorioretinal dystrophy. A combination of ataxia and myoclonus can be seen in many diseases including some mitochondrial disorders, sialidosis, ceroid lipofuscinosis, and related to a mutation in the cystatin B gene in Unverricht–Lundborg syndrome. Several inborn errors of metabolism can result in ataxia, in addition to other neurological and systemic features (Table 5.2).

Table 5.2. Some metabolic errors in which ataxia may be seen as a major feature

Aminoacidopathies: maple syrup urine disease, L-2 hydroxyglutaric acidemia, isovaleric acidemia

Urea cycle defects: ornithine transcarbamylase deficiency, citrullinemia

Lactic acidosis: Leigh's disease

Leukodystrophies: Alexander's disease, adrenoleukodystrophy, ataxia with central hypomyelination (vanishing white matter disease)

Lysosomal diseases: metachromatic leukodystrophy, Nieman–Pick C_1, hexosaminidase A deficiency

Glycosylation diseases: congenital disorders of glycosylation

Others: Wilson's disease, giant axonal neuropathy

Autosomal dominant ataxias (Table 5.3)

Clinical features [55,56]

The progressive autosomal dominant ataxias are usually labeled spinocerebellar ataxia (SCA) followed by a number to denote the gene locus (HUGO: www.gene.ucl.ac.uk/hugo/). SCA 3 is also known as Machado–Joseph disease (MJD), and dentatorubral-pallidoluysian atrophy (DRPLA) does not have an SCA designation. In addition, there are dominantly inherited episodic ataxia (EA) syndromes.

The SCAs exhibit many phenotypic similarities so that it is almost impossible to diagnose the genotype from the phenotype alone. The diseases are transmitted from generation to generation and penetrance, for the most part, is nearly complete. Anticipation in age at onset is seen in many of the diseases. The core clinical features seen in these diseases are ataxia of gait and limbs and dysarthria. Many eye movement abnormalities related to cerebellar pathology are seen as well, including nystagmus, abnormal pursuit, and saccadic dysmetria.

Patients often exhibit many other neurological signs that can evolve over the course of years. There may be noncerebellar oculomotor features such as slow saccades, oculomotor palsy, blepaharospasm, an ocular stare, and ptosis. Visual function may be compromised owing to a maculopathy (seen in SCA 7). There may be signs of brainstem disease such as facial atrophy and fasciculations, temporal muscle atrophy, tongue atrophy and fasciculations, and poor cough, as well as

Table 5.3. Autosomal dominant ataxias with known gene loci

Disease	Locus/gene	Mutation
SCA 1	6p/ataxin 1	CAG expansion (39–82)
SCA 2	12q/ataxin 2	CAG expansion (33–64)
MJD (SCA 3)	14q/ataxin 3	CAG expansion (54–86)
SCA 4	16q/unknown	Unknown
SCA 5	11p/unknown	Unknown
SCA 6	19p/CACNA1	CAG expansion (19–30)
SCA 7	3p/ataxin 7	CAG expansion (37–200)
SCA 8	13q	CTG expansion (107–127)
SCA 10	22q	ATTCT expansion (1000–4000)
SCA 11	15q/TTBK 2	Conventional mutations
SCA 12	5q/PPP2R2B	CAG expansion (66–78)
SCA 13	10q/KCNC 3	Conventional mutations
SCA 14	19q/PKC γ	Conventional mutations
SCA 15/16	8q23–24.1/ITPR 1	Conventional mutations
SCA 17	6q/TBP	CAG expansion (50–63)
SCA 27	/FGF 14	Conventional mutations
SCA 31	16q/puratrophin	TAGAA insertion
DRPLA	12p/atrophin	CAG expansion (54–79)
EA 1	12p/KCNA 1	Conventional mutations
EA 2	19p/CACNA1	Conventional mutations

SCA, spinocerebellar ataxia; MJD, Machado–Joseph disease; DRPLA, dentatorubral-pallidoluysian atrophy; CAG, cytosine–adenine–guanine; CTG, cytosine–thymine–guanine; ATTCT, adenine–thymidine–thymidine–cytosine–thymidine; numbers in ( ), expanded range.

dysphagia. Spasticity, brisk reflexes, and extensor plantar responses occur in many genotypes. Extrapyramidal signs may include an akinetic-rigid syndrome responsive to dopamine agonists, dystonia, and chorea. A peripheral neuropathy develops in some patients, leading to distal sensory loss, loss of deep tendon reflexes, and abnormal nerve conduction tests. Cerebral involvement may be prominent in some genotypes with myoclonus, seizures, and dementia.

Gene mutations and phenotype–genotype correlations

A variety of gene mutations are responsible for the dominant ataxias. The best-characterized ones are the unstable trinucleotide expansions involving cytosine–adenine–guanine (CAG) tracts. Unstable CAG expansions within coding regions of genes, inherited in a heterozygous fashion (i.e. only one allele has the expansion) are implicated in SCA 1, SCA 2, MJD, SCA 6, SCA 7, SCA 17, and DRPLA [57–65]. The proteins in SCA 1, SCA 2, MJD, SCA 7, and DRPLA are novel proteins and are labeled ataxin 1, ataxin 2, ataxin 3, ataxin 7, and atrophin, respectively; the SCA 6 expansion involves the alpha subunit of the PQ type calcium channel gene and the SCA 17 expansion involves the TATA-binding protein gene. An unstable CAG expansion in a promoter region of the *PPP2R2B* gene (chromosome 5) causes SCA 12 [65]. SCA 8 has been related to an unstable cytosine–thymine–guanine (CTG) expansion located in an untranslated region of the gene [66]. The relationship of this expansion to ataxia has been established only in one family to date. The same expansion has been documented in a sizable proportion of control chromosomes as well as in patients with many non-ataxic disorders. Thus, the presence of this mutation in any given patient with ataxia should be interpreted with caution and generally cannot be used for genetic counseling [67]. SCA 10 is caused by an unstable expansion of an intronic pentanucleotide repeat (ATTCT) [68]. Point mutations cause the EA syndromes: EA 1 in a potassium channel gene, *KCNA 1*, and EA 2 in the neuronal PQ type calcium channel gene, *CACNA 1A* [69,70]. More recently, many progressive SCAs related to conventional mutations have been described as well. These include mutations in the protein kinase C gamma gene for SCA 14 [71], in the fibroblast growth factor 14 gene for SCA 27 [72], in the β spectrin gene for SCA 5 [73], in a tau tubulin kinase gene (*TTBK 2*) in SCA 11 [74], in a potassium channel gene (*KCNC3*) in SCA 13 [75], and in the inositol triphosphate receptor 1 gene (*ITPR1*) in SCA 15/16 [76]. A duplication in chromosome 11 has been related to SCA 20 [77], and an insertion of a pentanucleotide repeat sequence related to a common form of ataxia in Japan known as SCA 31 [78].

The unstable CAG expansions may either contract or expand with intergenerational transmission; there is an overall tendency for them to expand, especially with paternal transmission. This at least partly accounts for the phenomenon of anticipation seen in many families. The age at onset usually has an inverse correlation with the number of repeats in the expanded allele. Earlier onset is also associated

with a more rapid course and a more florid phenotype.

Clinical experience is best with the genotypes that are common and have been known for some time such as SCA 1, SCA 2, MJD (SCA 3), SCA 6, and SCA 7 [79–83]. Age at onset for most disorders can range widely but typically is in the 30s for SCA 1, SCA 2, and SCA 3, but later for SCA 6. SCA 7 can have an adult onset, but it can also begin very early in childhood when it tends to produce a devastating disease with ataxia, dementia, and seizures; this can happen in a child when the affected parent (usually the father) has not yet developed symptoms. Anticipation in age at onset is seen in SCA 1, SCA 2, SCA 3, SCA 6, and SCA 7, but can be especially large in SCA 7 and in DRPLA. SCA 1, SCA 2, MJD, and SCA 7 tend to shorten the lifespan; SCA 6 patients usually have normal lifespans. Upper motor neuron signs are frequent in SCA 1, MJD, and SCA 7, rare in SCA 2, and variable in SCA 6 and SCA 12. Early occurrence of slow saccades is frequent in SCA 2 as well as in SCA 7; this tends to occur late in the disease in MJD and SCA 1, and slow saccades are almost never seen in SCA 6. Downbeat nystagmus is frequent in SCA 6, related to a CAG expansion in the calcium channel gene. Bulbar disease with facial and tongue atrophy and compromised cough are seen more often in SCA 1, SCA 2, SCA 7, and MJD. Features resembling Parkinson's disease have been reported in SCA 2, MJD, and SCA 17. Chorea-athetosis and dystonia are not uncommon in many SCAs late in the disease. Peripheral nerve involvement is prominent with generalized areflexia in SCA 2 and in some families with SCA 4, but can also be seen in MJD; it is less frequent in SCA 1 and uncommon in SCA 6 and SCA 7. Seizures occur in SCA 10 and also with childhood-onset in SCA 7 and DRPLA. Overt visual loss related to a maculopathy is confined to SCA 7, but is a variable feature. Among the ataxias where the clinical experience is more limited, SCA 4 presents with either pure cerebellar ataxia or ataxia with an axonal neuropathy [84]. Again, SCA 5 has cerebellar signs mostly and a slow course [85]; SCA 8 is a spastic ataxia [86]. SCA 11 causes a slowly progressive pure cerebellar syndrome [87]; SCA 12 has a more varied phenotype with tremor as a major feature, in addition to ataxia and bradykinesia [65]. SCA 13 is reported to cause childhood-onset ataxia that is very slowly progressive and associated with mental retardation, but in other families it causes pure ataxia [88]. SCA 14 causes ataxia and axial myoclonus in some families [65,89]. SCA 15/16 (which were found to be related to the same mutation) present with pure cerebellar ataxia [90], or with additional signs such as head tremor [91]; SCA 18 has axonal neuropathy [92]; and SCA 19 has myoclonus, tremor, and cognitive decline [93]. SCA 21 has been reported to have a slow course and has associated akinesia and cognitive deficit [94].

The EA syndromes are also genetically heterogeneous. EA 1 has very short episodes (minutes) of ataxia and is associated with skeletal myokymia in the interictal phase. The episodes of ataxia in EA 2 last for hours and may be associated with diplopia, vertigo, and migraine. EA 2 also often exhibits interictal cerebellar signs and may present with progressive ataxia without prior episodes.

Pathogenesis of dominant ataxias [95–96]

The CAG expansions in coding sequences, which cause many of the dominant ataxias, result in the production of mutated proteins with an extended glutamine tract, and it is believed that the presence of a longer-than-normal glutamine stretch within the protein confers added properties to the protein, such as an abnormal conformation, that is deleterious to neurons. In many of the polyglutamine ataxias, aggregates of the mutated protein can be found, either within neuronal nuclei or cytoplasm or both. These aggregates are being shown to have numerous interactions that may have pathogenic significance. Such interactions include recruitment of proteins important for cell survival, such as the ubiquitin-proteasome system and the heat-shock protein chaperone system, recruitment of the protein product of the normal allele, coaggregation of transcription factors and RNA binding properties, and interactions with splicing machinery. There is evidence that the aggregates themselves may not be necessary for neuronal toxicity. In SCA 1, it has been established that entry of the mutated protein into neuronal nuclei is essential for pathogenesis and such entry may require specific biochemical processing of the protein in the cytoplasm such as phosphorylation. Truncation of the protein by caspases may be another process that may enhance the toxicity of the mutated protein.

Other mechanisms probably operate in the dominant ataxias that do not have a polyglutamine mechanism. These may include a gain of function at the RNA level, as has been postulated for SCA 8, and

Table 5.4. Laboratory studies of value in persons with progressive ataxia

1. MRI and other imaging studies of the brain
2. Routine chemistries: thyroid, B12, metal levels
3. Cerebrospinal fluid examination, including IgG studies and possibly 14–3–3 studies
4. Peripheral and central electrophysiological studies
5. Immune studies: paraneoplastic antibodies, anti-GAD antibody, anti-gliadin antibody
6. Studies to detect inborn errors of metabolism
7. Gene-based tests

altered function of other key pathways important for cerebellar neuronal activity [97,98].

Genetic testing in inherited ataxias (Tables 5.1, 5.3, and 5.4)

Given the heterogeneity of the ataxias, obtaining the right gene test can be a difficult task [99]. One may have to exclude many acquired disorders with appropriate tests (Table 5.4). A genetic cause may be assumed under several circumstances. Singleton cases with early onset often are presumed to have an autosomal recessive mode of inheritance although mitochondrial and X-linked modes may also have to be considered. The later in life the onset among such singleton cases, the less likely that the disorder is a monogenic disease, although one can never be certain of this. Singleton patients with onset in young or middle life may still have a genetic cause, especially if the phenotype is distinctly reminiscent of one of the inherited ataxias. A clear recessive, dominant, or X-linked pattern of family history leads to an inescapable conclusion of a genetic cause. So how does one approach gene tests? I believe that one should look for the FA mutation in all cases of typical FA to confirm the diagnosis. Among this population, about 10% may be negative for this mutation, suggesting genetic heterogeneity. Ataxia with isolated vitamin E deficiency may present in a similar fashion; this is better established by vitamin E levels than a mutation search. The FA mutation should be investigated in all singleton and recessive patients, no matter what the age of onset, if a ready alternative explanation cannot be established. If FA and AVED are excluded, other less common recessive ataxias need to be considered, among them

AOA2, AOA 1, and *POLG 1* related ataxias. What about the dominant ataxia mutations in a sporadic case? In many series of cases, a few sporadic patients have tested positive for SCA 1, SCA 2, SCA 6, or MJD. There are no easy answers as to when to test for a dominant mutation in a sporadic case. If the family history is adequate over three generations and the case can truly be considered sporadic, the yield of such testing will be negligible, but wrong paternity is still a possibility. In this situation, one may consider a dominant ataxia panel if the phenotype is very close to one of the inherited ataxias. If there is clear evidence for a dominant inheritance, one can simply carry out the available dominant ataxia tests. Many clinicians will favor a sequential approach, using the phenotype as a clue, including the age at onset, overall course of disease in the family, other phenotypic features such as visual loss or epilepsy, etc. Despite this, some dominant ataxias will test negative for the available tests.

Many persons from families with ataxia will request predictive testing and occasionally prenatal testing. One has to be clear that before such testing can be offered to a person, the molecular diagnosis in that particular family should be established with no doubt. The testing protocols for such situations have generally followed those for Huntington's disease [100]. It is important to request the help of a geneticist or genetic counselor in many such situations.

Treatment of ataxias

At present, no effective curative treatment is available for any of the inherited ataxias; the topic has been reviewed recently [101,102]. Current treatment of these diseases remains mainly a rehabilitative approach using physical, occupational, and speech therapy, and other similar modalities. Medications that may give occasional and marginal symptomatic improvement in various aspects of cerebellar dysfunction include amantidine and buspirone for balance, clonazepam and propranolol for tremor, and gabapentin and baclofen for nystagmus. Associated spasticity can respond to anti-spasticity medications such as baclofen and tizanidine, and Parkinsonian symptoms may respond to dopaminergic drugs. Associated symptoms such as dysphagia, pain, anxiety, and depression may need to be managed as well. Disease-modifying therapies are under investigation and include antioxidants and drugs that may modify excitotoxicity or apoptosis.

References

1. Konigsmark BW, Weiner LP. The olivopontocerebellar atrophies: a review. *Medicine* 1970; **49**: 227–241.

2. Harding AE. *The Hereditary Ataxias and Related Disorders*. Edinburgh, UK: Churchill Livingstone, 1984.

3. Pandolfo M. Friedreich ataxia. *Semin Pediatr Neurol* 2003; **10**: 163–172.

4. Harding AE. Friedreich ataxia: A clinical and genetic study of 90 families with an analysis of early diagnosis criteria and intrafamilial clustering of clinical features. *Brain* 1981; **104**: 589–620.

5. Filla A, De Michele G, Cavalcanti F, *et al*. The relationship between trinucleotide (GAA) repeat length and clinical features in Friedreich ataxia. *Am J Hum Genet* 1996; **59**: 554–560.

6. Durr A, Cossee M, Agid Y, *et al*. Clinical and genetic abnormalities in patients with Friedreich ataxia. *N Engl J Med* 1996; **335**: 1169–1175.

7. Montermini L, Richter A, Morgan K, *et al*. Phenotypic variability in Friedreich ataxia: Role of the associated GAA triplet repeat expansion. *Ann Neurol* 1997; **41**: 675–682.

8. Wessel K, Schroth G, Diener HC, *et al*. Significance of MRI-confirmed atrophy of the cranial spinal cord in Friedreich ataxia. *Eur Arch Psychiatry Neurol Sci* 1989; **238**: 225–230.

9. Campuzano V, Montermini L, Molto MD, *et al*. Friedreich's ataxia: Autosomal recessive disease caused by an intronic GAA triplet repeat expansion. *Science* 1996; **271**: 1423–1427.

10. Cossee M, Durr A, Schmitt M, *et al*. Frataxin point mutations and clinical presentation of compound heterozygous Friedreich ataxia patients. *Ann Neurol* 1999; **45**: 200–206.

11. Lamont PJ, Davis MB, Wood NW. Identification and sizing of the GAA trinucleotide repeat expansion of Friedreich ataxia in 56 patients – clinical and genetic correlates. *Brain* 1997; **120**: 673–680.

12. McDaniel DO, Keats B, Vedanarayanan VV, *et al*. Interrupted sequence of trinucleotide GAA repeat expansion associated with extreme phenotypic variation in Friedreich's ataxia. *Mov Disord* 2001; **16**: 1153–1158.

13. McCabe DJ, Ryan F, Moore DP, *et al*. Typical Friedreich's ataxia without GAA expansions and GAA expansion without typical

Friedreich's ataxia. *J Neurol* 2000; **247**: 346–355.

14. Campuzano V, Montermini L, Lutz Y, *et al.* Frataxin is reduced in Friedreich ataxia patients and is associated with mitochondrial membranes. *Hum Mol Genet* 1997; **6**: 1771–1780.

15. Babcock M, de Silva D, Oaks R, *et al.* Regulation of mitochondrial iron accumulation by Yfh1, a putative homolog of frataxin. *Science* 1997; **276**: 1709–1712.

16. Sakamoto NK, Ohshima KL, Montermini LM, *et al.* Sticky DNA, a self-associated complex formed at long GAA-TTC repeats in intron 1 of the frataxin gene, inhibits transcription. *J Biol Chem* 2001; **276**: 27171–27177.

17. Cossee M, Puccion H, Gansmuller A, *et al.* Inactivation of the Friedreich ataxia mouse gene leads to early embryonic lethality without iron accumulation. *Hum Mol Genet* 2000; **9**: 1219–1226.

18. Wilson RB, Roof DM. Respiratory deficiency due to loss of mitochondrial DNA in yeast lacking the frataxin homologue. *Nat Genet* 1997; **16**: 352–357.

19. Bradley JL, Blake JC, Chamberlain PK, *et al.* Clinical, biochemical and molecular genetic correlations in Friedreich's ataxia. *Hum Mol Genet* 2000; **9**: 275–282.

20. Waldvogel D, van Gelderen P, Hallett M. Increased iron in the dentate nucleus of patients with Friedreich ataxia. *Ann Neurol* 1999; **46**: 123–125.

21. Patel PI, Isaya G. Friedreich ataxia: from GAA triplet-repeat expansion to frataxin deficiency. *Am J Hum Genet* 2001; **69**: 15–24.

22. Rotig A, de Lonlay P, Chretien D, *et al.* Aconitase and mitochondrial iron-sulfur protein deficiency in Friedreich ataxia. *Nat Genet* 1997; **17**: 215–217.

23. Emond M, Lepage G, Vanasse M, *et al.* Increased levels of plasma malondialdehyde in Friedreich ataxia. *Neurology* 2000; **55**: 1752–1753.

24. Schulz JB, Dehmer T, Schols L, *et al.* Oxidative stress in patients with Friedreich ataxia. *Neurology* 2000; **55**: 1719–1721.

25. LODi R, Cooper JM, Bradley JL. Deficit of in vivo mitochondrial ATP production in patients with Friedrich ataxia. *Proc Natl Acad Sci USA* 1999; **96**: 11492–11495.

26. Rustin P, von Kleist-Retzow JC, Chantrel-Groussard K, *et al.* Effect of idebenone on cardiomyopathy in Friedreich's ataxia: A preliminary study. *Lancet* 1999; **354**: 477–479.

27. Meir T, Buise G. Idebenone: an emerging therapy for Friedreich ataxia. *J Neurol* 2009; **256**: 25–30.

28. LODi R, Hart PE, Rajagopalan B, *et al.* Antioxidant treatment improves in vivo cardiac and skeletal muscle bioenergetics in patients with Friedreich's ataxia. *Ann Neurol* 2001; **49**: 590–596.

29. Cavalier L, Ouahchi K, Kayden HJ, *et al.* Ataxia with isolated vitamin E deficiency: heterogeneity of mutations and phenotypic variability in a large number of families. *Am J Hum Genet* 1998; **62**: 301–310.

30. Ouahchi K, Arita M, Kayden H, *et al.* Ataxia with isolated vitamin E deficiency is caused by mutations in the alpha-tocopheroal transfer protein. *Nat Genet* 1995; **9**: 141–145.

31. Gotoda T, Arita M, Arai H, *et al.* Adult-onset spinocerebellar dysfunction caused by a mutation in the gene for alpha-tocopherol-transfer protein.

N Engl J Med 1995; **333**: 1313–1318.

32. Sharp D, Blinderman L, Combs KA, *et al.* Cloning and gene defects in micosomal triglyceride transfer protein associated with abetalipoproteinaemia. *Nature* 1993; **365**: 65–69.

33. Kohlschutter A. Abetalipproteinemia. In Klockgether T, ed. *Handbook of Ataxia Disorders.* New York, NY, USA: Marcel Dekker, 2000; 205–221.

34. Perlman S, Becker-Catania S, Gatti RA. Ataxia-telangiectasia: diagnosis and treatment. *Semin Pediatr Neurol* 2003; **10**: 173–182.

35. Savitsky K, Bar-Shira A, Gilad S, *et al.* A single ataxia-telangiectasia gene with a product similar to PI-3 kinase. *Science* 1995; **268**: 1749–1753.

36. Becker-Catania SG, Chen G, Hwang MJ, *et al.* Ataxia-telangiectasia: phenotype/genotype studies of ATM protein expression, mutations, and radiosensitivity. *Mol Genet Metab* 2000; **70**: 122–133.

37. Mitui M, Campbell C, Coutinho G, *et al.* Independent mutational events are rare in the ATM gene: haplotype prescreening enhances mutation detection rate. *Hum Mutat* 2003; **22**: 43–50.

38. Aicardi J, Barbosa C, Andermann F, *et al.* Ataxia-ocular motor apraxia: a syndrome mimicking ataxia-telangiectasia. *Ann Neurol* 1988; **24**: 497–502.

39. Barbot C, Coutinho P, Chorao R, *et al.* Recessive ataxia with ocular apraxia: review of 22 Portuguese patients. *Arch Neurol* 2001; **58**: 201–205.

40. Date H, Onodera O, Tanak H, *et al.* Early-onset ataxia with ocular motor apraxia and hypoalbuminemia is caused by

mutations in a new HIT superfamily gene. *Nat Genet* 2001; **29**: 184–188.

41. Moreira MC, Barbot C, Tachi N, *et al.* The gene mutated in ataxia-ocular apraxia 1 encodes the new HIT/Zn-finger protein aprataxin. *Nat Genet* 2001; **29**: 189–193.

42. Takashima HC, Boerkoel F, John J, *et al.* Mutation of TDP1, encoding a topoisomerase I-dependent DNA damage repair enzyme in spinocerebellar ataxia with axonal neuropathy. *Nat Genet* 2002; **32**: 267–272.

43. Stewart GS, Maser RS, Stankovic T, *et al.* The DNA double-strand break repair gene hMRE11 is mutated in individuals with an ataxia-telangiectasia-like disorder. *Cell* 1999; **99**: 577–587.

44. Anheim M, Monga B, Fleury M, *et al.* Ataxia with oculomotor apraxia type 2: clinical, biological and genotype/phenotype correlation study of a cohort of 90 patients. *Brain* 2009; **132**: 2688–2698.

45. Moreira MC, Klur S, Watanabe M, *et al.* Senataxin, the ortholog of a yeast RNA helicase, is mutant in ataxia-ocular apraxia 2. *Nat Genet* 2004; **36**: 225–227.

46. Nemeth AH, Bochukova E, Dunne E, *et al.* Autosomal recessive cerebellar ataxia with oculomotor apraxia (ataxia-telangiectasia-like syndrome) is linked to chromosome 9q34. *Am J Hum Genet* 2000; **67**: 1320–1326.

47. Bouchard JP, Richter A, Mathieu J, *et al.* Autosomal recessive spastic ataxia of Charlevoix–Saguenay. *Neuromuscul Disord* 1998; **8**: 474–479.

48. Engert JC, Berube P, Mercier J, *et al.* ARSACS, a spastic ataxia common in northeastern Quebec, is caused by mutations in a new gene encoding an 11.5-kb ORF. *Nat Genet* 2000; **24**: 120–125.

49. Gucuyener K, Ozgul K, Paternotte C, *et al.* Autosomal recessive spastic ataxia of Charlevoix–Saguenay in two unrelated Turkish families. *Neuropediatrics* 2001; **32**: 142–146.

50. El Euch-Fayache G, Lalani I, Amouri R, *et al.* Phenotypic features and genetic findings in sacsin related autosomal recessive ataxia in Tunisia. *Arch Neurol* 2003; **60**: 982–988.

51. Hakonen AH, Heiskonen S, Juvonen V. Mitochondrial DNA polymerase W748S mutation a common cause of autosomal recessive ataxia with ancient European origin. *Am J Hum Genet* 2005; **77**: 430–441.

52. Bomar JM, Benke PJ, Slattery EL, *et al.* Mutations in a novel gene encoding a CRAL-TRIO domain cause human Cayman ataxia and ataxia/dystonia in the jittery mouse. *Nat Genet* 2003; **35**: 264–269.

53. Nikali K, Suomalainen A, Saharinen J, *et al.* Infantile onset spinocerebellar ataxia is caused by recessive mutations in mitochondrial proteins Twinkle and Twinky. *Hum Mol Genet* 2005; **14**: 2981–2990.

54. Dupré N, Gros-Louis F, Christian N, *et al.* Clinical and genetic study of autosomal recessive cerebellar ataxia type 1. *Ann Neurol* 2007; **62**: 93–98.

55. Gomez CM, Subramony SH. Dominantly inherited ataxias. *Semin Pediatr Neurol* 2003; **10**: 210–222.

56. Subramony SH. Genetics of inherited ataxias. *Continuum* 2005; **11**: 115–142.

57. Orr HT, Chung M, Banfi S, *et al.* Expansion of an unstable trinucleotide CAG repeat in spinocerebellar axtaxia type 1. *Nat Genet* 1993; **4**: 221–226.

58. Pulst S-M, Nechiporuk A, Nechiporuk T, *et al.* Moderate expansion of a normally biallelic trinucleotide repeat in spinocerebellar ataxia type 2. *Nat Genet* 1996; **14**: 269–276.

59. Sanpei K, Takano H, Igarashi S, *et al.* Identification of spinocerebellar ataxia type 2 gene using a direct identification of repeat expansion and cloning technique, DIRECT. *Nat Genet* 1996; **14**: 277–284.

60. Kawaguchi Y, Okamoto T, Taniwaki M, *et al.* CAG expansion in a novel gene for Machado–Joseph disease at chromosome 14q32.1. *Nat Genet* 1994; **8**: 221–224.

61. Zuchenko O, Bailey J, Bonnen P, *et al.* Autosomal dominant cerebellar ataxia (SCA 6) associated with small polyglutamine expansions in the alpha 1A-voltage-dependent calcium channel. *Nat Genet* 1997; **15**: 62–69.

62. David G, Abbas N, Stevanin G, *et al.* Cloning of the SCA 7 gene reveals a highly unstable CAG repeat expansion. *Nat Genet* 1997; **17**: 65–70.

63. Zuhlke C, Hellenbroich Y, Dalski A, *et al.* Different types of repeat expansions in TATA-binding protein gene are associated with a new form of inherited ataxia. *Eur J Hum Genet* 2001; **9**: 160–164.

64. Nagafuchi S, Yanagisawa H, Sato K, *et al.* Dentatorubral and pallidoluysian atrophy expansion of an unstable GAG trinucleotide of chromosome 12p. *Nat Genet* 1994; **6**: 14–18.

65. Holmes SE, O'Hearn EE, McInnis MG, *et al.* Expansion of a novel CAG trinucleotide repeat in the 5' prime region of PPP2R2B is associated with SCA 12. *Nat Genet* 1999; **23**: 391–392.

66. Koob MD, Moseley ML, Schut LJ, *et al.* An untranslated CTG expansion causes a novel form of spinocerebellar ataxia (SCA 8). *Nat Genet* 1999; **21**: 379–384.

67. Nance MA. Seeking clarity through the genetic lens. A work in progress. *Ann Neurol* 2003; **54**: 5–7.

68. Matsuura T, Yamagata T, Burgess DL, *et al.* Large expansion of the ATTCT pentanucleotide repeat in spinocerebellar ataxia type 10. *Nat Genet* 2000; **26**: 191–194.

69. Browne DL, Gancher ST, Nutt JG, *et al.* Episodic ataxia/myokymia syndrome is associated with point mutations in the human potassium channel gene KCNA1. *Nat Genet* 1994; **8**: 136–140.

70. Ophoff RA, Terwindt GM, Vergouwe MN, *et al.* Familial hemiplegic migraine and episodic ataxia type 2 are caused by mutations in the Ca^{2+} channel gene CACNL1A4. *Cell* 1996; **7**: 543–552.

71. Chen D-H, Brkanac Z, Verlinde CLMJ, *et al.* Missense mutations in the regulatory domain of PKC_γ: a new mechanism for dominant nonepisodic cerebellar ataxia. *Am J Hum Genet* 2003; **72**: 839–849.

72. van Swieten JC, Brusse E, de Graaf BM, *et al.* A mutation in the fibroblast growth factor 14 gene is associated with autosomal dominant cerebral ataxia. *Am J Hum Genet* 2003; **72**: 191–199.

73. Ikeda Y, Dick KA, Weatherspoon MR, *et al.* Spectrin mutations cause spinocerebellar ataxia type 5. *Nat Genet* 2006; **38**: 184–190.

74. Houlden H, Johnson J, Garner-Thorpe C, *et al.* Mutations in TTBK2, encoding a kinase implicated in tau phosphorylation, segregate with spinocerebellar ataxia type 11. *Nat Genet* 2007; **39**: 1434–1436.

75. Waters MF, Minassian NA, Stevanin G, *et al.* Mutations in voltage-gated potassium channel KCNC3 cause degenerative and developmental central nervous system phenotypes. *Nat Genet* 2006; **38**: 447–451.

76. Iwaki, A, Kawano Y, Miura S, *et al.* Heterozygous deletion of ITPR1 but not SUMF 1 in spinocerebellar ataxia type 16. *J Med Genet* 2008; **45**: 32–35.

77. Knight, MA, Hernandez D, Diede SJ, *et al.* A duplication at chromosome 11q12.2-11q12.3 is associated with spinocerebellar ataxia type 20. *Hum Mol Genet* 2008; **17**: 3847–3853.

78. Sato, N, Amino T, Kobayashi K, *et al.* Spinocerebellar ataxia type 31 is associated with "inserted" penta-nucleotide repeats containing (TGGAA)n. *Am J Hum Genet* 2009; **85**: 1–14.

79. Goldfarb LG, Vasconcelos O, Platonov FA, *et al.* Unstable triplet repeat and phenotypic variability of spinocerebellar ataxia type 1. *Ann Neurol* 1996; **39**: 500–506.

80. Orozco G, Nodarse A, Cordoves RC, *et al.* Autosomal dominant cerebellar ataxia: clinical analysis of 263 patients from a homogeneous population in Holguin, Cuba. *Neurology* 1990; **40**: 1369–1375.

81. Sequeiros J, Coutinho P. Epidemiology and clinical aspects of Machado–Joseph disease. In Harding AE, Duefel T, eds. *Advances in Neurology.* New York, NY, USA: Raven Press, 1993; 139–153.

82. Gomez CM, Thompson RM, Gammack JT, *et al.* Spinocerebellar ataxia type 6: gaze-evoked and vertical nystagmus, Purkinje cell degeneration, and variable age of onset. *Ann Neurol* 1997; **42**: 933–950.

83. Enevoldson TP, Sanders MD, Harding AE. Autosomal dominant cerebellar ataxia with pitmentary macular dystrophy. A clinical and genetic study of eight families. *Brain* 1994; **117**: 445–460.

84. Flanigan K, Gardner K, Alderson K, *et al.* Autosomal dominant spinocerebellar ataxia with sensory axonal neuropathy (SCA 4): clinical description and genetic localization to chromosome 16q22.1. *Am J Hum Genet* 1996; **59**: 392–399.

85. Schut LJ, Day JW, Clark HB, *et al.* Spinocerebellar ataxia type 5. In Klockgehter T, ed. *Handbook of Ataxia Disorders.* New York, NY, USA: Marcel–Dekker, 2000; 435–445.

86. Day JW, Schut LJ, Moseley ML, *et al.* Spinocerebellar ataxia type 8. Clinical features in a large family. *Neurology* 2000; **55**: 649–657.

87. Worth PF, Giunti P, Gardner-Thorpe C, *et al.* Autosomal dominant cerebellar ataxia type III: linkage in a large British family to a 7.6-cM region on chromosome 15q13–21.3. *Am J Hum Genet* 1999; **65**: 420–426.

88. Waters MF, Pulst SM. SCA13. *Cerebellum* 2008; **7**: 165–169.

89. Yamashita I, Sasaki H, Yabe I, *et al.* A novel locus for dominant cerebellar ataxia (SCA 14) maps to a 10.2-cM interval flanked by D19S206 and D19S605 on chromosome 19q13.4-qter. *Ann Neurol* 2000; **48**: 156–163.

90. Storey E, Gardner RJ, Knight MA, *et al.* A new autosomal dominant pure cerebellar ataxia. *Neurology* 2000; **57**: 1913–1915.

91. Miyoshi Y, Yamada T, Tanimura M, *et al.* A novel spinocerebellar ataxia (SCA 16) linked to chromosome 8q22.1–24.1. *Neurology* 2001; **57**, 96–100.

92. Brkanac Z, Fernandez M, Matsuhita M, *et al.* Autosomal dominant sensory/motor neuropathy with ataxia (SMNA): linkage to chromosome 7q22-q32. *Am J Med Genet* 2002; **114**: 450–457.

93. Schelhaas HJ, Ippel PF, Hageman G, *et al*. Clinical and genetic analysis of a four-generation family with distinct autosomal dominant cerebellar ataxia. *J Neurol* 2001; **248**: 113–120.

94. Devos S, Schraen-Maschke S, Vuillaume I, *et al*. Clinical features and genetic analysis of a new form of spinocerebellar axatia. *Neurology* 2001; **56**: 234–238.

95. Zoghbi HY, Orr HT. Glutamine repeats and neurodegeneration. *Annu Rev Neurosci* 2000; **23**: 217–247.

96. Duenas AM, Goold R, Giunti P. Molecular pathogenesis of nocerebellar ataxias. *Brain* 2006; **129**: 1357–1370.

97. Ranum LP, Day JW. Dominantly inherited, no-coding microsatellite expansion disorders. *Curr Opin Genet Dev* 2002; **12**: 266–271.

98. Schorge S, van de Leemput J, Singleton A, *et al*. Human ataxias: a genetic dissection of inositol triphosphate receptor (ITPR1)-dependent signaling: 2010; **33**: 211–219.

99. Nance M. Genetic testing in inherited ataxias. *Semin Pediatr Neurol* 2003; **10**: 223–231.

100. International Huntington Association, World Federation of Neurology. Ethical issues policy statement on Huntington's disease molecular genetics predictive test. *J Med Ethics* 1990; **27**: 34–38.

101. Perlman SL. Spinocerebellar degeneration. *Expert Opin Pharmacother* 2003; **4**: 1637–1641.

102. Perlman SL. Cerebellar ataxia. *Curr Treat Options Neurol* 2000; **2**: 215–224.

Huntington's disease

Edward J. Wild and Sarah J. Tabrizi

Introduction

Huntington's disease (HD) is a slowly progressive autosomal dominant neurodegenerative disorder. The onset is usually in adult life with a mean age of about 40 years, although juvenile onset and onset in the elderly are well described. The disease progresses inexorably, with death occurring 15 to 20 years from the time of onset. The prevalence is usually given as 4–10 per 100 000 in populations of Western European descent, but the true prevalence is likely to be significantly higher because of historical stigma and misdiagnosis [1]. HD has been described throughout the world.

Huntington's disease is named after George Huntington who originally described the disease in 1872. Dr Huntington was only 21 years of age and had recently graduated from Columbia University. He presented his paper before the Meigs and Mason Academy of Medicine at Middleport, Ohio on the February 15, 1872. It was published two months later in the Medical and Surgical Reporter of Philadelphia. His paper is cited to this day as one of the best and all-encompassing descriptions of the key features of HD [2]. From a young age, Huntington had observed patients with HD while traveling around on his father's medical practitioner's rounds in East Hampton, Long Island, New York. An extract from his original paper is given below:

"The hereditary chorea as I shall call it, is confined to certain and fortunately few families and has been transmitted to them as an heirloom from generations way back in the dim past. It is spoken of by those in whose veins the seeds of the disease are known to exist with a kind of horror and not at all alluded to except through dire necessity with it being mentioned as 'that disorder'. It is attended generally by all the symptoms of common chorea, only in an aggravated degree, hardly ever manifesting itself until adult life and then coming on gradually, but surely, increasing by degrees and often occupying years in its development until the hapless sufferer is but a quivering wreck of his former self.

There are three marked peculiarities in this disease: (1) its hereditary nature; (2) a tendency to insanity and suicide; and (3) its manifesting itself as a grave disease only in adult life.

"I have never known a recovery or even an amelioration of symptoms in this form of chorea; when once it begins it clings to the bitter end. No treatment seems to be of avail, and indeed nowadays its end is so well known to the sufferer and his friends that medical advice is seldom sought. It seems at least to be one of the incurables."

Huntington also astutely noted the hereditary nature of the disease and wrote *"If the thread is broken then the grandchildren of the original shakers may rest assured that they are free from the disease."* This was 120 years before the causative genetic mutation was identified in 1993 [3].

Molecular genetics of Huntington's disease

The HD locus was one of the first disease associated loci to be mapped using restriction fragment length polymorphisms [4]. This finding allowed presymptomatic detection of HD-allele carriers. It was 10 years later in 1993 that the gene responsible was discovered [3]. Exon amplification of cosmids in the chromosome 4p16.3 interval yielded "interesting transcript 15" (IT15) from a novel gene in which an expanded cytosine–adenine–guanine (CAG) repeat within the predicted open reading frame was associated with HD. The protein product was termed huntingtin. The polyglutamine expansion is located in exon 1 and starts at residue 18. Other than the poly-CAG tract, the gene lacked homology to any known genes. Genomic sequencing of the exon-intron boundaries indicated that IT15 (now called the *HTT* gene) spans 180 kb and contains 67 exons [5]. The predicted open reading frame yields a protein containing 3144 amino acid residues, with a predicted molecular mass of 348 kDa [6]. Studies have shown there is significant sequence

Table 6.1. CAG repeat thresholds in Huntington's disease

	Normal	Paternal meiotic instability	Reduced penetrance range	HD
CAG length	<27 Not pathogenic Not unstable	27 to 35 Not pathogenic May expand into disease range in future generations ('new mutations')	36 to 39 Pathogenic	≥40 Always causes HD

HD, Huntington's disease. Different CAG repeat ranges are seen in normal individuals (<27), in those with intermediate alleles (≤35), in the reduced penetrance range that may be pathogenic (36–39), and in those repeat lengths that are always pathogenic (≥40).

homology of *HTT* across a wide variety of mammalian species [7], and this high degree of conservation across species suggests that normal huntingtin is an essential protein. Indeed, homozygous huntingtin knockout in mice is embryonically lethal [8]. The HD gene was the second neurodegenerative disease found to be caused by an expanded CAG repeat (CAG repeat expansions were described in mutations in the androgen receptor causing spinal and bulbar muscular atrophy [SBMA] in 1991 [9]), and since then eight other neurodegenerative disorders – namely dentatorubral-pallidoluysian atrophy (DRPLA) and spinocerebellar ataxia (SCA) 1, 2, 3, 6, 7, 12, and 17 – have all been found to be because of CAG repeat expansions [10]. The codon CAG encodes the amino acid glutamine and, therefore, this group of diseases is often referred to as the polyglutamine disorders.

Detailed studies involving large numbers of patients with HD and controls showed that the normal huntingtin CAG repeat length is 10–35, with a mean of 18. Patients with HD with mutant huntingtin have CAG repeat lengths of 36–121 with a mean of 40 repeats [11] (Table 6.1). Adult-onset patients usually have an expansion between 40 and 55, with juvenile-onset patients having expansions above 60. CAG repeats above 40 are fully penetrant, although there is a borderline repeat range between 36 and 39 repeats where there is reduced penetrance. Rubinsztein *et al.* (1996) [12] studied 178 patients with HD worldwide, and found seven with 36 repeats (they found no cases with a lower number), and individuals with 36, 37, 38, and 39 repeats who did not have any signs of the disease (all aged >69 years old). They describe a 95-year-old man with 39 repeats who did not have the disease, which suggests the gene may not be fully penetrant in rare cases. Recent reports of individuals with manifest HD and repeat lengths below 36 remain controversial [13,14].

Anticipation and parent-of-origin effect

CAG repeat lengths vary from generation to generation, with both expansion and contraction of the number of repeats, but with a tendency for repeat lengths to increase [15]. The gender of the transmitting parent was found to be important in terms of repeat length expansion. When transmitted from the mother, repeat length increases or decreases up to seven CAG repeat lengths with an overall mean change of zero. When transmission occurs from the father, there is a tendency toward much larger expansions, with up to a doubling of paternal repeat length and expansions occurring much more than contractions, resulting in a mean intergenerational increase of four CAG repeats from paternal transmission [15–17]. The reasons for this are incompletely understood but genetic instability of the CAG repeat during spermatogenesis, perhaps from slippage of the DNA replication apparatus along CAG tracts, has been suggested [15,18]. The tendency of the CAG expansion to expand during transmission underlies the phenomenon of anticipation. Genetic anticipation describes the increasing severity of an inherited disease during intergenerational transmission and is a hallmark of HD and the other trinucleotide repeat disorders. The CAG repeat instability during paternal transmission is important in the development of large expansions associated with juvenile HD, and approximately 80% of juvenile HD patients with large CAG repeat lengths inherited the HD gene from the father [19].

Intermediate repeat alleles and new mutations

New mutations in HD were originally thought to be very rare, but it is now known that intermediate alleles with CAG repeat lengths between 27 and 35 may expand into the pathogenic range when transmitted through the paternal line as discussed previously (Table 6.1). This has important implications for the molecular epidemiology of HD, as the frequency of intermediate allele carriers is between 1.5% and 1.9% in the general population in Europe and the United States [20].

Correlation between CAG repeat and clinical disease

There is a direct correlation between the CAG repeat size and the age of onset, such that the larger the size of the repeat, the earlier the disease onset [11,21]. Most individuals with greater than 50 repeats develop the disease before the age of 30. The size of the CAG repeat itself allows some estimate of the age of onset in premanifest individuals [22]. However, this can be variable, and generally such estimates are confined to the research setting when estimating years-to-onset in premanifest gene carriers. In addition, it has been found that the CAG repeat number appears to govern the development rate of neuropathological changes directly [23], with more rapid degenerative changes seen with longer CAG repeat lengths. This may explain the earlier onset with longer CAG repeats. However, it is now known that the CAG repeat accounts for only 50%–70% of variation in the age of onset [24], so there is interest in modifying genes that affect age of onset, and identification of these modifiers, particularly those that lead to postponing age of onset, is an important area of study.

A study of the Venezuelan kindred, at the edge of Lake Maracaibo (see following section), revealed that both genetic and environmental factors modulate the age of onset of the disease [25]. A genome scan of 629 affected sib-pairs found linkage at 4p16 (LOD = 1.93), 6p21–23 (LOD = 2.29), and 6q24–26 (LOD = 2.28) [24]. Recent studies have identified numerous individual genes (including *PPARGC1A* and *GRIK2*) the polymorphisms of which appear to alter the age at onset, although as yet no study has revealed specific exploitable mechanisms for these apparent effects [26]. The CAG repeat does not predict the clinical phenotype nor the severity of clinical disease progression, and other modifying genes obviously play an important role in this respect.

Epidemiology

The prevalence of HD in populations of Western European descent is usually given as approximately 4–10 per 100 000 [19]. There are areas of particular

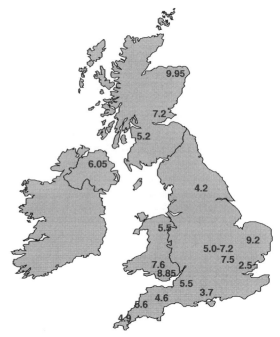

Figure 6.1. Huntington's disease in the UK. This map shows the result of different prevalence studies based on defined geographical regions [19]. (Adapted from Figure 6.5, p. 171 in *Huntington's Disease*, Bates, Harper, and Jones, eds, third edition, Oxford Medical Publications, with permission from Oxford University Press.)

high or low geographical incidence; for example, HD is rare in Japan, Finland, and South African black populations, and relatively little is known about its prevalence in the Middle East and most of Asia. Genealogical studies have shown that HD spread around the world because of migration from northwest Europe and there are regions of high incidence. The highest frequency in the world is in Venezuela at the edge of Lake Maracaibo with a prevalence of 700 per 100 000; the region is relatively isolated both socially and geographically and this has led to the high gene frequency in this small population. It was the systematic study of this small Venezuelan community in 1979 that was crucial in the linkage and cloning of the HD gene. There are regions of higher prevalence in the United Kingdom in South Wales, Northern Ireland, East Anglia, and parts of Scotland (Figure 6.1); the minimum prevalence overall in the United Kingdom is 4–10 per 100 000, which makes it one of the more common inherited neurological diseases in the United Kingdom after neurofibromatosis type 1, Charcot–Marie–Tooth disease, and Duchenne muscular dystrophy [19]. It is increasingly recognized that the true prevalence of HD is probably at least double the quoted values, because of historical inaccuracies in reporting owing to a combination of the stigma of having such a disease in the family, and underdiagnosis, especially in mild, late-onset cases and before the molecular genetic test. From a molecular epidemiology view, all cases of HD ultimately had an ancestral origin from healthy individuals carrying an intermediate repeat allele of between 29 and 35 repeats. The UK Huntington's Prediction Consortium has shown that only about 15% of those at risk undergo predictive testing [27].

Clinical features of Huntington's disease

HD onset has been described as between the ages of 2 and 87 years. HD can produce a wide range of phenotypic presentations and, as the disease progresses, the signs and symptoms often change [28].

Motor features

The onset of HD is often difficult to discern clearly and many patients have a history of psychiatric problems or mild cognitive symptoms prior to the onset of any motor problems. However, the definitive diagnosis of HD is usually made when patients are noted to have unequivocal motor abnormalities on examination. Early signs may be subtle and not noticed by the patient but may be obvious to the clinician; it is not an unusual situation for patients with evident chorea to present for predictive testing believing themselves to be entirely presymptomatic. Minor motor abnormalities that may be seen early in the disease are general restlessness, abnormal eye movements, hyperreflexia, impaired finger tapping, and fidgety movements of fingers, hands, and toes during stress or when walking. Eye movements are particularly important when assessing patients with very early disease, and oculomotor abnormalities are a cardinal feature of the disease and they are often the earliest motor sign. Saccadic abnormalities are characteristic and include delayed initiation of voluntary saccades, slowing of saccades (vertical worse than horizontal), and inability to suppress reflexive glances at novel stimuli. As the disease progresses, head thrusting is used to initiate saccades. Patients with HD often are unable to suppress blinking during saccades as they use blinking to initiate saccades. Pursuit is impaired with saccadic intrusions and, as the disease progresses, a characteristic sign is gaze impersistence with difficulty fixating on an object. All these oculomotor abnormalities are likely to represent disruption to frontostriatal control of eye movements [29]. As the disease progresses, patients develop more obvious extrapyramidal signs: chorea is seen in 90% of adult-onset patients with varying degrees of dystonia, parkinsonism, and bradykinesia. A key motor abnormality in HD is that of impairment of voluntary motor function with clumsiness and disturbances in fine motor control and motor speed. Gait disturbance is common, with impairment of postural reflexes making patients more prone to falling. Impairment of voluntary motor control is generally much more functionally disabling than the more visible hyperkinetic movement disorder. Common problems are dysarthria and dysphagia, and it is important always to ask directly about swallowing symptoms.

Cognitive features

Cognitive abnormalities are an invariable feature of HD and present early in the course of the disease; however, the severity varies greatly. Patients with HD have a very specific and characteristic cognitive dysfunction that is not a global disturbance and, in fact, many people feel that the term dementia is not appropriate. Many cognitive functions remain relatively intact even in the advanced stages of the disease. For example, language function is preserved with relatively little impairment of perceptual and spatial skills, which is in marked contrast to, say, Alzheimer's disease where these functions are lost early. Many of the cognitive changes in HD represent disruption to frontostriatal circuits and this is evident from the key cognitive abnormalities seen in these patients. They are most impaired in executive function with poor planning and judgment, impulsive behavior, disorganized actions, and difficulty coping with multiple tasks. Many patients exhibit psychomotor slowing with apathy, lack of self-care, and loss of initiative, which can make caring for these patients difficult. One of the most common symptoms that patients complain of early is visual and verbal memory problems in addition to common symptoms of poor concentration and attention.

Psychiatric features

It is the combination of psychiatric and cognitive features that causes the greatest disability, functional decline, and distress to relatives. Patients with HD with prominent psychiatric problems are often poorly catered for in our society because they fall between psychiatry and neurology, as well as between hospital and community care. Psychiatric symptoms are common and depression and anxiety particularly so [reviewed in 30]. It is very important to ask about these symptoms and treat them, as even a mild degree of depression exacerbates the other cognitive features of HD and can make patients even more withdrawn and unable to care for themselves. Irritability is also very common and some patients become aggressive. Common symptoms as the disease progresses are recurrent obsessions and compulsions, which can make life difficult for carers and relatives. Psychosis, despite being well recognized, in fact is relatively rare; it has been suggested that there are additional familial and genetic factors that predispose to schizophrenia-like symptoms in HD, as many such patients come from families with a high incidence of schizophrenia itself [31]. Mania is seen but patients more commonly present with hypomania – one study suggested that brief episodes of hypomania are seen in up to 10% of patients [32]. Suicide in HD is much higher than in the general population; Farrer et al. (1986) reported a 27.6% rate of attempted suicide in HD [33], and it has been found that risk factors for suicide in HD were similar to those seen in the general population; namely, loneliness, childlessness, single status, depression, and substance dependence [34]. Therefore, in the assessment of HD patients, questions regarding feelings about suicide are important in the appropriate context; medical treatment, strengthening social support, and psychological therapy will all have an impact on reducing this risk. It has been suggested that the incidence of alcohol and drug abuse is higher in the HD population, but a number of studies have not supported this view. However, aggressive management of drug and alcohol problems in HD is recommended as their deleterious effects rapidly compound the motor and cognitive symptoms of the disease. An important area that is often neglected is that of the psychosexual problems in HD, which are common. It is usually assumed that problems of hypersexuality are more common but systematic studies have reported that hyposexuality is, in fact, more prevalent, mainly owing to the motor and cognitive aspects of the disease [35].

Juvenile Huntington's disease

Juvenile cases are defined as those with an onset before the age of 20 years, associated with larger CAG repeats that usually are greater than 55. Juvenile HD patients have a more severe disease with a shorter life expectancy. The akinetic-rigid form of the disease (or Westphal variant) is more common in juvenile HD cases; patients typically have little chorea and are predominantly rigid and dystonic. Akinetic-rigid forms of the disease are well recognized in young adults (in their 20s) but are rare in older age groups. Juvenile HD patients also have a higher incidence of seizures than adult-onset patients [28].

United Huntington's disease rating scale

This rating scale, the UHDRS, is the most commonly used assessment scale for patients with HD. It comprises a motor rating scale (Figure 6.2a) [36]; a cognitive assessment that includes the digit symbols test, the color conflict Stroop test, and verbal fluency; a behavioral/psychiatric assessment, and a functional capacity assessment (Figure 6.2b) [37]. The total functional capacity shows good correlation with disease progression and is simple to administer [28]. The UHDRS is valuable in the clinical setting as it is administered rapidly and easily and provides a quantifiable measurement of disease status. The newer Short Behavioral Assessment is now felt to be superior to the UHDRS behavioral scale [35].

Neuropathology

In the early stages of disease, the brain can look normal macroscopically, but later there is marked cortical atrophy with ventricular dilation. There is severe atrophy of the caudate nucleus and the putamen to a lesser extent, with atrophy of the internal segment of the globus pallidus and substantia nigra pars reticulata. Histological examination reveals neuronal loss and gliosis in the neostriatum. The neuronal loss is selective with marked depletion of medium spiny neurons, and relative preservation of cholinergic interneurons and medium-size aspiny neurons [38]. The most well-recognized neuropathological classification is the Vonsattel grade. There are five grades: grade 0, in which HD brains show no gross or generalized microscopic abnormalities consistent with HD, despite premortem symptomatology and positive family history, progressing to grade 4, which shows extreme atrophy [39]. Microglial activation is also seen from early in the disease [40].

Investigations

Before the advent of genetic testing for HD, diagnosis was based on a combination of clinical evaluation

(a)

6. OCULAR PURSUIT

0 = normal
1 = jerky movement
2 = interrupted pursuits/full range
3 = incomplete range
4 = cannot pursue

Horizontal Vertical
☐ ☐

7. SACCADE INITIATION

0 = normal
1 = increased latency
2 = suppressible blinks or
 head movements to initiate
3 = unsuppressible head movements
4 = cannot initiate

Horizontal Vertical
☐ ☐

8. SACCADE VELOCITY

0 = normal
1 = mild slowing
2 = moderate slowing
3 = very slow, full range
4 = incomplete range

Horizontal Vertical
☐ ☐

9. DYSARTHRIA ☐

0 = normal
1 = unclear
2 = must repeat to be understood
3 = mostly incomprehensible
4 = mute

10. TONGUE PROTRUSION ☐

0 = maintains for 10 seconds
1 = less than 10 seconds
2 = less than 5 seconds
3 = cannot fully protrude
4 = cannot protrude tongue beyond lips

11. FINGER TAPS

0 = >= 15 taps/5 seconds
1 = mild slowing and/or reduced amplitude (11−14)
2 = moderate impairment, occasional arrests (7−10)
3 = severely impaired, frequent hesitation or arrests (3−6)
4 = cannot execute

12. PRONATION/SUPINATION

0 = normal
1 = mild slowing and/or irregular
2 = moderate slowing and irregular
3 = severe slowing and irregular
4 = cannot execute

Right Left
☐ ☐

13. LURIA ☐

0 = >4 in 10 seconds
1 = <4 in 10 seconds
2 = <4 in 10 seconds, needs verbal cues
3 = <4 in 10 seconds, errors despite cues
4 = cannot perform

14. RIGIDITY - ARMS

0 = normal
1 = slight or present only with activation
2 = mild-moderate
3 = severe, full range of motion
4 = severe with limited range

Right Left
☐ ☐

15. BRADYKINESIA ☐

0 = normal
1 = minimally slow (?normal)
2 = mild but clearly slow
3 = moderately slow, some hesitation
4 = markedly slow, long delays in initiation

16. MAXIMAL DYSTONIA

Trunk	RUE	LUE	RLE	LLE
☐	☐	☐	☐	☐
16a	16b	16c	16d	16e

0 = absent
1 = slight/intermittent
2 = mild/common or moderate/intermittent
3 = moderate/common
4 = marked/prolonged

17. MAXIMAL CHOREA

Face	BOL	Trunk	RUE	LUE	RLE	LLE
☐	☐	☐	☐	☐	☐	☐
17a	17b	17c	17d	17e	17f	17g

0 = absent
1 = slight/intermittent
2 = mild/common or moderate/intermittent
3 = moderate/common
4 = marked/prolonged

18. GAIT ☐

0 = normal gait, narrow base
1 = wide base and/or slow
2 = wide base and walks with difficulty
3 = walks only with assistance
4 = cannot walk

19. TANDEM ☐

0 = normal for 10 steps
1 = 1−3 deviations
2 = >3 deviations
3 = cannot complete task
4 = cannot attempt task

20. RETROPULSION/PULL ☐

0 = normal
1 = recovers spontaneously
2 = would fall if not caught
3 = tends to fall spontaneously
4 = cannot stand

Figure 6.2a. Motor subset of the United Huntington's disease rating scale (UHDRS) [36]. A motor score is generated with a maximum score of 124. (Reproduced with permission from John Wiley & Sons Ltd. © 1996 Movement Disorder Society.)

(b)

DOMAIN	LEVEL OF FUNCTIONING	SCORE
OCCUPATION	0 = unable 1 = marginal work only 2 = reduced capacity for usual job 3 = normal	70 ☐
FINANCES	0 = unable 1 = major assistance 2 = slight assistance 3 = normal	71 ☐
DOMESTIC CHORES	0 = unable 1 = impaired 2 = normal	72 ☐
ADL	0 = total care 1 = gross tasks only 2 = minimal impairment 3 = normal	74 ☐
CARE LEVEL	0 = full time skilled nursing 1 = home or chronic care 2 = home	75 ☐

Figure 6.2b. (cont.) **Total Functional Capacity (TFC) scale from the UHDRS.** A functional capacity score that ranges from 0 to 13 is generated. (Reproduced from Schoulson and Fahn (1979) [37] with permission from Lippincott, Williams, and Wilkins.)

and neuropathological examination. Now there is molecular diagnosis that allows definitive confirmation of the disease. Neuroimaging and cerebrospinal fluid examination are not useful diagnostically; patients often have normal magnetic resonance images early in the disease.

Differential diagnosis of Huntington's disease

The most common causes of inherited chorea are summarized in Table 6.2; however, this section will focus on those disorders that are phenocopies of HD (see Table 6.3). The wide availability of gene testing has allowed detailed genotype/phenotype studies in HD; it has also increased our understanding of disorders that present with a similar clinical picture to HD (HD phenocopies) with similar cognitive, psychiatric, and motor features, but which are HD-gene negative. From large genetic cohorts, HD phenocopies represent 1% of individuals with clinical signs of HD [41]. A 192-nucleotide insertion in the prion protein gene encoding eight octapeptide repeats was associated with an HD-like disease in a single family: this familial prion disease was called HD-like-1

(HDL-1) [42]. However, this family had prominent adult-onset seizures not characteristic of HD. HDL-2 (HD-like 2) is caused by a CAG/CTG expansion in the *Junctophilin-3* gene and is generally rare [43]; however, the rate is considerably higher among individuals of African ancestry and is almost as common as HD in black South Africans. An autosomal recessive, progressive neurodegenerative HD-like disorder was mapped to 4p15.3 and named HDL-3, but it has not been seen outside this pedigree [44]. Another autosomal dominant disease that mimics HD is DRPLA, which is also a polyglutamine disorder caused by a CAG repeat expansion in the atrophin-1 gene on chromosome 12; this often causes seizures as well [45]. Spinocerebellar ataxia 17 is an autosomal dominant polyglutamine disease caused by a CAG repeat expansion in the TATA-binding gene (*TBP*); this comprises ataxia, dementia, and chorea and may closely resemble HD; in fact, it has also been termed HDL-4 [46]. Other SCA disorders that may mimic HD are SCA 1 and SCA 3. In addition, inherited prion disorders caused by mutations in the prion protein gene (separate from the HDL-1 mutation) may cause HD phenocopies, as can neuro-acanthocytosis; autosomal recessive cases have been associated with mutations in the chorein gene on chromosome 9 [47]. In one HD phenocopy series, an atypical case of Friedreich's ataxia with chorea, cognitive impairment, and eye movement disorder was identified [48]. Lastly, a recently described disorder, neuroferritinopathy, caused by mutations in the ferritin light chain polypeptide,

has autosomal dominant inheritance and clinical features that overlap with HD [49].

Ultimately, of the 1% of patients with HD-like presentations who test negative for the HD genetic expansion, a genetic diagnosis is reached in only 3% of cases, with SCA 17 the most commonly found disorder (see Figure 6.3) [50].

Genetic counseling in HD

The discovery of the gene in 1993 allowed the accurate genetic diagnosis of HD, and also paved the way for precise presymptomatic or predictive testing for healthy people at risk of inheriting the disorder. This risk is dependent on the at-risk subject's age; for a person in early adult life with an affected parent, the risk is 50%, but by the time the person

Table 6.2. Inherited causes of chorea

- Huntington's disease
- Neuroacanthocytosis and McLeod syndrome
- Dentatorubro-pallidoluysian atrophy (DRPLA)
- Paroxysmal hyperkinesias
- Spinocerebellar ataxia type 1, 3, and 17
- Mitochondrial disorders (Leigh's syndrome)
- Inherited prion disease
- Wilson's disease
- Friedreich's ataxia
- Neurodegeneration with brain iron accumulation (NBIA), including pantothenate kinase associated neurodegeneration (PKAN, formerly Hallervorden–Spatz syndrome) and neuroferritinopathy
- Ataxia telangectasia
- Lysosomal storage diseases
- Amino acid disorders
- Benign hereditary chorea
- Tuberous sclerosis

Table 6.3. Autosomal dominant Huntington's disease phenocopies

- HDL1–octapeptide repeat insertion in prion protein gene – one family
- HDL2–Junctophilin-3
- Inherited prion diseases
- SCA1, SCA3, and SCA 17 ("HDL4")
- DRPLA
- Neuroacanthocytosis (may be AD/AR)
- Neuroferritinopathy

HD, Huntington's disease; SCA, spinocerebellar ataxia; DRPLA, dentatorubro-pallidoluysian atrophy.

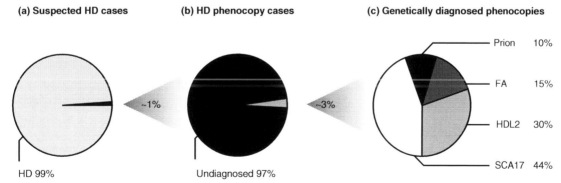

(a) Suspected HD cases   **(b) HD phenocopy cases**   **(c) Genetically diagnosed phenocopies**

~1%   ~3%

Prion 10%
FA 15%
HDL2 30%
SCA17 44%

HD 99%   Undiagnosed 97%

Figure 6.3. Relative frequencies of (a) Huntington's disease phenocopies, (b) successful genetic diagnosis, and (c) individual phenocopy syndromes. Percentages in (c) are derived from pooled results of published HD phenocopy cohort studies. HD, Huntington's disease; FA, Friedreich's ataxia; Prion, familial prion disease; HDL 2, HD-like disease, type 2; SCA, spinocerebellar ataxia. (Reproduced from Wild and Tabrizi (2007) [50] with permission from Lippincott, Williams, and Wilkins.)

71

Table 6.4. Risk for a healthy individual at 50% prior risk of Huntington's disease carrying the HD gene at different ages

Age (years)	Probability of an HD mutation
20	49.6
22.5	49.3
25	49.0
27.5	48.4
30	47.6
32.5	46.6
35	45.5
37.5	44.2
40	42.5
42.5	40.3
45	37.8
47.5	34.8
50	31.5
52.5	27.8
55	24.8
57.5	22.1
60	18.7
62.5	15.2
65	12.8
67.5	10.8
70	6.2
72.5	4.6

HD, Huntington's disease. (Reproduced from Harper and Newcombe (1992) [51] with permission from BMJ Publishing Group Ltd.)

reaches the age of 65 years and is still asymptomatic, the risk of a positive test has dropped considerably to about 13% (see Table 6.4). The risk for a healthy subject at 50% prior risk of inheriting the HD gene at different ages is shown in Table 6.4; this is based on the life-table analysis of South Wales data [51]. Issues can arise when an at-risk person has an allele with a reduced penetrance CAG repeat size between 36 and 39 (reduced penetrance allele). In our practice, the issue of reduced penetrance is discussed and explained to the patient. The risks to their offspring are also discussed, as men with 36–39 CAG repeat length alleles, although at less risk of developing the disease themselves, may pass on alleles with larger expansions (>40) owing to paternal somatic instability and, thereby, produce an affected offspring.

Predictive testing for HD

Prior to the availability of the genetic test, surveys suggested that 80% of those with a family history of the disease would take up predictive testing, but the demand has been lower than expected. In countries where genetic counseling and testing is widely available, the takeup of predictive testing for HD is less than 20% of those at risk. The reasons most commonly given for desiring a test were relieving uncertainty, planning for the future, planning a family, and the need to inform children [52]. Predictive genetic testing for HD is offered using the internationally agreed Huntington's disease protocol [53], and it is most important that predictive testing for HD is offered by specialized centers with the necessary expertise and professional support. The HD predictive testing guidelines recommend that individuals at risk are seen for two to four counseling sessions spread over a three-month period, before disclosure of the test results. This is to allow the person to consider all possible benefits and harms for them personally and for others close to them. What is absolutely clear from the extensive research that has been carried out in this area is the importance of providing accurate information, pre- and post-test counseling and support, and for mechanisms to be in place to ensure adequate safeguards against discrimination and breaches of confidentiality. An informed, competent adult should be free to make his/her own decision, but in certain circumstances, such as when the patient is depressed, testing should be delayed. It is generally agreed that it is unethical to perform presymptomatic testing on children below the age of 18 (or age of majority in the respective country) for an adult-onset, untreatable, neurodegenerative condition such as HD [54].

There are numerous issues relating to insurance, employment, and genetic discrimination of persons at risk of HD, and these issues will become even more pertinent as more genetic information becomes available about our risk of diseases. This is a topic that is often in the news, as illustrated in the case of a woman in Germany who was refused employment as a teacher because of a family history of HD [55]. This subject has been reviewed in detail [55,56].

Prenatal testing and preimplantation genetic diagnosis in Huntington's disease

A prospective parent who knows he/she may have inherited the HD gene can choose prenatal diagnosis in the first trimester. This is carried out by direct mutation analysis of a sample of fetal DNA, taken at about 10 weeks' gestation by chorionic villus sampling. This test is performed with the expectation that the pregnancy will be terminated if a fetus is found to have the genetic mutation. Only a minority of those at risk of HD use prenatal diagnosis to prevent transmission of the disease [55]. The decision to take up prenatal testing for an adult-onset disorder is not easy, and the development of disease modifying therapies in HD is likely to reduce the demand for prenatal testing further.

Preimplantation genetic diagnosis (PGD) is an evolving technique that provides a practical alternative to prenatal testing and termination of pregnancy and has been used in over a thousand cases [reviewed in 57]. Samples for genetic testing are obtained by extracting a single cell from a three-day embryo generated by in vitro fertilization. Only embryos that are shown to be free of the genetic disorder are implanted into the uterus to establish pregnancy. This procedure is available for HD at-risk couples, but the number of specialist centers offering PGD is still small, and as with all assisted reproduction technologies, the chance of a treatment resulting in a successful birth is only 10%–20% per cycle, and commonly several cycles of treatment are necessary.

Diagnostic testing in Huntington's disease

Diagnostic testing for HD usually is undertaken by neurologists when patients present with the neurological signs and symptoms of the disease. Adequate genetic counseling and informed consent in these situations is equally important. In some instances there may be no known family history of HD, so the diagnosis comes as a huge shock to the person and their family. In these situations, it is ideal to involve partners and other family members early in the diagnostic counseling process, as a confirmatory result of HD has profound implications for siblings and offspring.

Pathophysiology of Huntington's disease (Figure 6.4)

Huntingtin protein is expressed widely in the central nervous system (CNS) and peripheral tissues and in most intracellular compartments. Although its normal function is incompletely understood, it is known to be involved in vesicular transport, cytoskeletal anchoring, neuronal transport, postsynaptic signaling, cytoprotection, and transcriptional regulation [reviewed in 58].

The interactions of the mutant protein are diverse, and numerous derangements contribute synergistically to its detrimental effects [reviewed in 59]. Mechanisms involving toxic gain-of-function and dominant-negative effects (where the mutant protein interferes with the function of the normal protein) have been suggested to contribute to HD. The main mechanisms of dysfunction are felt to be gene transcriptional dysregulation, disordered protein folding, and deficient protein degradation (Figure 6.4).

Many transcription factors with key roles in neuronal function and survival interact with both wild-type and mutant huntingtin [reviewed in 60]. Huntingtin also binds directly to DNA, altering the function of gene promoters in a polyglutamine-dependent manner [61]. Among the specific pathways deranged are the cAMP-responsive element (CRE) and specificity protein 1 (SP1) pathways, critical to neuronal survival [60], and neuron-restrictive silencer element (NRSE), which enables trophic support of the striatum by brain-derived neurotrophic factor (BDNF) [62]. Mutant huntingtin activates the IκB/NFκB system, an important transcriptional activator of inflammatory genes [63]. Microarray studies confirm widespread derangement of gene expression in HD [64].

The ubiquitin-proteasome system (UPS) degrades unwanted small proteins into amino acids. Mutant huntingtin aggregates are ubiquitinated, indicating that they are targeted for removal by the proteasome but cannot be degraded by it [65]. The UPS is almost completely inhibited in the presence of polyglutamine-containing mutant huntingtin fragments [66]. Huntingtin aggregates sequester key chaperone proteins the presence of which may otherwise enhance cell survival [67]. The autophagy pathway can degrade proteins that the proteasome cannot, including mutant huntingtin aggregates, which appear to activate autophagy directly [68].

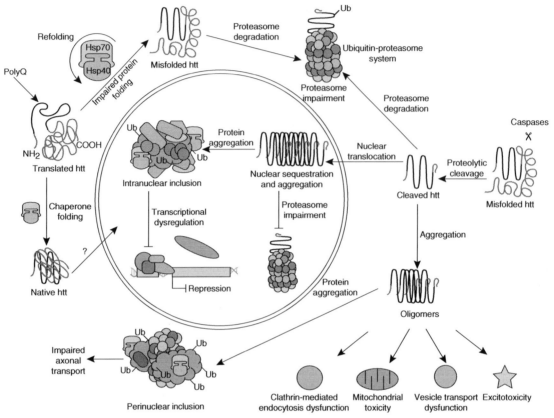

Figure 6.4. Model for Huntington's disease cellular pathogenesis. The HD mutation causes a conformational change and abnormal folding of the protein, which can be ameliorated by molecular chaperones. In the cytoplasm, full-length mutant huntingtin can interfere with brain-derived neurotrophic factor (BDNF) vesicular transport on microtubules. It can also undergo proteolytic cleavage, both in the cytoplasm and in the nucleus, which may involve several steps. The N-terminus with the expanded repeat can assume a beta-sheet structure. Toxicity in the cytoplasm may involve soluble monomers or oligomers or possibly insoluble aggregates. Cytoplasmic aggregates accumulate in perinuclear or neuritic regions and are ubiquitinated. The mutant protein translocates to the nucleus, where it forms intranuclear inclusions, although these are not primarily responsible for toxicity. Nuclear toxicity is believed to be caused by interference with gene transcription, leading to loss of transcription of neuroprotective molecules such as BDNF. htt, huntingtin; Ub, ubiquitin. (Adapted from Landles and Bates (2004) [59], with modifications after Ross and Tabrizi (2011) [58], with permission from Macmillan Publishers Ltd.)

Proteolytic processing of huntingtin seems to have a key role in pathogenesis, with a toxic N-terminal fragment of the mutant protein, containing the expanded polyglutamine tract, being cleaved from the full-length protein. This cleavage is performed by caspase enzymes, specifically caspases 3 and 6, and prevention of caspase 6 cleavage prevents neurodegeneration and clinical decline, possibly through prevention of nuclear entry [69,70]. Other apparent effects of mutant huntingtin include impairments of endocytosis [71], mitochondrial function [72], and vesicular trafficking [73].

Neurons are inextricably linked with the glial cells that outnumber them ten-fold, regulating the CNS milieu, performing immune functions, and modulating neurotransmission. Increasingly, glial cells are recognized as having critical roles in neurodegeneration [74]. The enzyme kynurenine monooxygenase (KMO), from a microglial pathway linked to oxidative damage, was shown to be a therapeutic target in yeast and mouse models of HD [75,76]. Parallel CNS and peripheral pathways of inflammatory activation, thought to be a result of the expression of mutant huntingtin in immune cells, have been linked with HD pathogenesis [77]. Non-neuronal and peripheral cellular dysfunction in HD are areas of considerable interest in the search for therapeutic targets.

Management of patients with Huntington's disease

Patients with HD have different needs as the disease progresses and the care of this group of patients is best managed with a multidisciplinary approach. Most clinics are run by a combination of clinical geneticists, neurologists, neuropsychiatrists, psychologists, nurse specialists, with additional input from dieticians, physical therapists, and speech and language therapists. Access to clinical research programs is also empowering for many patients. Throughout Western Europe and the United States, there are important HD patient organizations that have done much to drive care of patients with HD. In the United Kingdom, the Huntington's disease association (HDA; www.hda. org.uk) employs specialist HD regional care advisors who advise on management of all aspects of HD including issues with insurance, employment, and finances. The UK HDA also publishes several useful booklets on management of various symptoms and challenges in HD.

Management of psychiatric symptoms

Psychiatric symptoms often cause a great deal of distress to both patients and relatives but are among the most amenable to treatment and should be actively managed. Much of our current practice is based on anecdotal evidence of efficacy. The most useful drugs for depression are the serotonin-selective reuptake inhibitors, and although there have not been any detailed randomized studies, anecdotal reports and our own practice suggest that citalopram and mirtazapine are particularly effective in this group of patients, especially if anxiety is a cofactor in the depressive symptoms. The newer anti-psychotics have replaced older drugs such as haloperidol and chlorpromazine owing to the adverse side-effect profile of the older drugs. The most commonly used newer anti-psychotics with good efficacy include risperidone, olanzapine, and quetiapine. These drugs are best started at the lowest possible dose and titrated up slowly if necessary. These newer anti-psychotics have an improved side-effect profile in terms of extrapyramidal symptoms and are also useful for severe anxiety or aggressive and impulsive behavior. Mood-stabilizing drugs such as valproate and carbamazepine are useful for symptoms of mania. Benzodiazepines are useful for short-term treatment of anxiety although they may be used for long-term management of agitation, which may occur as the disease progresses into the advanced stages. Non-pharmacological management of psychiatric symptoms is also important and, despite the degenerative nature of HD, many patients do benefit from a cognitive behavioral therapeutic approach, particularly in early disease, as well as counseling support for both the patient and their caregivers.

Management of cognitive symptoms

The most important aspects of management are to maintain the patient's safety and quality of life. As the disease progresses, patients become less able to maintain their own selfcare and domestic chores such as cooking, washing, and shopping become difficult. Care of these patients requires an integrated care package with the involvement of social services, the general practitioner, and their caregivers. A fairly common problem in practice is patients with little insight who insist that they are able to care for themselves or where there are employment or safety issues, and formal neuropsychological and clinical assessment is important in these cases to help advise on optimum management and care.

Management of motor symptoms

Although a very common feature of the disease, chorea is seldom the most functionally disabling motor symptom. It causes cosmetic embarrassment to some patients but many do not notice the severity of their chorea. Best agreed practice is to use antichoreic medication sparingly as no drug is particularly efficacious, and a balance has to be struck as their motor side-effects may contribute to functional disability. For chorea that is functionally disabling, drugs such as sulpiride, olanzapine, and risperidone are useful. Tetrabenazine is also an effective option [78], but the side-effect of depression has to be considered. Impairment of voluntary motor function and gait disturbances are difficult to treat but patients benefit from physical therapy assessments and advice. Dopaminergic stabilizing drugs may hold some potential for these problems but have yet to be tested in widespread use. As the disease progresses, falls are a common problem and walking aids and adapted wheelchairs often become necessary. In the later stages of the disease, the chorea lessens and patients become more rigid and dystonic. Here, anti-spasticity drugs such as baclofen and clonazepam have some efficacy, although there is no drug that is greatly beneficial at this stage and the importance of safe bedding, specialist mattresses, and good nursing become paramount. Patients with juvenile HD and young adults with prominent parkinsonian features may benefit from treatment with levodopa with a peripheral dopa-decarboxylase inhibitor.

A significant and often early problem in HD is speech and swallowing impairment, and this should be asked about specifically. Dysarthria contributes to communication difficulties. As the disease advances, patients become mute, which often causes great frustration for both the patient and carers. Early referral to speech and language therapists is recommended as exercises may be useful in the early to moderately advanced cases, and electronic communication aids patients with more advanced disease. Dysphagia with choking episodes is reported even in patients with early disease and, as the disease advances, management of swallowing problems is one of the main areas that need to be addressed. In early disease, impulsive, disordered eating causes dysphagia whereas in later disease, mechanical disintegration of swallowing is usually to blame. It is important that patients have input from therapists who can advise about modified diets and maneuvers to minimize the likelihood of aspiration.

Other management issues in Huntington's disease

Weight loss is common in HD, and the etiology is likely to be multifactorial, including poor nutritional intake, swallowing problems, and increased resting energy expenditure. However, the mutant protein is expressed in every tissue, and it is now clear that there is peripheral pathology in HD; the weight loss, therefore, is likely to be related to the disease process itself. It is important that patients maintain their weight as slower disease progression has been associated with higher premorbid body mass index [79].

An often ignored problem is dental care and hygiene, which contributes to comorbidity in HD with problems with dental decay and may worsen dysarthria and dysphagia; many patients with HD do not go to the dentist because of their motor symptoms as their movements can make dental care difficult. However, patients can have dental treatment under mild sedation and many dentists are able to treat such patients.

There are many issues relating to the palliative care of patients with advanced disease. The main goals in patient care at this stage are to minimize pain and suffering, provide appropriate nursing care, and ensure adequate nutrition. The issues of gastrostomy feeding tubes, treatment of recurrent infections, and end-of-life decisions become important and need a skilled team of carers to address them. Such matters should be approached sensitively, early in the disease, so that patients and their loved ones can make informed decisions and these decisions can be documented for future reference.

Therapeutic developments in Huntington's disease

Therapeutic trials in patients with HD looking for disease-modifying effects are challenging for a number of reasons. Disease progression is relatively slow, and the current widely used UHDRS is not sensitive enough to measure progression over relatively short periods of time; it has high measurement variability, particularly in the behavioral/psychiatric assessment, and it cannot distinguish effects on disease progression from symptomatic benefit. In addition, patients present with variable clinical phenotypes (differing burdens of motor, cognitive, and psychiatric symptoms), which can make comparative wide-scale assessments difficult. Thus, there is a need for biomarkers in HD that could be used to track disease progression. The ability to identify those destined to develop HD through a reliable genetic test, often many years in advance, is a great asset in the search for effective therapies, as treatments given before gene carriers develop symptoms might delay disease onset before there is significant neurological disability or neuronal loss. Markers capable of detecting disease-related changes in HD gene carriers will be essential for the development of such treatments [reviewed in 80]. A number of major international research programs have made significant progress toward identifying a battery of biomarkers to track disease progression in HD [81–83].

Our increased understanding of HD pathogenesis has come from the development of both cell models and a number of transgenic mouse models of the disease. A detailed discussion of experimental therapeutics in transgenic mouse models of HD is outside the scope of this chapter but the topic has been well reviewed [84]. The most widely studied mouse model of HD is the R6/2 HD [85]. This mouse model is popular because it has a well-characterized homogenous phenotype and

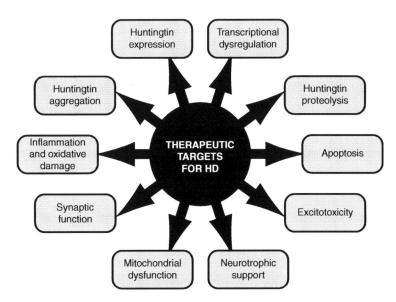

Figure 6.5. Targets for therapeutics in Huntington's disease illustrating the different pathophysiological processes that have been found to influence neuronal death in HD. (Adapted from Beal and Ferrante (2004) [84], with permission from Macmillan Publishers Ltd. © 2004.)

has been used in many preclinical drug trials [84]. Recently, primate and sheep transgenic models of HD have been developed which, with their large and more developed brains, are likely to be of value in bringing therapies to human patients [86,87].

There are numerous plausible therapeutic targets in HD, based on our understanding of the different pathogenic pathways resulting in neuronal death (summarized in Figure 6.5).

Classes of compounds from preclinical studies that significantly prolonged survival in HD mouse models include those that target transcriptional dysregulation, such as histone deacetylase inhibitors [88]; caspase inhibitors [89]; drugs to promote autophagy [68]; KMO inhibitors [76] drugs that provide or mimic neurotrophic support [90], and neuroprotective drugs targeting mitochondrial dysfunction and excitotoxicity [91]. There is great interest in the potential of gene silencing therapies, using RNA interference or antisense oligonucleotides to switch off the mutant huntingtin gene as a potential therapeutic strategy [reviewed in 92]. A useful overview of promising therapeutic avenues is by Munos-Sanjuan and Bates, 2011 [93].

A number of possible neuroprotective agents have been trialled in patients with HD and findings to date are the subject of a recent Cochrane Review [94]. These include coenzyme Q and remacemide [95], lamotrigine [96], idebenone [97], baclofen [98], riluzole [99], amantadine [100], creatine [101], minocycline [102], and eicosopentanoic acid [103]. All yielded essentially negative results, and this may have been in part because of the fact that many of them were underpowered in terms of patient numbers to detect a significant change in UHDRS scores. This emphasizes the need for reliable biomarkers in HD (see previous discussion). Fetal stem cell transplantation has shown promise but is currently limited by technical and ethical concerns. In one study, three of five patients maintained or slightly improved motor and cognitive function after transplantation but the improvement was not sustained [104].

Currently, there are several large clinical trials ongoing, including high-dose creatine, coenzyme Q10, and memantine (summarized at huntingtonstudy-group.org and clinicaltrials.gov). It may be that a combination of therapeutic agents that target the different disease mechanisms in HD will have greater efficacy, rather like the combined chemotherapy approach used in cancer treatment, and current research suggests significant progress is being made toward this goal.

Recommended further reading

Huntington's disease edited by Bates G, Harper P, and Jones L. Oxford Medical Publications. Third edition. November 2002 ISBN 0198510608. This book is an outstanding source of information including historical, clinical, genetic, and scientific reviews.

Useful websites

hdbuzz.net	HDBuzz – making the latest HD research news available to patients and family members in plain language
hdfoundation.org	Hereditary disease foundation, USA
www.hda.org.uk	UK Huntington's disease association
hdsa.org	Huntington's Disease Society of America
euro-hd.net	European HD Network – the European research and clinical care collaboration with specific information on contacts and availability of multidisciplinary clinics in each country
huntington-study-group.org	Huntington Study Group – a US-based multicenter trials group
hdresearch.ucl.ac.uk	An interactive website on Huntington's disease research from University College London
hdresearchcrossroads.org	A site for researchers to consolidate the latest information on therapeutic targets in HD
chdifoundation.org	The CHDI Foundation Inc., a major non-profit funder and driver of HD research globally

Useful addresses in the United Kingdom

Huntington's Disease Association

Huntington's Disease Association
Down Stream Building
1 London Bridge
London SE1 9BG
England, UK
Telephone: +44(0)151 482 1199
Fax: +44(0)151 482 1199
Email:info@hda.org.uk
The UK HDA also publishes several useful booklets on management issues in HD aimed at patients and physicians.

UK Huntington's disease network

This is a network of clinicians, scientists, and nurses involved in both the care of patients and research into HD.
The co-ordinating center is in Cardiff and contact details are:
Academic Dept. Neurology
C2-B2 Corridor
University of Wales College of Medicine, Heath Park
Cardiff CF14 4XN
Wales, UK
Telephone: 029 20743454

References

1. Rawlins M. Huntington's disease out of the closet? *Lancet* 2010; **376**: 1372–1373.

2. Huntington G. On Chorea. *Medical and Surgical Reporter*, 1872; **26**: 317–321.

3. The Huntington's Disease Collaborative Research Group. A novel gene containing a trinucleotide repeat that is expanded and unstable on Huntington's disease chromosomes. *Cell* 1993; **72**: 971–983.

4. Gusella JF, Wexler NS, Conneally PM, *et al*. A polymorphic DNA marker genetically linked to Huntington's disease. *Nature* 1983; **306**: 234–238.

5. Ambrose CM, Duyao MP, Barnes G, *et al*. Structure and expression of the Huntington's disease gene: evidence against simple inactivation due to an expanded CAG repeat. *Somat Cell Mol Genet* 1994; **20**: 27–38.

6. Hoogeveen AT, Willemsen R, Meyer N, *et al*. Characterization and localization of the Huntington disease gene product. *Hum Mol Genet* 1993; **2**: 2069–2073.

7. Rubinsztein DC, Amos W, Leggo J, *et al*. Mutational bias provides a model for the evolution of Huntington's disease and predicts a general increase in disease prevalence. *Nat Genet* 1994; **7**: 525–530.

8. Duyao MP, Auerbach AB, Ryan A, *et al*. Inactivation of the mouse Huntington's disease gene homolog Hdh. *Science* 1995; **269**: 407–410.

9. La Spada AR, Wilson EM, Lubahn DB, Harding AE, Fischbeck KH. Androgen receptor gene mutations in X-linked spinal and bulbar muscular atrophy. *Nature* 1991; **352**: 77–79.

10. Everett CM, Wood NW. Trinucleotide repeats and neurodegenerative disease. *Brain* 2004; **127**: 2385–2405.

11. Snell RG, MacMillan JC, Cheadle JP, *et al*. Relationship between trinucleotide repeat expansion and phenotypic

variation in Huntington's disease. *Nat Genet* 1993; **4**: 393–397.

12. Rubinsztein DC, Leggo J, Coles R, *et al*. Phenotypic characterization of individuals with 30–40 CAG repeats in the Huntington disease (HD) gene reveals HD cases with 36 repeats and apparently normal elderly individuals with 36–39 repeats. *Am J Hum Genet* 1996; **59**: 16–22.

13. Kenney C, Powell S, Jankovic J. Autopsy-proven Huntington's disease with 29 trinucleotide repeats. *Mov Disord* 2007; **22**: 127–130.

14. Semaka A, Warby S, Leavitt BR, Hayden MR. Re: autopsy-proven Huntington's disease with 29 trinucleotide repeats. *Mov Disord* 2008; **23**: 1794–1795.

15. Kremer B, Almqvist E, Theilmann J, *et al*. Sex-dependent mechanisms for expansions and contractions of the CAG repeat on affected Huntington disease chromosomes. *Am J Hum Genet* 1995; **57**: 343–350.

16. Zuhlke C, Reiss O, Bockel B, Lange H, Thies U. Mitotic stability and meiotic variability of the (CAG)n repeat in the Huntington disease gene. *Hum Mol Genet* 1993; **2**: 2063–2067.

17. Ranen NG, Stine OC, Abbott MH, *et al*. Anticipation and instability of IT-15 (CAG)n repeats in parent–offspring pairs with Huntington disease. *Am J Hum Genet* 1995; **57**: 593–602.

18. Pearson CE. Slipping while sleeping? Trinucleotide repeat expansions in germ cells. *Trends Mol Med* 2003; **9**: 490–495.

19. Harper PS. The epidemiology of Huntington's disease. In Bates G, Harper PS, and Jones L ed., *Huntington's Disease*. Oxford, UK: Oxford Medical Publications, 2002.

20. Goldberg YP, McMurray CT, Zeisler J, *et al*. Increased instability of intermediate alleles in families with sporadic Huntington disease compared to similar sized intermediate alleles in the general population. *Hum Mol Genet* 1995; **4**: 1911–1918.

21. Duyao M, Ambrose C, Myers R, *et al*. Trinucleotide repeat length instability and age of onset in Huntington's disease. *Nat Genet* 1993; **4**: 387–392.

22. Langbehn DR, Brinkman RR, Falush D, Paulsen JS, Hayden MR. A new model for prediction of the age of onset and penetrance for Huntington's disease based on CAG length. *Clin Genet* 2004; **65**: 267–277.

23. Penney JB Jr, Vonsattel JP, MacDonald ME, Gusella JF, Myers RH. CAG repeat number governs the development rate of pathology in Huntington's disease. *Ann Neurol* 1997; **41**: 689–692.

24. Li JL, Hayden MR, Almqvist EW, *et al*. A genome scan for modifiers of age at onset in Huntington disease: the HD MAPS study. *Am J Hum Genet* 2003; **73**: 682–687.

25. Wexler NS, Lorimer J, Porter J, *et al*. Venezuelan kindreds reveal that genetic and environmental factors modulate Huntington's disease age of onset. *Proc Natl Acad Sci USA* 2004; **101**: 3498–3503.

26. Gusella JF, MacDonald ME. Huntington's disease: the case for genetic modifiers. *Genome Med* 2009; **1**: 80.

27. Harper PS, Lim C, Craufurd D. Ten years of presymptomatic testing for Huntington's disease: the experience of the UK Huntington's Disease Prediction Consortium. *J Med Genet* 2000; **37**: 567–571.

28. Kremer B. Clinical neurology of Huntington's disease. In Bates G, Harper PS, and Jones L ed. *Huntington's Disease*. Oxford, UK: Oxford Medical Publications, 2002.

29. Lasker AG, Zee DS. Ocular motor abnormalities in Huntington's disease. *Vision Res* 1997; **37**: 3639–3645.

30. Craufurd D, Snowden J. Neuropsychological and neuropsychiatric aspects of Huntington's disease. In Bates G, Harper PS, and Jones L ed. *Huntington's Disease*. Oxford, UK: Oxford Medical Publications, 2002.

31. Lovestone S, Hodgson S, Sham P, Differ AM, Levy R. Familial psychiatric presentation of Huntington's disease. *J Med Genet* 1996; **33**: 128–131.

32. Folstein SE, Chase GA, Wahl WE, McDonnell AM, Folstein MF. Huntington disease in Maryland: clinical aspects of racial variation. *Am J Hum Genet* 1987; **41**: 168–179.

33. Farrer LA. Suicide and attempted suicide in Huntington disease: implications for preclinical testing of persons at risk. *Am J Med Genet* 1986; **24**: 305–311.

34. Lipe H, Schultz A, Bird TD. Risk factors for suicide in Huntingtons disease: a retrospective case controlled study. *Am J Med Genet* 1993; **48**: 231–233.

35. Craufurd D, Thompson JC, Snowden JS. Behavioral changes in Huntington disease. *Neuropsychiatry Neuropsychol Behav Neurol* 2001; **14**: 219–226.

36. The Huntington Study Group. Unified Huntington's disease rating scale: reliability and consistency. *Mov Disord* 1996; **11**: 136–142.

37. Shoulson I, Fahn S. Huntington disease: clinical care and evaluation. *Neurology* 1979; **29**: 1–3.

38. Ferrante RJ, Kowall NW, Beal MF, *et al*. Selective sparing of a class of striatal neurons in Huntington's disease. *Science* 1985; **230**: 561–563.

39. Vonsattel J-P, Myers RH, Stevens TJ, *et al*. Neuropathological

classification of Huntington's disease. *J Neuropathol Exp Neurol* 1985; **44**: 559–577.

40. Sapp E, Kegel KB, Aronin N, *et al.* Early and progressive accumulation of reactive microglia in the Huntington disease brain. *J Neuropathol Exp Neurol* 2001; **60**: 161–172.

41. Andrew SE, Goldberg YP, Kremer B, *et al.* Huntington disease without CAG expansion: phenocopies or errors in assignment? *Am J Hum Genet* 1994; **54**: 852–863.

42. Moore RC, Xiang F, Monaghan J, *et al.* Huntington disease phenocopy is a familial prion disease. *Am J Hum Genet* 2001; **69**: 1385–1388.

43. Margolis RL, O'Hearn E, Rosenblatt A, *et al.* A disorder similar to Huntington's disease is associated with a novel CAG repeat expansion. *Ann Neurol* 2001; **50**: 373–380.

44. Kambouris M, Bohlega S, Al-Tahan A, Meyer BF, *et al.* Localization of the gene for a novel autosomal recessive neurodegenerative Huntington-like disorder to 4p15.3. *Am J Hum Genet* 2000; **66**: 445–452.

45. Koide R, Ikeuchi T, Onodera O, *et al.* Unstable expansion of CAG repeat in hereditary dentatorubral-pallidoluysian atrophy (DRPLA). *Nat Genet* 1994; **6**: 9–13.

46. Stevanin G, Fujigasaki H, Lebre A-S, *et al.* Huntington's disease-like phenotype due to trinucleotide repeat expansions in the TBP and JPH3 genes. *Brain* 2003; **126**: 1599–1603.

47. Ueno S, Maruki Y, Nakamura M, *et al.* The gene encoding a newly discovered protein, chorein, is mutated in chorea-acanthocytosis. *Nat Genet* 2001; **28**: 121–122.

48. Wild EJ, Mudanohwo EE, Sweeney MG, *et al.* Huntington's disease phenocopies are clinically and genetically heterogeneous. *Mov Disord* 2008; **23**: 716–720.

49. Curtis AR J, Fey C, Morris CM, *et al.* Mutation in the gene encoding ferritin light polypeptide causes dominant adult-onset basal ganglia disease. *Nat Genet* 2001; **28**: 350–354.

50. Wild EJ, Tabrizi SJ. Huntington's disease phenocopy syndromes. *Curr Opin Neurol* 2007; **20**: 681–687.

51. Harper PS, Newcombe RG. Age at onset and life table risks in genetic counselling for Huntington's disease. *J Med Genet* 1992; **29**: 239–242.

52. Meiser B, Dunn S. Psychological impact of genetic testing for Huntington's disease: an update of the literature. *J Neurol Neurosurg Psychiatry* 2000; **69**: 574–578.

53. International Huntington Association and World Federation of Neurology Research Group on Huntington's Chorea. Guidelines for the molecular genetics predictive test in Huntington's disease. *Neurology* 1994; **44**: 1533–1536.

54. British Medical Association. *Human Genetics: Choice and Responsibility.* Oxford, UK: Oxford University Press, 1998.

55. Harper PS, Gevers S, de Wert G, *et al.* Genetic testing and Huntington's disease: issues of employment. *Lancet Neurol* 2004; **3**: 249–252.

56. Tibben A. Genetic counselling and presymptomatic testing. In Bates G, Harper PS, and Jones L ed. *Huntington's Disease.* Oxford, UK: Oxford Medical Publications, 2002.

57. Geraedts JP, De Wert GM. Preimplantation genetic diagnosis. *Clin Genet* 2009; **76**: 315–325.

58. Ross CA, Tabrizi SJ. Huntington's disease: from molecular pathogenesis to clinical treatment. *Lancet Neurol* 2011; **10**: 83–98.

59. Landles C, Bates GP. Huntingtin and the molecular pathogenesis of Huntington's disease. *EMBO Rep* 2004; **5**: 958–963.

60. Sugars KL, Rubinsztein DC. Transcriptional abnormalities in Huntington disease. *Trends Genet* 2003; **19**: 233–238.

61. Benn CL, Sun T, Sadri-Vakili G, *et al.* Huntingtin modulates transcription, occupies gene promoters in vivo, and binds directly to DNA in a polyglutamine-dependent manner. *J Neurosci* 2008; **28**: 10720–10733.

62. Zuccato C, Tartari M, Crotti A, *et al.* Huntingtin interacts with REST/NRSF to modulate the transcription of NRSE-controlled neuronal genes. *Nat Genet* 2003; **35**: 76–83.

63. Khoshnan A, Ko J, Watkin EE, *et al.* Activation of the I kappa B kinase complex and nuclear factor kappa B contributes to mutant huntingtin neurotoxicity. *J Neurosci* 2004; **24**: 7999–8008.

64. Hodges A, Strand AD, Aragaki AK, *et al.* Regional and cellular gene expression changes in human Huntington's disease brain. *Hum Mol Genet* 2006; **15**: 965–977.

65. Ciechanover A, Brundin P. The ubiquitin proteasome system in neurodegenerative diseases: sometimes the chicken, sometimes the egg. *Neuron* 2003; **40**: 427–446.

66. Bence NF, Sampat RM, Kopito RR. Impairment of the ubiquitin-proteasome system by protein aggregation. *Science* 2001; **292**: 1552–1555.

67. Hay DG, Sathasivam K, Tobaben S, *et al.* Progressive decrease in chaperone protein levels in a mouse model of Huntington's disease and induction of stress proteins as a therapeutic approach. *Hum Mol Genet* 2004; **13**: 1389–1405.

68. Ravikumar B, Vacher C, Berger Z, et al. Inhibition of mTOR induces autophagy and reduces toxicity of polyglutamine expansions in fly and mouse models of Huntington disease. *Nat Genet* 2004; **36**: 585–595.

69. Graham RK, Deng Y, Slow EJ, et al. Cleavage at the caspase-6 site is required for neuronal dysfunction and degeneration due to mutant huntingtin. *Cell* 2006; **125**: 1179–1191.

70. Warby SC, Doty CN, Graham RK, et al. Activated caspase-6 and caspase-6-cleaved fragments of huntingtin specifically colocalize in the nucleus. *Hum Mol Genet* 2008; **17**: 2390–2404.

71. Li S-H, Li X-J. Huntingtin-protein interactions and the pathogenesis of Huntington's disease. *Trends Genet* 2004; **20**: 146–154.

72. Panov AV, Gutekunst CA, Leavitt BR, et al. Early mitochondrial calcium defects in Huntington's disease are a direct effect of polyglutamines. *Nat Neurosci* 2002; **5**: 731–736.

73. Zala D, Colin E, Rangone H, et al. Phosphorylation of mutant huntingtin at S421 restores anterograde and retrograde transport in neurons. *Hum Mol Genet* 2008; **17**: 3837–3846.

74. Lobsiger CS, Cleveland DW. Glial cells as intrinsic components of non-cell-autonomous neurodegenerative disease. *Nat Neurosci* 2007; **10**: 1355–1360.

75. Giorgini F, Guidetti P, Nguyen Q, Bennett SC, Muchowski PJ, et al. A genomic screen in yeast implicates kynurenine 3-monooxygenase as a therapeutic target for Huntington disease. *Nat Genet* 2005; **37**: 526–531.

76. Zwilling D, Huang SY, Sathyasaikumar KV, et al. Kynurenine 3-monooxygenase inhibition in blood ameliorates neurodegeneration. *Cell* 2011; **145**: 863–874.

77. Björkqvist M, Wild EJ, Thiele J, et al. A novel pathogenic pathway of immune activation detectable before clinical onset in Huntington's disease. *J Exp Med* 2008; **205**: 1869–1877.

78. The Huntington Study Group. Tetrabenazine as antichorea therapy in Huntington disease: a randomized controlled trial. *Neurology* 2006; **66**: 366–372.

79. Myers RH, Sax DS, Koroshetz WJ, et al. Factors associated with slow progression in Huntington's disease. *Arch Neurol* 1991; **48**: 800–804.

80. Wild EJ, Tabrizi SJ. Biomarkers for Huntington's disease. *Expert Opin Med Diagn* 2008; **2**: 47–62.

81. Tabrizi SJ, Langbehn DR, Leavitt BR, et al. Biological and clinical manifestations of Huntington's disease in the longitudinal TRACK-HD study: cross-sectional analysis of baseline data. *Lancet Neurol* 2009; **8**: 791–801.

82. Tabrizi SJ, Scahill RI, Durr A, et al. Biological and clinical changes in premanifest and early stage Huntington's disease in the TRACK-HD study: the 12-month longitudinal analysis. *Lancet Neurol* 2011; **10**: 31–42.

83. Paulsen JS, Langbehn DR, Stout JC, et al. Detection of Huntington's disease decades before diagnosis: the Predict-HD study. *J Neurol Neurosurg Psychiatry* 2008; **79**: 874–880.

84. Beal MF, Ferrante RJ. Experimental therapeutics in transgenic mouse models of Huntington's disease. *Nat Rev Neurosci* 2004; **5**: 373–384.

85. Mangiarini L, Sathasivam K, Seller M, et al. Exon 1 of the HD gene with an expanded CAG repeat is sufficient to cause a progressive neurological phenotype in transgenic mice. *Cell* 1996; **87**: 493–506.

86. Yang S-H, Cheng P-H, Banta H, et al. Towards a transgenic model of Huntington's disease in a non-human primate. *Nature* 2008; **453**: 921–924.

87. Jacobsen JC, Bawden CS, Rudiger SR, et al. An ovine transgenic Huntington's disease model. *Hum Mol Genet* 2010; **15**: 1873–1882.

88. Butler R, Bates GP. Histone deacetylase inhibitors as therapeutics for polyglutamine disorders. *Nat Rev Neurosci* 2006; **7**: 784–796.

89. Ona VO, Li M, Vonsattel JPG, et al. Inhibition of caspase-1 slows disease progression in a mouse model of Huntington's disease. *Nature* 1999; **399**: 263–267.

90. Borrell-Pagès M, Canals JM, Cordelières FP, et al. Cystamine and cysteamine increase brain levels of BDNF in Huntington disease via HSJ1b and transglutaminase. *J Clin Invest* 2006; **116**: 1410–1424.

91. Ferrante RJ, Andreassen OA, Dedeoglu A, et al. Therapeutic effects of coenzyme Q10 and remacemide in transgenic mouse models of Huntington's disease. *J Neurosci* 2002; **22**: 1592–1599.

92. Sah DWY, Aronin N. Oligonucleotide therapeutic approaches for Huntington disease. *J Clin Invest* 2011; **121**: 500–507.

93. Munoz-Sanjuan I, Bates GP. The importance of integrating basic and clinical research toward the development of new therapies for Huntington disease. *J Clin Invest* 2011; **121**: 476–483.

94. Mestre T, Ferreira J, Coelho MM, Rosa M, Sampaio C. Therapeutic interventions for disease progression in Huntington's disease. *Cochrane Database Syst Rev* 2009: CD006455.

95. The Huntington Study Group. A randomized, placebo-controlled trial of coenzyme Q10 and

remacemide in Huntington's disease. *Neurology* 2001; 57: 397–404.

96. Kremer B, Clark CM, Almqvist EW, *et al.* Influence of lamotrigine on progression of early Huntington disease: a randomized clinical trial. *Neurology* 1999; 53: 1000–1011.

97. Ranen NG, Peyser CE, Coyle JT, *et al.* A controlled trial of idebenone in Huntington's disease. *Mov Disord* 1996; 11: 549–554.

98. Shoulson I, Odoroff C, Oakes D, *et al.* A controlled clinical trial of baclofen as protective therapy in early Huntington's disease. *Ann Neurol* 1989; 25: 252–259.

99. Seppi K, Mueller J, Bodner T, *et al.* Riluzole in Huntington's disease (HD): an open label study with one year follow up. *J Neurol* 2001; 248: 866–869.

100. O'Suilleabhain P, RB. Dewey RB Jr. A randomized trial of amantadine in Huntington disease. *Arch Neurol* 2003; 60: 996–998.

101. Tabrizi SJ, Blamire AM, Manners DN, *et al.* High-dose creatine therapy for Huntington disease: a 2-year clinical and MRS study. *Neurology* 2005; 64: 1655–1656.

102. Bonelli RM, Hodl AK, Hofmann P, Kapfhammer HP. Neuroprotection in Huntington's disease: a 2-year study on minocycline. *Int Clin Psychopharmacol* 2004; 19: 337–342.

103. Huntington Study Group TREND-HD Investigators. Randomized controlled trial of ethyl-eicosapentaenoic acid in Huntington disease: the TREND-HD study. *Arch Neurol* 2008; 65: 1582–1589.

104. Bachoud-Levi AC, Gaura V, Brugieres P, *et al.* Effect of fetal neural transplants in patients with Huntington's disease 6 years after surgery: a long-term follow-up study. *Lancet Neurol* 2006; 5: 303–309.

Parkinsonism

Vincenzo Bonifati

Introduction

The term parkinsonism defines the combination of two or more of four cardinal motor signs: brady-kinesia (slowness of movement), resting tremor, muscular rigidity, and postural instability [1–3]. This etiologically heterogeneous syndrome might be the clinical correlate of dysfunctions at various levels in the basal ganglia, and especially in the substantia nigra and striatum, caused by processes as different as neurodegeneration, inflammation, toxicity (including iatrogenic causes), tissue infiltration/compression (tumors), and ischemia.

Parkinson's disease (PD) is the principal form of parkinsonism, characterized clinically by the association of this syndrome with a progressive course and a positive response to dopamine replacement therapy, and pathologically by dopaminergic neuronal loss in the substantia nigra and other brain areas, and with the formation of cytoplasmic inclusions called Lewy bodies (LB) or Lewy neurites in the surviving neurons [4,5]. Parkinson's disease is the second most common neurodegenerative disease after Alzheimer's disease (AD), with a prevalence of more than 1% after the age of 65 years, and an increasing public health problem in the aging population [6].

It is important to recognize that brain LB pathology is not a specific feature of PD, but it is observed in many conditions, including Alzheimer's disease, LB dementia, progressive supranuclear palsy, neurodegeneration with iron accumulation type 1, and importantly, in some elderly individuals who died without neurological symptoms [7]. The current clinicopathological definition of PD, therefore, is capturing the overlap of two spectra: that of levodopa-responsive progressive parkinsonian syndromes and that of LB-associated conditions.

The role of genetics versus environment in the etiology of PD has been a matter of debate for more than a century, with alternating fortunes. Strong support for the environmental theories came from the occurrence of postencephalitic parkinsonism after the pandemic of influenza in the early 1900s, and after the more recent discovery of permanent parkinsonism in humans caused by 1-methyl-4-phenyl-1,2,3,6-tetrahydropyridine (MPTP) [8], a substance similar to widely used pesticides. However, the disease has survived the era of the postencephalitic cohort, and despite the epidemiological association of PD with environmental factors such as rural living and occupational exposure to pesticides, a putative MPTP-like toxin causing PD has not been identified to date.

Clinical genetics of PD

Familial aggregation of PD has long been noted [9,10], reemerging consistently in the subsequent surveys [11,12] until recently [13,14], and supporting a role for genetic factors. Studies in PD twins, however, have produced conflicting results. According to the largest of such studies [15], the pattern of concordance in monozygotic versus dizygotic twins differs critically on the basis of PD onset age, in keeping with a prominent role for genetic factors in early onset cases (before 50 years of age, according to that study), but has a negligible role in late-onset PD, which represents the vast majority of cases. However, the study was based on a cross-sectional, clinical survey. The period elapsing before a co-twin develops clinically overt PD, becoming concordant, can be as long as 20 years [16], indicating that a longer followup is important in studying PD twins. Moreover, if positron emission tomography (PET) is used to assess the integrity of the nigrostriatal dopaminergic system, the concordance between monozygotic twins appeared significantly higher than that of dizygotic twins, once again supporting the role of genetic factors [17].

Parkinson's disease appears as a sporadic disorder in most patients. However, in a significant percentage of cases (10%–15% in most studies), the disease runs in families without a clear-cut Mendelian pattern of inheritance. Recent segregation analyses found evidence for a major gene with reduced, age-related penetrance [13]. However, these studies might be biased toward segregation patterns consistent with major genes depending on the ascertainment strategy, and the observed scenario is also compatible with the common PD form being a complex trait determined by several genetic as well as non-genetic factors. A general caveat in the segregation analyses is that they consider PD as one entity, while it is clear today that the disease is etiologically highly heterogeneous.

Large families have indeed been identified, in which the PD phenotype is transmitted as a Mendelian trait, with either autosomal dominant or recessive inheritance, and the causative mutation is known in many of these forms. Several elements might hide a Mendelian pattern of inheritance in most cases of PD. The possible age-related (perhaps incomplete) penetrance of the underlying mutation, combined with the censoring effect of mortality owing to other causes, might lead to the disease skipping generations. Other important issues are the possible varying phenotypical expressivity (which may overlap with LB disease), and the small size of the families in modern times, at least in Western countries.

A distinct but related issue is that, even in the rare Mendelian forms, there is large intrafamilial variation in onset age and phenotypical features [18], strongly suggesting that other factors also play important modifying roles. In this sense, PD is undoubtedly a complex trait, determined by the interplay of several components, which might include genetic as well as non-genetic factors.

Genome-wide molecular genetics of Parkinson's disease

The era of genome-wide approaches to the dissection of PD etiology was initiated recently, despite this disease being long considered non-genetic in nature. Nonetheless, in the last 10 years, family-based linkage analysis and positional cloning have led to the identification of several loci and genes for PD (Table 7.1). The implication of these discoveries for both the scientific and the clinical communities is profound [19–21]. Some of these Mendelian forms are very rare, but their importance resides in the identification of novel molecular players and pathways, which

might be crucial in the pathogenesis of the common PD form. Extensive investigations on the first of such monogenic forms (PARK1/α-synuclein and PARK2/parkin) are delineating protein misfolding and a defective protein quality control system as central themes in these forms and in PD in general. For the more recently identified forms, like PARK6/PINK1, PARK7/DJ-1, and PARK8/LRRK2, the pathogenetic mechanisms and relationships to common PD are less clear, and these forms might unravel the involvement of novel pathways. Some Mendelian forms, including those caused by mutations in the parkin and especially the LRRK2 gene, are frequent enough to have relevance for clinical practice.

Current technology for mRNA expression profiling at the level of whole transcriptome (expression microarrays) may also contribute soon to the identification of susceptibility genes for PD and to dissecting the molecular pathways leading to PD [22–24].

In the following sections, I discuss the genetics of the Mendelian forms of PD identified to date, focusing on five genes (α-synuclein, parkin, DJ-1, PINK1, and LRRK2) that have been associated conclusively with this disease. Other chromosomal loci (including PARK3, PARK10, PARK11) have been identified by genome-wide approaches, and these regions might harbor further (although still unknown) genes for PD. For a few other genes (including UCH-L1, NR4A2, SNCAIP, HtrA2/Omi, and GBA), there is weaker evidence of association with PD, but this is not based on genome-wide approaches. These loci and genes are also briefly discussed.

SNCA/α-synuclein (PARK1)

This autosomal dominant form of PD with LB pathology is caused by mutations in the SNCA gene on chromosome 4q21-q23, encoding the α-synuclein protein [25]. Mutations in the SNCA gene are rare, and they include missense variants and whole-locus multiplications [26]. Three missense mutations are known today: A53T, found in about fifteen families of Greek ancestry; A30P, identified in a single German family [27]; and E46K, recently identified in one Spanish family [28]. Triplications or duplications of the whole α-synuclein locus have been found to date in five kindreds (of Iowan, Swedish, French, and Italian origin) [26,29–31]. The multiplications are probably more frequent than missense mutations, but they are also rare, being present in about 1% of

Table 7.1. Current catalog of genes and loci for Parkinson's disease

Locus	Map position	Gene	Inheritance	Pathology
A				
PARK1	4q21–q23	*SNCA (α-synuclein)*	Dominant	LB+
PARK8	12p11–q13	*LRRK2*	Dominant	Pleomorphic (LB+, tau+, ub+)
PARK2	6q25–q27	*parkin*	Recessive	Mostly lb-
PARK6	1p36–p35	*PINK1*	Recessive	Unknown
PARK7	1p36	*DJ-1*	Recessive	Unknown
PARK9*	1p36	*ATP13A2*	Recessive	Unknown
B				
PARK3	2p13	Unknown	Dominant	LB+
PARK10	1p32	Unknown	Unclear	Unknown
PARK11	2q36–q37	Unknown	Unclear	Unknown
Pending	Xq	Unknown	Unclear	Unknown
C				
PARK5	4p14	*UCHL1*	Unclear	Unknown
Pending	2q22–q23	*NR4A2 (NURR1)*	Unclear	Unknown
Pending	5q23	*SNCAIP (synphilin-1)*	Unclear	Unknown
Pending	2p12	*HTRA2 (OMI)*	Unclear	Unknown
Pending	1q21	*GBA*	Unclear	Unknown

A – loci and genes implicated in Parkinson's disease (PD) with conclusive evidence from genome-wide linkage screens.
B – further loci identified in genome-wide linkage screens.
C – genes proposed to be implicated in PD causation in studies adopting a candidate-gene approach.
Note: The PARK4 locus (chromosome 4p15) has been removed from the catalog because a mutation of the *α-synuclein* gene (locus triplication) is associated with PD in the family, which initially provided evidence for the existence of PARK4.
* PARK9 is associated with atypical phenotype, which might be unrelated to PD.

the families compatible with autosomal dominant inheritance (5 positive families out of more than 400 screened). Intriguingly, the presence of a dosage effect is suggested by the observation that duplications are associated with the classical PD phenotype, whereas triplications lead to a more severe phenotype, which is closer to diffuse LB disease. These findings support the view that PD and LB disease represent different parts of the same neurodegenerative spectrum [30,31].

The discovery of *α-synuclein* gene mutations in PARK1 led to the identification of α-synuclein protein as one of the major components of LB, as well as of the glial cytoplasmic inclusions in multiple system atrophy [32]. Over-expressing wild-type or mutant human α-synuclein in transgenic animals yields varying degrees of biochemical, pathological, and clinical abnormalities reminiscent of PD, once again implicating α-synuclein in the pathogenesis of the disease in general [33–35].

The discovery that α-synuclein locus multiplications cause familial PD confirms and extends the results of the studies in transgenic animals, showing that the overexpression of wild-type α-synuclein is associated with neurodegeneration in humans. Although mutations in its gene are rare, α-synuclein protein plays a central role in PD. In keeping with this view, studies also suggest that allelic variation in the α-synuclein promoter modulates susceptibility to the sporadic form of PD [36,37].

The phenotypical spectrum associated with missense mutations in *α-synuclein* is broad. Some cases are similar to classical PD, but more often the phenotype is more aggressive, and it includes additional features (dementia, myoclonus, and severe autonomic dysfunctions), making the picture closer to LB disease than to PD. In addition, a wide variability of onset ages may be observed in the same family, suggesting the existence of genetic and/or non-genetic modifiers [18].

α-Synuclein is abundant in neurons and enriched in the presynaptic compartment [38]. Although its function remains unknown, it might be involved in synaptic plasticity, and regulation of size and turnover of synaptic vesicles. α-Synuclein oligomers are believed to represent the precursors of higher order aggregates (fibrils), which are assembled in vivo in the filamentous structures seen in LB.

In different neurodegenerative diseases, the oligomers, rather than the mature fibrils, might be the real neurotoxic molecules [39]. The regulation of the levels of monomeric, oligomeric, or fibrillar α-synuclein in neurons appears critical, and this regulation might be altered in the common PD forms owing to an increased α-synuclein expression or decreased clearance, or both. The pathways for degradation of normal and misfolded α-synuclein are poorly understood, but a recent study suggests that the system of the chaperone mediated autophagy and the lysosomes (rather than the ubiquitin–proteasome system) play the most important role [40].

How monomeric, oligomeric, or fibrillar α-synuclein exerts neurotoxicity remains unclear, but several possibilities have been suggested [41,42], including a direct inhibition of the proteasome system, an impairment of mitochondrial function, derangement in cellular trafficking, and damage or functional impairment of synaptic vesicles. Recent data suggest that α-synuclein protects the presynaptic terminals in cooperation with another protein, termed cysteine-string protein-alpha (CSPalpha) [43]; disturbances of this neuroprotective function might be relevant for PD pathogenesis.

Any kind of selective interaction between α-synuclein and dopamine has the potential to explain the relative selectivity of the PD pathology. As an example, the oxidative metabolite dopamine quinone can form adducts with α-synuclein, and these adducts inhibit the conversion of α-synuclein oligomers to higher aggregates, further reinforcing the toxicity associated with the oligomers [44].

LRRK2/dardarin (PARK8)

A novel locus for autosomal dominant PD, mapping to the centromeric region of chromosome 12, was identified in a large Japanese pedigree with late-onset PD (51±6 years) [45]. Linkage to the PARK8 region has since been confirmed in two white families with dominantly inherited neurodegeneration, suggesting PARK8 to be an important locus [46].

Leucine-rich repeat kinase 2 (*LRRK2*) has been identified as the gene causing PARK8 [47,48]. This gene possesses 51 exons, and it encodes a large protein, also termed dardarin, which contains 2527 amino acids and has an unknown function. The protein belongs to a group, termed ROCO, within the Ras/GTPase superfamily, and is characterized by the presence of two conserved domains: Roc (for Ras in complex proteins) and COR (C terminus of Roc), together with other domains such as ankyrin and leucine-rich repeat regions, a WD40 domain, and a protein kinase catalytic domain (Figure 7.1) [48]. The discovery of *LRRK2* gene mutations in PARK8 establishes a novel, important link between the dardarin protein and neurodegeneration.

Owing to the large size of the *LRRK2* gene, a comprehensive mutation screening of the entire coding region (51 exons) has been performed in very few studies only. The results show that mutations in this gene account for ~10% of the autosomal dominant PD families, therefore representing a common genetic cause of the disease [48–52].

One mutation, Gly2019Ser, replacing a very conserved residue in the kinase domain of dardarin, is particularly important. This mutation was initially identified by several groups as a common cause of the disease, being detected not only in ~5%–6% of familial PD but also in ~1%–2% of sporadic PD in European and US populations [53–57]. More recently, it became clear that the prevalence of Gly2019Ser is population specific [58]: very rare in Asia, [59] low in Northern Europe [54], high in Italy [60,61], Spain [62], and Portugal [63], but extremely high among Arab patients from North Africa [64] and Ashkenazi Jews [65] (also suggesting likely regions of origin of the mutation). The low penetrance (~30%) estimated for this (and possibly other) *LRRK2* gene mutations and the censor effects likely explain the high Gly2019Ser prevalence among patients with sporadic PD, particularly if they are of Arab and Ashkenazi Jewish ethnicity, and its (rare)

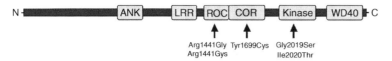

Figure 7.1. Schematic representation of the human LRRK2 protein, its known functional domains, and five mutations associated with Parkinson's disease and considered as definitely disease-causing.
ANK, ankyrine-like repeats; LRR, leucine-rich repeat; ROC, Ras of complex proteins (GTPase); COR, C-terminus of ROC; WD40, WD40-like domain.

occurrence in controls (especially among the younger individuals) [64,65]. For the same reasons, the Gly2019Ser mutation may also be found in European and US populations among sporadic PD patients or in familial cases without a clear pattern of autosomal dominant inheritance (unclear familial pattern) [58,60]. Haplotype analyses revealed that most carriers of this mutation among patients originating from Europe, North Africa, and the Middle East inherited it from a single, very old founder chromosome [56,60,66,67].

The exact prevalence and penetrance of the Gly2019Ser mutation in the different populations must be explored further; earlier figures of penetrance obtained in selected samples of dominant families were likely overestimated, and values should be calculated in unselected, consecutive series, ideally from population-based studies. Whether and when Gly2019Ser testing might be used for genetic counseling should await a much deeper understanding of the mechanisms of the disease caused by this and other mutations in *LRRK2*, and of the factors governing their penetrance. However Gly2019Ser represents the first common pathogenic mutation identified in PD, and it establishes, for the first time, the proof-of-principle for a genetic determinant frequently involved in the classical, late-onset, sporadic forms of PD.

A different variant located in the WD40 domain, Gly2385Arg, is a common polymorphism in the Chinese population, and it is significantly more frequent among PD cases than ethnically matched controls [68]. This finding has been confirmed in an large independent sample [69]. If the association is further replicated, Gly2385Arg would represent the first identified genetic risk factor for the common PD form in the Asian population.

Overall, the clinical characteristics of patients with *LRRK2* gene mutations (particularly those with the common Gly2019Ser mutation) are very similar, if not indistinguishable, from those of classical PD [55,60,61,64,65]. Functional neuroimaging studies of patients with *LRRK2* mutations confirm a typical pattern of nigrostriatal abnormality, as observed in the common form of PD [51,57,70,71].

Another very important aspect is the wide pathological spectrum associated with *LRRK2* mutations. Dopaminergic neuronal cell loss and gliosis in the substantia nigra are the common features in the patients carrying *LRRK2* mutations, and this is likely the pathological substrate of the parkinsonism. However, in addition to cell loss and gliosis, a wide range of inclusions has been observed (~30 cases have come to autopsy to date). Most cases (particularly those carrying the Gly2019Ser mutation) do have typical LB pathology, ranging from the brainstem type to the diffuse type [72–74]. However, some do not display any type of inclusions, or only tau-positive pathology, or ubiquitin-positive cytoplasmic and nuclear inclusions [45,48,75,76]. The elucidation of the function of the dardarin protein might provide important insights for understanding the pathogenesis of PD and the overlap between different neurodegenerative spectra [77]. These findings also challenge the validity of the current clinicopathological definition of PD [78]. The role of the dardarin protein in biology and pathology is currently the object of intensive investigation. Initial in vitro studies suggest that dardarin does have kinase activity, which seems increased by the PD-causing mutations, and the kinase activity correlates with cytotoxicity [79–83]. Protein kinases are good targets for small molecule drugs, and modulating the activity of the dardarin protein could become an innovative therapeutic strategy for all patients with PD.

Parkin (PARK2)

A common form of autosomal recessive parkinsonism with early onset is caused by mutations in the *parkin* gene [84]. More than 70 mutations in this gene have been identified worldwide [85–90]. In addition to point mutations, large genomic rearrangements (leading to exon deletions and multiplications) are frequently detected, in the homozygous or heterozygous state, indicating the importance of gene dosage techniques for a sensitive screening of the *parkin* gene.

The results of large and comprehensive studies indicate that mutations in this gene are found in about 50% of the familial PD cases compatible with recessive inheritance and onset before the age of 45 years, and in about 15% of the sporadic cases with onset before 45 years of age [85,87]. Most of the sporadic PD cases with *parkin* gene mutations have a very early onset (before the age of 30 years) [85,87]. *Parkin* mutations are, therefore, a major cause of early onset PD.

The involvement of the *parkin* gene in late-onset PD has been explored to a lesser extent, as patients with early onset and/or recessive inheritance were preselected in most of the mutational screening performed to date [85–87]. However, recent studies implicate *parkin* in a smaller fraction of late-onset familial PD compatible with recessive inheritance [88,89].

In some PD cases, only a single heterozygous *parkin* gene mutation has been found, raising the question of whether single heterozygous *parkin* mutations are sometimes sufficient to cause PD. The genetic evidence suggests that most *parkin* mutations are recessive, but in some cases the second mutation escapes detection by current methods. However, it is still possible that a few *parkin* gene mutations are dominant and thus cause disease in the heterozygous state. More genetic and functional studies are required to clarify the role of single heterozygous *parkin* mutations in both early and late-onset PD. The same debate concerns the interpretation of single heterozygous mutations found in the *PINK1* and *DJ-1* genes.

The pathology associated with mutations in *parkin* has been studied in a few brains only. The commonly observed features are neuronal loss and gliosis in the substantia nigra pars compacta and locus coeruleus with deposition of extraneuronal melanin in the substantia nigra [91]. However, LB were present in two of these brains [92,93], whereas another showed few atypical α-synuclein-positive inclusions [94]. Tau-positive inclusions were also found in the neurons and astrocytes in some of these brains.

PET studies with fluorodopa in patients with *parkin* gene mutations revealed a pattern of marked presynaptic dopaminergic dysfunction, including left–right asymmetry (although less pronounced than in classical PD), and a rostrocaudal gradient (the putamen being more severely affected than the caudate nucleus) [95]. In addition, postsynaptic dopaminergic dysfunctions have been reported [96].

The parkin protein has 465 amino acids and it is widely expressed in neurons and glial cells, where it is localized in several subcellular compartments. The protein contains an N-terminal domain homologous to ubiquitin and two RING finger domains separated by an IBR (in-between-RING) domain in the C-terminal part. The parkin protein has ubiquitin–ligase activity [97]. Covalent attachment of multiple copies of the ubiquitin polypeptide (polyubiquitylation) tags proteins for proteasomal degradation, and this is a fundamental mechanism for the protein quality control system. Furthermore, monoubiquitylation is involved in other cell processes, including regulation of gene expression and protein sorting. Whatever the normal role of the parkin protein is, PARK2 is a classical recessive disease in most cases, suggesting that the loss of parkin function is pathogenic. Several disease causing missense mutations in parkin abolish the ubiquitin–ligase activity. Thus, a major hypothesis is that the accumulation of non-ubiquitylated substrates in the brain of patients with *parkin* gene mutations might be important in the pathogenesis of this form. Yeast two-hybrid screens and other approaches have provided several putative interactors and substrates of parkin (reviewed in [98]). However, the role of these proteins as parkin interactors in vivo remains unclear, and the known association between parkin and the chaperone Hsp70 could mediate the interaction with a variety of misfolded targets, perhaps explaining the apparent broad substrate specificity of parkin.

The discovery of an interaction between parkin and a brain-specific, glycosylated form of α-synuclein [99], as well as between parkin and synphilin-1 [100], has important potential implications for PD in general, as these interactions link parkin to α-synuclein, another protein which is central in the pathogenesis of PD. This interaction might be relevant for the deposition of ubiquitylated α-synuclein in LB. To the extent that parkin activity is essential for LB formation, the parkin defect would explain the absence of LB in the brain of patients with *parkin* gene mutations. The link between parkin and α-synuclein has been supported in recent studies, which suggested parkin to be a modifier of the α-synuclein-induced neurodegeneration in cell cultures and in transgenic drosophila, once again suggesting that parkin is implicated in the pathogenesis of PD in general [101,102]. In keeping with these studies, recent data suggest that a different, posttranslational modification of parkin, S-nitrosylation, inhibits its ubiquitin–ligase activity. As nitrosative stress and S-nitrosylation of parkin also occurs in the brains of PD patients, this mechanism might contribute to the disease pathogenesis [103,104].

Two of the proposed parkin substrates, cyclin-E and p38, suggest additional and intriguing links between parkin activity and protection of neurons from apoptosis [105,106]. The links between parkin, mitochondria, and apoptosis are supported by findings in the drosophila *parkin* knockout model [107]. Furthermore, the later stages in PD display evidence of mitochondrial derangement, oxidative stress, and apoptosis, suggesting further links to the pathogenesis of classical PD. On the other hand, the available *parkin* knockout mice models fail to fully reproduce the pathology of human disease caused by *parkin* gene mutation, but they suggest a role for *parkin* in the regulation of nigrostriatal dopaminergic neurotransmission [108–110]. In one of these mice, there is loss of catecholaminergic neurons in the locus coeruleus and loss of brain norepinephrine [110].

The clinical phenotype associated with *parkin* mutations in humans (the parkin disease) is characterized by early onset parkinsonism, good and prolonged response to levodopa (and other dopaminergic drugs), and a benign, slow course. The average onset age is in the early 30s in European patients, but late-onset cases have been described in patients of up to 70 years of age. Motor fluctuations and levodopa-induced dyskinesias are present, whereas marked cognitive or vegetative disturbances seem rare.

The age of disease onset is the most important predictor of mutations in *parkin* in that the earlier the onset, the higher the likelihood of mutations being present. There are no specific clinical features that distinguish patients with *parkin* mutations from other early onset PD forms [88]. However, symmetrical onset, dystonia at onset and hyperreflexia, slower progression of the disease, and a tendency toward a greater response to levodopa might be more frequent among patients with *parkin* mutations. The phenotypical spectrum overlaps with classical PD for late-onset cases, and with levodopa-responsive dystonia for early onset ones. Rare atypical presentations have also been described, and a wide variability in onset age and phenotype is observed even within the same

families. In conclusion, mutations in the *parkin* gene represent a frequent cause of familial early onset and isolated juvenile parkinsonism.

DJ-1 (PARK7)

A different form of autosomal recessive, early onset parkinsonism maps to chromosome 1p36 [111,112], and is caused by mutations in the *DJ-1* gene [113]. The screening of large series of patients with early onset PD delineated mutations in the *DJ-1* gene (which include missense, truncating, splice site mutations, and large deletions) as a rare cause of the disease, being implicated in about 1%–2% of these cases [114–118]. An extensive review on the genetics and the molecular biology of PARK7/*DJ-1* has been published [119]. The most significant findings from the recent studies include the resolution of the crystal structure of the human DJ-1 protein, and the discovery that it exists as a homodimer. The function of DJ-1 remains largely unknown, but evidence from genetic and biochemical studies in cell-based systems suggests a role as an antioxidant and/or a molecular chaperone which, according to recent reports, may extend to the α-synuclein protein [119–123]. A functional interaction between DJ-1 and parkin has also been proposed [124]. If confirmed, these functions would make DJ-1 an important player in the current pathogenetic scenarios of classical PD as well.

Furthermore, the different newly discovered interactions of the DJ-1 protein with mitochondria [125,126], cytosolic RNA-binding protein complexes, and nuclear transcriptional cofactors [127], as well as cytosolic proteins linked to apoptosis, such as PTEN and Daxx [128,129], are delineating a possible involvement of DJ-1 in several other pathways, which might be important for the survival of dopaminergic neurons and for the pathogenesis of PD [119].

The pathology of PARK7 remains unknown, and LB from classical PD are not stained by the currently available DJ-1 antibodies; however, DJ-1 immunoreactivity is markedly increased in the insoluble fraction of brain extracts from patients with classical LB-positive PD, and also those with diffuse LB disease [124]. Moreover, DJ-1 immunoreactivity is found in pathological tau inclusions in different tauopathies [130,131], and in glial inclusions in multiple system atrophy [131,132], suggesting further links between seemingly different diseases and a role of DJ-1 in their pathogenesis. A recent report has expanded the genetic and clinical spectra of DJ-1-related neurodegeneration, by the identification of homozygous *DJ-1* gene mutations in an Italian consanguineous family with early onset parkinsonism, dementia, and amyotrophic lateral sclerosis complex [133].

Different *DJ-1* knockout mice models have been generated [134–136]; these mice are viable and fertile, and they display normal numbers of brain dopaminergic neurons; however, they show marked abnormalities in several neurophysiological paradigms, which point to alterations in the central dopaminergic pathways, and they also develop age-related motor hypoactivity and hypersensitivity to MPTP. How the mice phenotype relates to the neurodegeneration seen in humans with *DJ-1* gene mutations remains unclear, but the DJ-1 protein likely plays an important role in the physiology of the brain dopaminergic systems. Therefore, further elucidating the role of DJ-1 might lead to a better understanding of the pathogenesis of classical PD and other common neurodegenerative disorders. More recently, the DJ-1-related neurodegeneration was modeled in transgenic drosophila [137–140]. These studies provided further evidence that the loss of DJ-1 function impairs the neuronal defenses against oxidative stressors, including environmental agents (such as paraquat and rotenone) linked to PD in humans.

Moreover, the phosphatidylinositol 3-kinase (PI3K)/Akt-signaling pathway appears to be activated in the molecular cascade of DJ-1 [139]. This is of particular interest because it might link DJ-1, PINK1, and parkin in a common pathway underlying autosomal recessive, early onset PD [128]. The occurrence of single heterozygous mutations in the *DJ-1* and *PINK1* genes in a Chinese family with early onset PD, and an interaction between the DJ-1 and PINK1 proteins detected in vitro, are potentially important findings that suggest a digenic inheritance of early onset PD and provide further evidence of a functional interaction between the protein products of the different PD-causing genes [141].

PINK1 (PARK6)

A genome-wide scan and homozygosity mapping in a large consanguineous kindred from Sicily (Italy) yielded significant linkage to the 1p36–p35 region [142]. In this family, four individuals had PD of early onset (range: 32–48 years). Linkage to the PARK6 region was subsequently confirmed in independent European and Asian families [143,144]. The pathology of this form remains unknown. Pathogenic mutations in the *PINK1* gene (PTEN-induced putative kinase 1) were later identified in PARK6-linked families [145]. The *PINK1* gene encodes a 581 amino acid protein with a mitochondrial targeting peptide at the N terminus, and a putative Ser/Thr kinase domain. The function of PINK1 remains unknown, but studies in overexpressing cell systems showed that the protein is localized to the mitochondria, and might protect cells from mitochondrial stress [145–149]. These findings are especially intriguing because mitochondrial abnormalities and oxidative stress have been linked to PD pathogenesis on the basis of previous extensive biochemical and pathological evidence [150,151].

Soon after the initial cloning, other studies provided independent confirmation that *PINK1* gene mutations cause PARK6 [152,153]. More recent analysis of large series of patients showed that *PINK1* gene mutations are less frequent than *parkin* mutations, but more common than *DJ-1* mutations [154–159]. We found homozygous *PINK1* mutations in ~4% of 90 Italian patients with sporadic early onset PD, and single heterozygous mutations in another 4% of cases [157]. The frequency of *PINK1* mutations may be higher in Italian early onset PD patients than in patients from Northern Europe, and higher in the Asian population than in Caucasians. The varying frequency of mutations in a given gene between populations is an emerging concept not only for *PINK1*-related parkinsonism but also for the other monogenic forms of PD; this issue has important implications for the diagnostic workup and counseling of patients. As observed in the studies on the *parkin* and *DJ-1* genes, in some cases a single heterozygous *PINK1* mutation has been identified despite intensive screening, raising the question of whether single heterozygous mutations are pathogenic [157,158,160].

The clinical phenotype in *PINK1*-related disease appears broad, and in some cases, very similar to the phenotype of *parkin*- and *DJ-1*-related disease [152,157,159]. No clinical features allow cases with *PINK1* mutations to be distinguished from those with mutations in the genes *parkin* or *DJ-1*, or those without mutations in these three genes. Genetic testing is, therefore, essential for an accurate diagnosis and distinction between the different recessive forms of early onset parkinsonism.

The PINK1-related neurodegeneration has recently been modelled in transgenic knockout drosophila [140,161,162]. The resulting phenotypes are very similar to those observed in *parkin* knockout flies, and rescue experiments suggest that parkin and PINK1 proteins are functionally linked, with PINK1 acting upstream of parkin. This supports the view that the same molecular pathway underlies the different forms of recessive, early onset PD.

The other loci for Mendelian and common forms of Parkinson's disease

Parkinsonism (sometimes with a good levodopa response) may be the prominent clinical feature in other inherited neurodegenerative diseases, which are usually associated with multisystemic neurological involvement, such as the chromosome 17-linked fronto-temporal dementia and parkinsonism (FTDP-17) [163,164], the spinocerebellar ataxias type 2 and type 3 (especially among patients of Asian and African origin) [165,166], the disease caused by mutations in the mitochondrial DNA polymerase (POLG) [167], the rapid-onset dystonia–parkinsonism (RDP, DYT12, caused by mutations in the gene encoding the ATPase alpha-3 subunit ATP1A3) [168], and the X-linked dystonia–parkinsonism of the Filipinos (lubag, DYT3) [169].

A different locus for autosomal dominant PD (PARK3) maps to chromosome 2p13 in kindreds of European ancestry [170]. The phenotypical spectrum is wide, encompassing typical PD of late onset (average onset age of 59 years) and LB pathology, but also cases with dementia in addition to parkinsonism, and presence of neurofibrillary tangles and senile plaques in addition to LB pathology. On the basis of haplotype analysis, a low penetrance (40%) was estimated in PARK3 families [170]. Linkage to the 2p13 region has not been replicated in other kindreds, and the gene defective at the PARK3 locus remains unknown. More recently, two genome-wide scans of affected sib-pairs found suggestive evidence for linkage of PD and PD onset age to the PARK3 region [171,172], confirming that an important genetic determinant of PD risk and/or a modifier of disease onset age might reside in this region. Recent analyses suggested a role for the sepiapterin reductase gene,

located within the PARK3 region and implicated in dopamine synthesis, in modifying PD risk or disease onset age [173,174].

PARK9 is the name assigned to a different recessive locus mapping to the 1p36 region in a consanguineous family from Jordan [175]. Five siblings were affected with a multisystemic neurodegenerative disease (Kufor–Rakeb syndrome), clinically quite different from PD and more closely resembling the pallidopyramidal degenerations, with juvenile onset (below the age of 20 years), akinetic-rigid parkinsonism with good levodopa response, pyramidal tract dysfunction, supranuclear gaze paresis, and cognitive deterioration [176]. The pathology of PARK9 remains unexplored, but neuroimaging showed progressive brain atrophy.

A second pedigree originating from Chile with a very similar phenotype yielded significant linkage to the same chromosomal region [177], and recessive mutations in the *ATP13A2* gene, encoding a large transmembrane protein with putative ATP-ase activity and lysosomal localization, were recently identified in the two previously mentioned PARK9-linked kindreds [177]. The function of the protein encoded by the gene *ATP13A2* remains unknown but, intriguingly, the ATP13A2 mRNA is highly expressed in the substantia nigra, and it appears to be upregulated in the brain of patients with the classical late-onset PD form [177]. Although the phenotype displayed by the original PARK9-linked families is different from classical PD, the identification of the molecular bases of this rare disease might have implications for unraveling the pathogenesis of the common PD forms. Whether *ATP13A2* gene mutations are also associated with forms of pure, early onset PD remains unknown.

It is likely that other Mendelian forms of PD will be identified in the future as most of the previous loci have been excluded in additional pedigrees. For example, we have recently obtained suggestive evidence in a Cuban family for linkage to chromosome 19 segregating clinically typical PD of late-onset [178].

In addition to the studies in single Mendelian families, five genome-wide scans in large series of small families, each containing at least one pair of relatives affected with classical PD, have been completed (reviewed in [172,179,180]) The most important results of these studies have been the detection of a significant linkage to three novel regions, on chromosomes 1p32 (PARK10) and 2q36–q37

(PARK11), and on the Xq chromosome (official locus name pending) [181–183]. Therefore, these regions might harbor susceptibility genes for classical, late-onset PD. In addition to these significant findings, a series of chromosomal regions with interesting or suggestive positive LOD scores has been generated, and the analysis of larger datasets might identify further genuine linkages [179,180].

Other proposed susceptibility genes for PD

UCHL1 (ubiquitin carboxy-terminal hydrolase L1) is an abundant neuronal protein, also found in LB, encoded by the *UCHL1* gene. Its function in vivo is probably to stabilize the neuronal levels of mono-meric ubiquitin [184]. Although linkage to the *UCHL1* gene region has not emerged in any genome-wide scans performed in PD, direct sequen-cing of the gene revealed a heterozygous missense mutation (Ile93Met) in two German siblings with classical PD and a positive family history suggesting autosomal dominant inheritance and incomplete penetrance [185]. The UCHL1 locus was assigned the PARK5 name. In that family, pathological studies were not available. Subsequent screening of this gene has consistently been negative, suggesting that Ile93-Met is either an extremely rare cause of PD or even a neutral polymorphism. Association between PD risk and a different polymorphic variant (Ser18Tyr) remains controversial [186,187].

The *NR4A2* (*NURR1*) gene, located at 2q22–q23, encodes a member of the nuclear receptor superfam-ily of transcription factors that is highly expressed in fetal and adult dopaminergic (DA) neurons. This protein is important for the genesis and maintenance of DA neurons, as *NR4A2* knockout mice display agenesis of these neurons. Evidence for association between an intronic *NR4A2* polymorphism and PD remains controversial. Linkage to the chromosomal region containing this gene was not found in genome scans. However, two mutations in the non-coding exon 1 of *NR4A2* (-291Tdel and -245T→G) were identified in the single heterozygous state in patients with familial PD and a dominant pattern of inherit-ance [188]. Onset age (54±7 years) and other clinical features were those of typical PD, but the associated pathology remains unknown. The screening of *NR4A2* exon 1 in independent large samples was negative, indicating that mutations in this gene

(at least those located in exon 1) are extremely rare in PD [189–192]. More recently, a single missense mutation was found in one sporadic PD case, but the pathogenic significance of this finding remains unclear [193].

Synphilin-1 is an α-synuclein interacting protein [194] of unknown function. Like α-synuclein, synphi-lin-1 is enriched in presynaptic terminals and associates with synaptic vesicles. Immunoreactivity for synphilin-1 is present in LB and glial cytoplasmic inclusions, sug-gesting that deposition of this protein is a feature of synucleinopathies [195,196]. Synphilin-1 is encoded by the *SNCAIP* gene, on chromosome 5q23, a possible candidate linkage region emerging in different genome screens of late-onset PD. A single heterozygous missense mutation (R621C) has recently been identified in two sporadic German patients with late-onset PD [197]. However, further work is needed to clarify whether this or different genetic variants in *SNCAIP* influence the susceptibility to PD.

The *HtrA2* (Omi) gene encodes a mitochondrial serine protease, which is released into the cytosol in response to apoptotic stimuli. This gene represents an attractive candidate for PD, mainly because *HtrA2* knockout mice display a neurodegenerative pheno-type that includes parkinsonian features [198]. More-over, the HtrA2 locus on chromosome 2p13 maps to a region very close to (but distinct from) the PARK3 locus. A single heterozygous missense mutation (Gly399Ser) in the *HtrA2* gene was detected in four German patients with sporadic PD, while a different polymorphic variant (Ala141Ser) was more frequent in PD than in controls [199]. Interestingly, both variants displayed defective activation of the HtrA2 protein in vitro. Screenings of the *HtrA2* gene in different samples of PD cases have not been published to date.

Mutations in the *GBA* gene, encoding the enzyme glucosidase beta acid (glucocerebrosidase), cause Gaucher disease, an autosomal recessive lysosomal storage disorder characterized by an accumulation of glucocerebrosides. The occurrence of parkinsonism and LB among Gaucher disease patients and their relatives led to the screening of the *GBA* gene in PD.

A strong association between *GBA* heterozygous and homozygous missense mutations and PD was reported among Ashkenazi Jewish patients, suggest-ing that carrying GBA missense alleles is a risk factor for PD in that population (OR 7.0, 95% CI 4.2–11.4, P<0.001) [200]. Evidence for such a strong association was not found in other series of patients of Jewish or different ethnicity [201–203], but comprehensive studies of this gene in large samples are still lacking. Recently, a high prevalence of *GBA* gene mutations (23%) has been reported among patients with LB dementia [204]. If these results are confirmed, *GBA* mutations will represent an important risk factor for α-synucleinopathies (PD and LB disease). Lysosomes are important for the degradation of the α-synuclein protein [40,205,206] and the association between mutations in *GBA* and α-synucleinopathies provide genetic support for a role of lysosomal abnormality in the pathogenesis of these diseases.

Allelic association studies

Several studies addressed the problem of the genetic bases of PD through the strategy of allelic association analysis in candidate genes and a case-control study design. However, the results of most of these studies have been inconclusive (reviewed in [207]). Allelic association studies are prone to false-positive results, mainly owing to small sample sizes, population stratification, and genotyping errors. Therefore, replication in independent, large samples is mandatory. Nevertheless, there is initial evidence from recent studies performed in large series of cases and controls that allelic variants in several nuclear and mitochondrial genes modify the susceptibility to or onset age of PD; these include the genes encoding the microtubule associated protein tau, dopamine beta-hydroxylase, glutathione S-transferase omega-1 (GSTO1), fibroblast growth factor 20 (FGF20), and glucocerebrosidase (GBA), among others [200, 208–212].

The discovery of very large numbers of single nucleotide polymorphisms (SNPs) scattered over the human genome, together with the evolution of the technology of DNA microarray (DNA chips), make it possible today to test hundreds of thousands of genetic markers in one experiment at affordable costs. This, in turn, allows allelic association studies to be performed at the level of the whole genome (genome-wide association, GWA), and in large samples of cases and controls [213–217]. It is likely in the near future that more and more studies will adopt this strategy. Genetically isolated populations might be particularly useful in this endeavor [218].

The implications of the genetic findings for clinical practice

Mutations in two of the PD-related genes now known, *parkin* and *LRRK2*, are frequent enough to have relevance in the diagnostic workup of PD cases. Figure 7.2 contains a simple algorithm to orient clinicians to when to perform gene testing in PD patients and which genes to test.

Parkin gene mutations are common in familial and sporadic cases of early onset [85,87–89]. An early onset (especially before the age of 40 years) and/or the presence of a family history compatible with recessive inheritance are critical to prioritize patients for testing of the *parkin* gene. The presence of consanguinity between parents of the patient may also suggest the presence of a recessive mechanism of inheritance in cases presenting without any family history of PD. Owing to the wide spectrum of mutations, the screening of *parkin* is difficult, and it should always include gene copy analysis in addition to sequencing. If *parkin* gene mutations are not found, screening for the *PINK1* gene should be done next, and if *PINK1* is negative, *DJ-1* screening may also be considered.

Emerging data delineate mutations in the *LRRK2* gene as the cause of up to 10% of the familial late-onset autosomal dominant PD forms, and also of a few sporadic cases [47–56]. It is important to be aware that, owing to their low and age-related penetrance, some *LRRK2* mutations (such as Gly2019Ser, Arg1441Gly, and Arg1441Cys) might also be found in patients without a family history for PD, or in those with familial PD but without a clear Mendelian pattern of inheritance. Moreover, these mutations are found in cases with both early and late-onset PD. Because of these reasons, screening for the most common *LRRK2* Gly2019Ser mutations might become relevant in the diagnostic workup for all patients with PD, particularly in the populations in which the frequency of a given mutation is high [58,64,65].

It is likely that other Mendelian forms of PD and the causative genes will be identified in the future, and these discoveries hold the promise of yielding further significant steps forward in the field. From the clinical standpoint, the importance of genetic testing for PD patients is expected to increase in the near future, also raising important ethical issues (see [219–222] for a detailed discussion of the issue of genetic testing in PD).

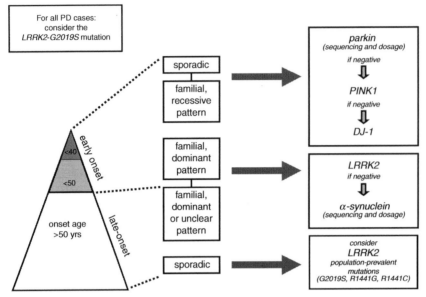

For all PD cases:
consider the
LRRK2-G2019S mutation

sporadic

familial,
recessive
pattern

familial,
dominant
pattern

familial,
dominant
or unclear
pattern

sporadic

early onset
<40
<50

onset age
>50 yrs

late-onset

parkin
(sequencing and dosage)

if negative

PINK1

if negative

DJ-1

LRRK2

if negative

α-synuclein
(sequencing and dosage)

consider
LRRK2
population-prevalent
mutations
(G2019S, R1441G, R1441C)

Figure 7.2. Algorithm for orienting the genetic screening of patients with Parkinson's disease.

Apart from the complexity of diagnostic screening, the genetic counseling of patients with *parkin* or *LRRK2* gene mutations and of their relatives is difficult because of the broad phenotypical spectrum associated, including a very large intrafamilial variance of onset ages and phenotypes, and because we do not always understand if and how a given mutation is pathogenic. Whether and when gene testing may be used for genetic counseling should await a much deeper understanding of the mechanisms of the disease caused by these mutations, and of the factors governing their penetrance. In the case of *parkin* and the other genes for recessive PD forms (*PINK1* and *DJ-1*), there is the additional, unsolved question of the role of the single heterozygous mutant alleles. In any case, owing to the potentially important implications for the psychological and social lives of the patient and the relatives, the genetic testing for diagnostic and especially predictive purposes should be considered only in the framework of a multidisciplinary team of professional experts, including neurologists, medical geneticists, and psychologists.

Acknowledgments

I thank Ruud Koppenol for artwork. This study was supported by grants from the Internationaal Parkinson Fonds (the Netherlands), the Hersenstichting Nederland, the National Parkinson Foundation (USA), and the Erasmus MC, Rotterdam (the Netherlands).

References

1. Fahn S. Description of Parkinson's disease as a clinical syndrome. *Ann NY Acad Sci* 2003; **991**: 1–14.

2. Hughes AJ, Daniel SE, Kilford L, Lees AJ. Accuracy of clinical diagnosis of idiopathic Parkinson's disease: a clinico-pathological study of 100 cases. *J Neurol Neurosurg Psychiatry* 1992; **55**: 181–184.

3. Gelb DJ, Oliver E, Gilman S. Diagnostic criteria for Parkinson disease. *Arch Neurol* 1999; **56**: 33–39.

4. Lang AE, Lozano AM. Parkinson's disease. First of two parts. *N Engl J Med* 1998; **339**: 1044–1053.

5. Lang AE, Lozano AM. Parkinson's disease. Second of two parts. *N Engl J Med* 1998; **339**: 1130–1143.

6. de Rijk MC, Launer LJ, Berger K, *et al.* Prevalence of Parkinson's disease in Europe: a collaborative study of population-based cohorts. Neurologic Diseases in the Elderly Research Group. *Neurology* 2000; **54**: S21–S23.

7. Parkkinen L, Kauppinen T, Pirttila T, *et al.* Alpha-synuclein pathology does not predict extrapyramidal symptoms or dementia. *Ann Neurol* 2005; **57**: 82–91.

8. Langston JW, Ballard P, Tetrud JW, Irwin I. Chronic Parkinsonism in humans due to a product of meperidine-analog synthesis. *Science* 1983; **219**: 979–980.

9. Mjones H. Paralysis agitans: a clinical and genetic study. *Acta Psychiatr Neurol* 1949; **25** (Suppl 54): 1–195.

10. Martin WE, Young WI, Anderson VE. Parkinson's disease. A genetic study. *Brain* 1973; **96**: 495–506.

11. Bonifati V, Fabrizio E, Vanacore N, *et al.* Familial Parkinson's disease: a clinical genetic analysis. *Can J Neurol Sci* 1995; **22**: 272–279.

12. Lazzarini AM, Myers RH, Zimmerman TR Jr, *et al.* A clinical genetic study of Parkinson's disease: evidence for dominant transmission. *Neurology* 1994; **44**: 499–506.

13. Maher NE, Currie LJ, Lazzarini AM, *et al.* Segregation analysis of Parkinson disease revealing evidence for a major causative gene. *Am J Med Genet* 2002; **109**: 191–197.

14. Sveinbjornsdottir S, Hicks AA, Jonsson T, *et al.* Familial aggregation of Parkinson's disease in Iceland. *N Engl J Med* 2000; **343**: 1765–1770.

15. Tanner CM, Ottman R, Goldman SM, *et al.* Parkinson disease in twins: an etiologic study. *JAMA* 1999; **281**: 341–346.

16. Dickson D, Farrer M, Lincoln S, *et al.* Pathology of PD in monozygotic twins with a 20-year discordance interval. *Neurology* 2001; **56**: 981–982.

17. Piccini P, Burn DJ, Ceravolo R, *et al.* The role of inheritance in sporadic Parkinson's disease: evidence from a longitudinal study of dopaminergic function in twins. *Ann Neurol* 1999; **45**: 577–582.

18. Golbe LI, Di Iorio G, Sanges G, *et al.* Clinical genetic analysis of Parkinson's disease in the Contursi kindred. *Ann Neurol* 1996; **40**: 767–775.

19. Dawson TM, Dawson VL. Molecular pathways of neurodegeneration in Parkinson's disease. *Science* 2003; **302**: 819–822.

20. Bonifati V, Oostra BA, Heutink P. Unraveling the pathogenesis of Parkinson's disease – the contribution of monogenic forms. *Cell Mol Life Sci* 2004; **61**: 1729–1750.

21. Vila M, Przedborski S. Genetic clues to the pathogenesis of Parkinson's disease. *Nat Med* 2004; **10**: S58–62.

22. Scherzer CR, Jensen RV, Gullans SR, Feany MB. Gene expression changes presage neurodegeneration in a Drosophila model of Parkinson's disease. *Hum Mol Genet* 2003; **12**: 2457–2466.

23. Grunblatt E, Mandel S, Jacob-Hirsch J, *et al.* Gene expression profiling of parkinsonian substantia nigra pars compacta; alterations in ubiquitin-proteasome, heat shock protein, iron and oxidative stress regulated proteins, cell adhesion/cellular matrix and vesicle trafficking genes. *J Neural Transm* 2004; **111**: 1543–1573.

24. Moran LB, Duke DC, Deprez M, *et al.* Whole genome expression profiling of the medial and lateral substantia nigra in Parkinson's disease. *Neurogenetics* 2006; 7: 1–11.

25. Polymeropoulos MH, Lavedan C, Leroy E, *et al.* Mutation in the alpha-synuclein gene identified in families with Parkinson's disease. *Science* 1997; **276**: 2045–2047.

26. Singleton AB, Farrer M, Johnson J, *et al.* alpha-Synuclein locus triplication causes Parkinson's disease. *Science* 2003; **302**: 841.

27. Kruger R, Kuhn W, Muller T, *et al.* Ala30Pro mutation in the gene encoding alpha-synuclein in Parkinson's disease. *Nat Genet* 1998; **18**: 106–108.

28. Zarranz JJ, Alegre J, Gomez-Esteban JC, *et al.* The new mutation, E46K, of alpha-synuclein causes parkinson and Lewy body dementia. *Ann Neurol* 2004; **55**: 164–173.

29. Farrer M, Kachergus J, Forno L, *et al.* Comparison of kindreds with parkinsonism and alpha-synuclein genomic multiplications. *Ann Neurol* 2004; **55**: 174–179.

30. Ibanez P, Bonnet AM, Debarges B, *et al.* Causal relation between alpha-synuclein gene duplication and familial Parkinson's disease. *Lancet* 2004; **364**: 1169–1171.

31. Chartier-Harlin MC, Kachergus J, Roumier C, *et al.* Alpha-synuclein locus duplication as a cause of familial Parkinson's disease. *Lancet* 2004; **364**: 1167–1169.

32. Spillantini MG, Goedert M. The alpha-synucleinopathies: Parkinson's disease, dementia with Lewy bodies, and multiple system atrophy. *Ann NY Acad Sci* 2000; **920**: 16–27.

33. Zoghbi HY, Botas J. Mouse and fly models of neurodegeneration. *Trends Genet* 2002; **18**: 463–471.

34. Springer W, Kahle PJ. Mechanisms and models of alpha-synuclein-related neurodegeneration. *Curr Neurol Neurosci Rep* 2006; **6**: 432–436.

35. Whitworth AJ, Wes PD, Pallanck LJ. Drosophila models pioneer a new approach to drug discovery for Parkinson's disease. *Drug Discov Today* 2006; **11**: 119–126.

36. Pals P, Lincoln S, Manning J, *et al.* alpha-Synuclein promoter confers susceptibility to Parkinson's disease. *Ann Neurol* 2004; **56**: 591–595.

37. Maraganore DM, de Andrade M, Elbaz A, *et al.* Collaborative analysis of alpha-synuclein gene promoter variability and Parkinson disease. *JAMA* 2006; **296**: 661–670.

38. Goedert M. Alpha-synuclein and neurodegenerative diseases. *Nat Rev Neurosci* 2001; **2**: 492–501.

39. Bucciantini M, Giannoni E, Chiti F, *et al.* Inherent toxicity of aggregates implies a common mechanism for protein misfolding diseases. *Nature* 2002; **416**: 507–511.

40. Cuervo AM, Stefanis L, Fredenburg R, *et al.* Impaired degradation of mutant alpha-synuclein by chaperone-mediated autophagy. *Science* 2004; **305**: 1292–1295.

41. Dawson TM, Dawson VL. Rare genetic mutations shed light on the pathogenesis of Parkinson disease. *J Clin Invest* 2003; **111**: 145–151.

42. Dauer W, Przedborski S. Parkinson's disease: mechanisms and models. *Neuron* 2003; **39**: 889–909.

43. Chandra S, Gallardo G, Fernandez-Chacon R, *et al.* Alpha-synuclein cooperates with CSPalpha in preventing neurodegeneration. *Cell* 2005; **123**: 383–396.

44. Conway KA, Rochet JC, Bieganski RM, Lansbury PT Jr. Kinetic stabilization of the alpha-synuclein protofibril by a dopamine-alpha-synuclein adduct. *Science* 2001; **294**: 1346–1349.

45. Funayama M, Hasegawa K, Kowa H, *et al.* A new locus for Parkinson's disease (PARK8) maps to chromosome 12p11.2-q13.1. *Ann Neurol* 2002; **51**: 296–301.

46. Zimprich A, Muller-Myhsok B, Farrer M, *et al.* The PARK8 locus in autosomal dominant parkinsonism: confirmation of linkage and further delineation of the disease-containing interval. *Am J Hum Genet* 2004; **74**: 11–19.

47. Paisan-Ruiz C, Jain S, Evans EW, *et al.* Cloning of the gene containing mutations that cause PARK8-linked Parkinson's disease. *Neuron* 2004; **44**: 595–600.

48. Zimprich A, Biskup S, Leitner P, *et al.* Mutations in LRRK2 cause autosomal-dominant parkinsonism with pleomorphic pathology. *Neuron* 2004; **44**: 601–607.

49. Berg D, Schweitzer K, Leitner P, *et al.* Type and frequency of mutations in the LRRK2 gene in familial and sporadic Parkinson's disease. *Brain* 2005; **128**: 3000–3011.

50. Di Fonzo A, Tassorelli C, De Mari M, *et al.* Comprehensive analysis of the LRRK2 gene in sixty families with Parkinson's disease. *Eur J Hum Genet* 2006; **14**: 322–331.

51. Khan NL, Jain S, Lynch JM, *et al.* Mutations in the gene LRRK2 encoding dardarin (PARK8) cause familial Parkinson's disease: clinical, pathological, olfactory and functional imaging and genetic data. *Brain* 2005; **128**: 2786–2796.

52. Mata IF, Kachergus JM, Taylor JP, *et al.* Lrrk2 pathogenic substitutions in Parkinson's disease. *Neurogenetics* 2005; **6**: 171–177.

53. Di Fonzo A, Rohe CF, Ferreira J, *et al.* A frequent LRRK2 gene mutation associated with autosomal dominant Parkinson's disease. *Lancet* 2005; **365**: 412–415.

54. Gilks WP, Abou-Sleiman PM, Gandhi S, *et al.* A common LRRK2 mutation in idiopathic Parkinson's disease. *Lancet* 2005; **365**: 415–416.

55. Nichols WC, Pankratz N, Hernandez D, *et al.* Genetic screening for a single common LRRK2 mutation in familial Parkinson's disease. *Lancet* 2005; **365**: 410–412.

56. Kachergus J, Mata IF, Hulihan M, *et al.* Identification of a novel LRRK2 mutation linked to autosomal dominant Parkinsonism: evidence of a common founder across European populations. *Am J Hum Genet* 2005; **76**: 672–680.

57. Hernandez DG, Paisan-Ruiz C, McInerney-Leo A, *et al.* Clinical and positron emission tomography of Parkinson's disease caused by LRRK2. *Ann Neurol* 2005; **57**: 453–456.

58. Bonifati V. Parkinson's disease: The LRRK2-G2019S mutation: opening a novel era in Parkinson's disease genetics. *Eur J Hum Genet* 2006; **14**: 1061–1062.

59. Lu CS, Simons EJ, Wu-Chou YH, *et al.* The LRRK2 I2012T, G2019S, and I2020T mutations are rare in Taiwanese patients with sporadic Parkinson's disease. *Parkinsonism Relat Disord* 2005; **11**: 521–522.

60. Goldwurm S, Di Fonzo A, Simons EJ, *et al.* The G6055A (G2019S) mutation in LRRK2 is frequent in both early and late onset Parkinson's disease and originates from a common ancestor. *J Med Genet* 2005; **42**: e65.

61. Goldwurm S, Zini M, Di Fonzo A, *et al.* LRRK2 G2019S mutation and Parkinson's disease: a clinical, neuropsychological and neuropsychiatric study in a large Italian sample. *Parkinsonism Relat Disord* 2006; **12**: 410–419.

62. Gaig C, Ezquerra M, Marti MJ, *et al.* LRRK2 mutations in Spanish patients with Parkinson disease: frequency, clinical features, and incomplete penetrance. *Arch Neurol* 2006; **63**: 377–382.

63. Bras JM, Guerreiro RJ, Ribeiro MH, *et al.* G2019S dardarin substitution is a common cause of Parkinson's disease in a Portuguese cohort. *Mov Disord* 2005; **20**: 1653–1655.

64. Lesage S, Durr A, Tazir M, *et al.* LRRK2 G2019S as a cause of Parkinson's disease in North African Arabs. *N Engl J Med* 2006; **354**: 422–423.

65. Ozelius LJ, Senthil G, Saunders-Pullman R, *et al.* LRRK2 G2019S as a cause of Parkinson's disease in Ashkenazi Jews. *N Engl J Med* 2006; **354**: 424–425.

66. Lesage S, Leutenegger A-L, Ibanez P, *et al.* LRRK2 Haplotype analyses in European and North African families with Parkinson's disease: a common founder for the G2019S mutation dating from the 13th century. *Am J Hum Genet* 2005; **77**: 330–332.

67. Zabetian CP, Hutter CM, Yearout D, *et al.* LRRK2 G2019S in families with Parkinson disease who originated from Europe and the Middle East: evidence of two distinct founding events beginning two millennia ago. *Am J Hum Genet* 2006; **79**: 752–758.

68. Di Fonzo A, Wu-Chou YH, Lu CS, *et al.* A common missense variant in the LRRK2 gene, Gly2385Arg, associated with Parkinson's disease risk in Taiwan. *Neurogenetics* 2006; **7**: 133–138.

69. Tan EK, Zhao Y, Skipper L, *et al.* The LRRK2 Gly2385Arg variant is associated with Parkinson's disease: genetic and functional evidence. *Hum Genet* 2006; **120**: 857–863.

70. Adams JR, van Netten H, Schulzer M, *et al.* PET in LRRK2 mutations: comparison to sporadic Parkinson's disease and evidence for presymptomatic compensation. *Brain* 2005; **128**: 2777–2785.

71. Isaias IU, Benti R, Goldwurm S, *et al.* Striatal dopamine transporter binding in Parkinson's disease associated with the LRRK2 Gly2019Ser mutation. *Mov Disord* 2006; **21**: 1144–1147.

72. Ross OA, Toft M, Whittle AJ, *et al.* Lrrk2 and Lewy body disease. *Ann Neurol* 2006; **59**: 388–393.

73. Giasson BI, Covy JP, Bonini NM, *et al.* Biochemical and pathological characterization of Lrrk2. *Ann Neurol* 2006; **59**: 315–322.

74. Papapetropoulos S, Singer C, Ross OA, *et al.* Clinical heterogeneity of the LRRK2 G2019S mutation. *Arch Neurol* 2006; **63**: 1242–1246.

75. Wszolek ZK, Vieregge P, Uitti RJ, *et al.* German-Canadian family (Family A) with parkinsonism, amyotrophy, and dementia – longitudinal observations. *Parkinsonism Relat Disord* 1997; **3**: 125–139.

76. Wszolek ZK, Pfeiffer RF, Tsuboi Y, *et al.* Autosomal dominant parkinsonism associated with variable synuclein and tau pathology. *Neurology* 2004; **62**: 1619–1622.

77. Bonifati V. The pleomorphic pathology of inherited Parkinson's disease: lessons from LRRK2. *Curr Neurol Neurosci Rep* 2006; **6**: 355–357.

78. Uitti RJ, Calne DB, Dickson DW, Wszolek ZK. Is the neuropathological 'gold standard' diagnosis dead? Implications of clinicopathological findings in an autosomal dominant neurodegenerative disorder. *Parkinsonism Relat Disord* 2004; **10**: 461–463.

79. Smith WW, Pei Z, Jiang H, *et al.* Kinase activity of mutant LRRK2 mediates neuronal toxicity. *Nat Neurosci* 2006; **9**: 1231–1233.

80. Smith WW, Pei Z, Jiang H, *et al.* Leucine-rich repeat kinase 2 (LRRK2) interacts with parkin, and mutant LRRK2 induces neuronal degeneration. *Proc Natl Acad Sci USA* 2005; **102**: 18676–18681.

81. West AB, Moore DJ, Biskup S, *et al.* Parkinson's disease-associated mutations in leucine-rich repeat kinase 2 augment kinase activity. *Proc Natl Acad Sci USA* 2005; **102**: 16842–16847.

82. Gloeckner CJ, Kinkl N, Schumacher A, *et al.* The Parkinson disease causing LRRK2 mutation I2020T is associated with increased kinase activity. *Hum Mol Genet* 2006; **15**: 223–232.

83. Greggio E, Jain S, Kingsbury A, *et al.* Kinase activity is required for the toxic effects of mutant LRRK2/dardarin. *Neurobiol Dis* 2006; **23**: 329–341.

84. Kitada T, Asakawa S, Hattori N, *et al.* Mutations in the parkin gene cause autosomal recessive juvenile parkinsonism. *Nature* 1998; **392**: 605–608.

85. Lucking CB, Durr A, Bonifati V, *et al.* Association between early-onset Parkinson's disease and mutations in the parkin gene. *N Engl J Med* 2000; **342**: 1560–1567.

86. Hedrich K, Marder K, Harris J, *et al.* Evaluation of 50 probands with early-onset Parkinson's disease for Parkin mutations. *Neurology* 2002; **58**: 1239–1246.

87. Periquet M, Latouche M, Lohmann E, *et al.* Parkin mutations are frequent in patients with isolated early-onset parkinsonism. *Brain* 2003; **126**: 1271–1278.

88. Lohmann E, Periquet M, Bonifati V, et al. How much phenotypic variation can be attributed to parkin genotype? *Ann Neurol* 2003; **54**: 176–185.

89. Foroud T, Uniacke SK, Liu L, et al. Heterozygosity for a mutation in the parkin gene leads to later onset Parkinson disease. *Neurology* 2003; **60**: 796–801.

90. Hedrich K, Eskelson C, Wilmot B, et al. Distribution, type, and origin of Parkin mutations: review and case studies. *Mov Disord* 2004; **19**: 1146–1157.

91. Mori H, Kondo T, Yokochi M, et al. Pathologic and biochemical studies of juvenile parkinsonism linked to chromosome 6q. *Neurology* 1998; **51**: 890–892.

92. Farrer M, Chan P, Chen R, et al. Lewy bodies and parkinsonism in families with parkin mutations. *Ann Neurol* 2001; **50**: 293–300.

93. Pramstaller PP, Schlossmacher MG, Jacques TS, et al. Lewy body Parkinson's disease in a large pedigree with 77 Parkin mutation carriers. *Ann Neurol* 2005; **58**: 411–422.

94. Sasaki S, Shirata A, Yamane K, Iwata M. Parkin-positive autosomal recessive juvenile parkinsonism with alpha-synuclein-positive inclusions. *Neurology* 2004; **63**: 678–682.

95. Thobois S, Ribeiro MJ, Lohmann E, et al. Young-onset Parkinson disease with and without parkin gene mutations: a fluorodopa F 18 positron emission tomography study. *Arch Neurol* 2003; **60**: 713–718.

96. Scherfler C, Khan NL, Pavese N, et al. Striatal and cortical pre- and postsynaptic dopaminergic dysfunction in sporadic parkin-linked parkinsonism. *Brain* 2004; **127**: 1332–1342.

97. Shimura H, Hattori N, Kubo S, et al. Familial Parkinson disease gene product, parkin, is a ubiquitin-protein ligase. *Nat Genet* 2000; **25**: 302–305.

98. Feany MB, Pallanck LJ. Parkin: a multipurpose neuroprotective agent? *Neuron* 2003; **38**: 13–16.

99. Shimura H, Schlossmacher MG, Hattori N, et al. Ubiquitination of a new form of alpha-synuclein by parkin from human brain: implications for Parkinson's disease. *Science* 2001; **293**: 263–269.

100. Chung KK, Zhang Y, Lim KL, et al. Parkin ubiquitinates the alpha-synuclein-interacting protein, synphilin-1: implications for Lewy-body formation in Parkinson disease. *Nat Med* 2001; **7**: 1144–1150.

101. Petrucelli L, O 'Farrell C, Lockhart PJ, et al. Parkin protects against the toxicity associated with mutant alpha-synuclein: proteasome dysfunction selectively affects catecholaminergic neurons. *Neuron* 2002; **36**: 1007–1019.

102. Yang Y, Nishimura I, Imai Y, et al. Parkin suppresses dopaminergic neuron-selective neurotoxicity induced by Pael-R in Drosophila. *Neuron* 2003; **37**: 911–924.

103. Chung KK, Thomas B, Li X, et al. S-nitrosylation of parkin regulates ubiquitination and compromises parkin's protective function. *Science* 2004; **304**: 1328–1331.

104. Yao D, Gu Z, Nakamura T, et al. Nitrosative stress linked to sporadic Parkinson's disease: S-nitrosylation of parkin regulates its E3 ubiquitin ligase activity. *Proc Natl Acad Sci USA* 2004; **101**: 10810–10814.

105. Staropoli JF, McDermott C, Martinat C, et al. Parkin is a component of an SCF-like ubiquitin ligase complex and protects postmitotic neurons from kainate excitotoxicity. *Neuron* 2003; **37**: 735–749.

106. Corti O, Hampe C, Koutnikova H, et al. The p38 subunit of the aminoacyl-tRNA synthetase complex is a Parkin substrate: linking protein biosynthesis and neurodegeneration. *Hum Mol Genet* 2003; **12**: 1427–1437.

107. Greene JC, Whitworth AJ, Kuo I, et al. Mitochondrial pathology and apoptotic muscle degeneration in Drosophila parkin mutants. *Proc Natl Acad Sci USA* 2003; **100**: 4078–4083.

108. Goldberg MS, Fleming SM, Palacino JJ, et al. Parkin-deficient mice exhibit nigrostriatal deficits but not loss of dopaminergic neurons. *J Biol Chem* 2003; **278**: 43628–43635.

109. Itier JM, Ibanez P, Mena MA, et al. Parkin gene inactivation alters behaviour and dopamine neurotransmission in the mouse. *Hum Mol Genet* 2003; **12**: 2277–2291.

110. Von Coelln R, Thomas B, Savitt JM, et al. Loss of locus coeruleus neurons and reduced startle in parkin null mice. *Proc Natl Acad Sci USA* 2004; **101**: 10744–10749.

111. van Duijn CM, Dekker MC, Bonifati V, et al. Park7, a novel locus for autosomal recessive early-onset parkinsonism, on chromosome 1p36. *Am J Hum Genet* 2001; **69**: 629–634.

112. Bonifati V, Breedveld GJ, Squitieri F, et al. Localization of autosomal recessive early-onset parkinsonism to chromosome 1p36 (PARK7) in an independent dataset. *Ann Neurol* 2002; **51**: 253–256.

113. Bonifati V, Rizzu P, van Baren MJ, et al. Mutations in the DJ-1 gene associated with autosomal recessive early-onset parkinsonism. *Science* 2003; **299**: 256–259.

114. Abou-Sleiman PM, Healy DG, Quinn N, et al. The role of pathogenic DJ-1 mutations in Parkinson's disease. *Ann Neurol* 2003; **54**: 283–286.

115. Hague S, Rogaeva E, Hernandez D, *et al.* Early-onset Parkinson's disease caused by a compound heterozygous DJ-1 mutation. *Ann Neurol* 2003; **54**: 271–274.

116. Hedrich K, Djarmati A, Schafer N, *et al.* DJ-1 (PARK7) mutations are less frequent than Parkin (PARK2) mutations in early-onset Parkinson disease. *Neurology* 2004; **62**: 389–394.

117. Hering R, Strauss KM, Tao X, *et al.* Novel homozygous p.E64D mutation in DJ1 in early onset Parkinson disease (PARK7). *Hum Mutat* 2004; **24**: 321–329.

118. Djarmati A, Hedrich K, Svetel M, *et al.* Detection of Parkin (PARK2) and DJ1 (PARK7) mutations in early-onset Parkinson disease: Parkin mutation frequency depends on ethnic origin of patients. *Hum Mutat* 2004; **23**: 525.

119. Bonifati V, Oostra BA, Heutink P. Linking DJ-1 to neurodegeneration offers novel insights for understanding the pathogenesis of Parkinson's disease. *J Mol Med* 2004; **82**: 163–174.

120. Martinat C, Shendelman S, Jonason A, *et al.* Sensitivity to oxidative stress in DJ-1-deficient dopamine neurons: an ES-derived cell model of primary parkinsonism. *PLoS Biol* 2004; **2**: e327.

121. Taira T, Saito Y, Niki T, *et al.* DJ-1 has a role in antioxidative stress to prevent cell death. *EMBO Rep* 2004; **5**: 213–218.

122. Shendelman S, Jonason A, Martinat C, *et al.* DJ-1 is a redox-dependent molecular chaperone that inhibits alpha-synuclein aggregate formation. *PLoS Biol* 2004; **2**: e362.

123. Zhou W, Zhu M, Wilson MA, *et al.* The oxidation state of DJ-1 regulates its chaperone activity toward alpha-synuclein. *J Mol Biol* 2006; **356**: 1036–1048.

124. Moore DJ, Zhang L, Troncoso J, *et al.* Association of DJ-1 and parkin mediated by pathogenic DJ-1 mutations and oxidative stress. *Hum Mol Genet* 2005; **14**: 71–84.

125. Canet-Aviles RM, Wilson MA, Miller DW, *et al.* The Parkinson's disease protein DJ-1 is neuroprotective due to cysteine-sulfinic acid-driven mitochondrial localization. *Proc Natl Acad Sci USA* 2004; **101**: 9103–9108.

126. Zhang L, Shimoji M, Thomas B, *et al.* Mitochondrial localization of the Parkinson's disease related protein DJ-1: implications for pathogenesis. *Hum Mol Genet* 2005; **14**: 2063–2073.

127. Xu J, Zhong N, Wang H, *et al.* The Parkinson's disease-associated DJ-1 protein is a transcriptional co-activator that protects against neuronal apoptosis. *Hum Mol Genet* 2005; **14**: 1231–1241.

128. Kim RH, Peters M, Jang Y, *et al.* DJ-1, a novel regulator of the tumor suppressor PTEN. *Cancer Cell* 2005; 7: 263–273.

129. Junn E, Taniguchi H, Jeong BS, *et al.* Interaction of DJ-1 with Daxx inhibits apoptosis signal-regulating kinase 1 activity and cell death. *Proc Natl Acad Sci USA* 2005; **102**: 9691–9696.

130. Rizzu P, Hinkle DA, Zhucareva V, *et al.* DJ-1 colocalizes with tau inclusions: a link between parkinsonism and dementia. *Ann Neurol* 2004; **55**: 113–118.

131. Meulener MC, Graves CL, Sampathu DM, *et al.* DJ-1 is present in a large molecular complex in human brain tissue and interacts with alpha-synuclein. *J Neurochem* 2005; **93**: 1524–1532.

132. Neumann M, Muller V, Gorner K, *et al.* Pathological properties of the Parkinson's disease-associated protein DJ-1 in alpha-synucleinopathies and tauopathies: relevance for multiple system atrophy and Pick's disease. *Acta Neuropathol* 2004; **107**: 489–496.

133. Annesi G, Savettieri G, Pugliese P, *et al.* DJ-1 mutations and parkinsonism-dementia-amyotrophic lateral sclerosis complex. *Ann Neurol* 2005; **58**: 803–807.

134. Kim RH, Smith PD, Aleyasin H, *et al.* Hypersensitivity of DJ-1-deficient mice to 1-methyl-4-phenyl-1,2,3,6-tetrahydropyrindine (MPTP) and oxidative stress. *Proc Natl Acad Sci USA* 2005; **102**: 5215–5220.

135. Chen L, Cagniard B, Mathews T, *et al.* Age-dependent motor deficits and dopaminergic dysfunction in DJ-1 null mice. *J Biol Chem* 2005; **280**: 21418–21426.

136. Goldberg MS, Pisani A, Haburcak M, *et al.* Nigrostriatal dopaminergic deficits and hypokinesia caused by inactivation of the familial Parkinsonism-linked gene DJ-1. *Neuron* 2005; **45**: 489–496.

137. Meulener M, Whitworth AJ, Armstrong-Gold CE, *et al.* Drosophila DJ-1 mutants are selectively sensitive to environmental toxins associated with Parkinson's disease. *Curr Biol* 2005; **15**: 1572–1577.

138. Menzies FM, Yenisetti SC, Min KT. Roles of Drosophila DJ-1 in survival of dopaminergic neurons and oxidative stress. *Curr Biol* 2005; **15**: 1578–1582.

139. Yang Y, Gehrke S, Haque ME, *et al.* Inactivation of Drosophila DJ-1 leads to impairments of oxidative stress response and phosphatidylinositol 3-kinase/Akt signaling. *Proc Natl Acad Sci USA* 2005; **102**: 13670–13675.

140. Yang Y, Gehrke S, Imai Y, *et al.* Mitochondrial pathology and muscle and dopaminergic neuron degeneration caused by

99

inactivation of Drosophila Pink1 is rescued by Parkin. *Proc Natl Acad Sci USA* 2006; **103**: 10793–10798.

141. Tang B, Xiong H, Sun P, *et al.* Association of PINK1 and DJ-1 confers digenic inheritance of early-onset Parkinson's disease. *Hum Mol Genet* 2006; **15**: 1816–1825.

142. Valente EM, Bentivoglio AR, Dixon PH, *et al.* Localization of a novel locus for autosomal recessive early-onset parkinsonism, PARK6, on human chromosome 1p35-p36. *Am J Hum Genet* 2001; **68**: 895–900.

143. Valente EM, Brancati F, Ferraris A, *et al.* PARK6-linked parkinsonism occurs in several European families. *Ann Neurol* 2002; **51**: 14–18.

144. Hatano Y, Sato K, Elibol B, *et al.* PARK6-linked autosomal recessive early-onset parkinsonism in Asian populations. *Neurology* 2004; **63**: 1482–1485.

145. Valente EM, Abou-Sleiman PM, Caputo V, *et al.* Hereditary early-onset Parkinson's disease caused by mutations in PINK1. *Science* 2004; **304**: 1158–1160.

146. Petit A, Kawarai T, Paitel E, *et al.* Wild-type PINK1 prevents basal and induced neuronal apoptosis, a protective effect abrogated by Parkinson disease-related mutations. *J Biol Chem* 2005; **280**: 34025–34032.

147. Beilina A, Van Der Brug M, Ahmad R, *et al.* Mutations in PTEN-induced putative kinase 1 associated with recessive parkinsonism have differential effects on protein stability. *Proc Natl Acad Sci USA* 2005; **102**: 5703–5708.

148. Silvestri L, Caputo V, Bellacchio E, *et al.* Mitochondrial import and enzymatic activity of PINK1 mutants associated to recessive parkinsonism. *Hum Mol Genet* 2005; **14**: 3477–3492.

149. Muqit MM, Abou-Sleiman PM, Saurin AT, *et al.* Altered cleavage and localization of PINK1 to aggresomes in the presence of proteasomal stress. *J Neurochem* 2006; **98**: 156–169.

150. Jenner P. Oxidative stress in Parkinson's disease. *Ann Neurol* 2003; **53**: S26–S36; discussion S36–S28.

151. Beal MF. Mitochondria, oxidative damage, and inflammation in Parkinson's disease. *Ann NY Acad Sci* 2003; **991**: 120–131.

152. Rohe CF, Montagna P, Breedveld G, *et al.* Homozygous PINK1 C-terminus mutation causing early-onset parkinsonism. *Ann Neurol* 2004; **56**: 427–431.

153. Hatano Y, Li Y, Sato K, *et al.* Novel PINK1 mutations in early-onset parkinsonism. *Ann Neurol* 2004; **56**: 424–427.

154. Valente EM, Salvi S, Ialongo T, *et al.* PINK1 mutations are associated with sporadic early-onset parkinsonism. *Ann Neurol* 2004; **56**: 336–341.

155. Healy DG, Abou-Sleiman PM, Gibson JM, *et al.* PINK1 (PARK6) associated Parkinson disease in Ireland. *Neurology* 2004; **63**: 1486–1488.

156. Rogaeva E, Johnson J, Lang AE, *et al.* Analysis of the PINK1 gene in a large cohort of cases with Parkinson disease. *Arch Neurol* 2004; **61**: 1898–1904.

157. Bonifati V, Rohe CF, Breedveld GJ, *et al.* Early-onset parkinsonism associated with PINK1 mutations: frequency, genotypes, and phenotypes. *Neurology* 2005; **65**: 87–95.

158. Klein C, Djarmati A, Hedrich K, *et al.* PINK1, Parkin, and DJ-1 mutations in Italian patients with early-onset parkinsonism. *Eur J Hum Genet* 2005; **13**: 1086–1093.

159. Ibanez P, Lesage S, Lohmann E, *et al.* Mutational analysis of the PINK1 gene in early-onset parkinsonism in Europe and North Africa. *Brain* 2006; **129**: 686–694.

160. Abou-Sleiman PM, Muqit MM, McDonald NQ, *et al.* A heterozygous effect for PINK1 mutations in Parkinson's disease? *Ann Neurol* 2006; **60**: 414–419.

161. Clark IE, Dodson MW, Jiang C, *et al.* Drosophila pink1 is required for mitochondrial function and interacts genetically with parkin. *Nature* 2006; **441**: 1162–1166.

162. Park J, Lee SB, Lee S, *et al.* Mitochondrial dysfunction in Drosophila PINK1 mutants is complemented by parkin. *Nature* 2006; **441**: 1157–1161.

163. Heutink P. Untangling tau-related dementia. *Hum Mol Genet* 2000; **9**: 979–986.

164. Rademakers R, Cruts M, van Broeckhoven C. The role of tau (MAPT) in frontotemporal dementia and related tauopathies. *Hum Mutat* 2004; **24**: 277–295.

165. Furtado S, Payami H, Lockhart PJ, *et al.* Profile of families with parkinsonism-predominant spinocerebellar ataxia type 2 (SCA2). *Mov Disord* 2004; **19**: 622–629.

166. Gwinn-Hardy K, Singleton A, O'Suilleabhain P, *et al.* Spinocerebellar ataxia type 3 phenotypically resembling parkinson disease in a black family. *Arch Neurol* 2001; **58**: 296–299.

167. Davidzon G, Greene P, Mancuso M, *et al.* Early-onset familial parkinsonism due to POLG mutations. *Ann Neurol* 2006; **59**: 859–862.

168. de Carvalho Aguiar P, Sweadner KJ, Penniston JT, *et al.* Mutations in the Na^+/K^+-ATPase alpha3 gene ATP1A3 are associated with rapid-onset dystonia parkinsonism. *Neuron* 2004; **43**: 169–175.

169. Evidente VG, Advincula J, Esteban R, et al. Phenomenology of Lubag or X-linked dystonia-parkinsonism. Mov Disord 2002; 17: 1271–1277.

170. Gasser T, Muller-Myhsok B, Wszolek ZK, et al. A susceptibility locus for Parkinson's disease maps to chromosome 2p13. Nat Genet 1998; 18: 262–265.

171. DeStefano AL, Lew MF, Golbe LI, et al. PARK3 influences age at onset in Parkinson disease: a genome scan in the GenePD study. Am J Hum Genet 2002; 70: 1089–1095.

172. Martinez M, Brice A, Vaughan JR, et al. Genome-wide scan linkage analysis for Parkinson's disease: the European genetic study of Parkinson's disease. J Med Genet 2004; 41: 900–907.

173. Karamohamed S, DeStefano AL, Wilk JB, et al. A haplotype at the PARK3 locus influences onset age for Parkinson's disease: the GenePD study. Neurology 2003; 61: 1557–1561.

174. Sharma M, Mueller JC, Zimprich A, et al. The sepiapterin reductase gene region reveals association in the PARK3 locus: analysis of familial and sporadic Parkinson's disease in European populations. J Med Genet 2006; 43: 557–562.

175. Hampshire DJ, Roberts E, Crow Y, et al. Kufor–Rakeb syndrome, pallido-pyramidal degeneration with supranuclear upgaze paresis and dementia, maps to 1p36. J Med Genet 2001; 38: 680–682.

176. Williams DR, Hadeed A, al-Din AS, et al. Kufor Rakeb disease: autosomal recessive, levodopa-responsive parkinsonism with pyramidal degeneration, supranuclear gaze palsy, and dementia. Mov Disord 2005; 20: 1264–1271.

177. Ramirez A, Heimbach A, Grundemann J, et al. Hereditary parkinsonism with dementia is caused by mutations in ATP13A2, encoding a lysosomal type 5 P-type ATPase. Nat Genet 2006; 38: 1184–1191.

178. Bertoli Avella AM, Giroud Benitez JL, Bonifati V, et al. Suggestive linkage to chromosome 19 in a large Cuban family with late-onset Parkinson's disease. Mov Disord 2003; 18: 1240–1249.

179. Bonifati V, Heutink P. Chromosome 1 and other hotspots for Parkinson 's disease genes. In Molecular Mechanisms of Parkinson 's Disease. Madame Curie Bioscience Database [Internet]. Austin, TX, USA: Landes Bioscience, 2000. Bookshelf ID: NBK6225.

180. Bertoli-Avella AM, Dekker MC, Aulchenko YS, et al. Evidence for novel loci for late-onset Parkinson's disease in a genetic isolate from the Netherlands. Hum Genet 2006; 119: 51–60.

181. Hicks AA, Petursson H, Jonsson T, et al. A susceptibility gene for late-onset idiopathic Parkinson's disease. Ann Neurol 2002; 52: 549–555.

182. Pankratz N, Nichols WC, Uniacke SK, et al. Significant linkage of Parkinson disease to chromosome 2q36–37. Am J Hum Genet 2003; 72: 1053–1057.

183. Pankratz N, Nichols WC, Uniacke SK, et al. Genome-wide linkage analysis and evidence of gene-by-gene interactions in a sample of 362 multiplex Parkinson disease families. Hum Mol Genet 2003; 12: 2599–2608.

184. Osaka H, Wang YL, Takada K, et al. Ubiquitin carboxy-terminal hydrolase L1 binds to and stabilizes monoubiquitin in neuron. Hum Mol Genet 2003; 12: 1945–1958.

185. Leroy E, Boyer R, Auburger G, et al. The ubiquitin pathway in Parkinson's disease. Nature 1998; 395: 451–452.

186. Maraganore DM, Lesnick TG, Elbaz A, et al. UCHL1 is a Parkinson's disease susceptibility gene. Ann Neurol 2004; 55: 512–521.

187. Healy DG, Abou-Sleiman PM, Casas JP, et al. UCHL-1 is not a Parkinson's disease susceptibility gene. Ann Neurol 2006; 59: 627–633.

188. Le WD, Xu P, Jankovic J, et al. Mutations in NR4A2 associated with familial Parkinson disease. Nat Genet 2003; 33: 85–89.

189. Zimprich A, Asmus F, Leitner P, et al. Point mutations in exon 1 of the NR4A2 gene are not a major cause of familial Parkinson's disease. Neurogenetics 2003; 4: 219–220.

190. Wellenbrock C, Hedrich K, Schafer N, et al. NR4A2 mutations are rare among European patients with familial Parkinson's disease. Ann Neurol 2003; 54: 415.

191. Levecque C, Destee A, Mouroux V, et al. Assessment of Nurr1 nucleotide variations in familial Parkinson's disease. Neurosci Lett 2004; 366: 135–138.

192. Nichols WC, Uniacke SK, Pankratz N, et al. Evaluation of the role of Nurr1 in a large sample of familial Parkinson's disease. Mov Disord 2004; 19: 649–655.

193. Grimes DA, Han F, Panisset M, et al. Translated mutation in the Nurr1 gene as a cause for Parkinson's disease. Mov Disord 2006; 21: 906–909.

194. Engelender S, Kaminsky Z, Guo X, et al. Synphilin-1 associates with alpha-synuclein and promotes the formation of cytosolic inclusions. Nat Genet 1999; 22: 110–114.

195. Wakabayashi K, Engelender S, Yoshimoto M, et al. Synphilin-1 is present in Lewy bodies in Parkinson's disease. Ann Neurol 2000; 47: 521–523.

196. Murray IJ, Medford MA, Guan HP, *et al*. Synphilin in normal human brains and in synucleinopathies: studies with new antibodies. *Acta Neuropathol* 2003; **105**: 177–184.

197. Marx FP, Holzmann C, Strauss KM, *et al*. Identification and functional characterization of a novel R621C mutation in the synphilin-1 gene in Parkinson's disease. *Hum Mol Genet* 2003; **12**: 1223–1231.

198. Martins LM, Morrison A, Klupsch K, *et al*. Neuroprotective role of the Reaper-related serine protease HtrA2/Omi revealed by targeted deletion in mice. *Mol Cell Biol* 2004; **24**: 9848–9862.

199. Strauss KM, Martins LM, Plun-Favreau H, *et al*. Loss of function mutations in the gene encoding Omi/HtrA2 in Parkinson's disease. *Hum Mol Genet* 2005; **14**: 2099–2111.

200. Aharon-Peretz J, Rosenbaum H, Gershoni-Baruch R. Mutations in the glucocerebrosidase gene and Parkinson's disease in Ashkenazi Jews. *N Engl J Med* 2004; **351**: 1972–1977.

201. Toft M, Pielsticker L, Ross OA, *et al*. Glucocerebrosidase gene mutations and Parkinson disease in the Norwegian population. *Neurology* 2006; **66**: 415–417.

202. Sato C, Morgan A, Lang AE, *et al*. Analysis of the glucocerebrosidase gene in Parkinson's disease. *Mov Disord* 2005; **20**: 367–370.

203. Clark LN, Nicolai A, Afridi S, *et al*. Pilot association study of the beta-glucocerebrosidase N370S allele and Parkinson's disease in subjects of Jewish ethnicity. *Mov Disord* 2005; **20**: 100–103.

204. Goker-Alpan O, Giasson BI, Eblan MJ, *et al*.

Glucocerebrosidase mutations are an important risk factor for Lewy body disorders. *Neurology* 2006; **67**: 908–910.

205. Lee HJ, Khoshaghideh F, Patel S, Lee SJ. Clearance of alpha-synuclein oligomeric intermediates via the lysosomal degradation pathway. *J Neurosci* 2004; **24**: 1888–1896.

206. Webb JL, Ravikumar B, Atkins J, *et al*. Alpha-synuclein is degraded by both autophagy and the proteasome. *J Biol Chem* 2003; **278**: 25009–25013.

207. Foltynie T, Sawcer S, Brayne C, Barker RA. The genetic basis of Parkinson's disease. *J Neurol Neurosurg Psychiatry* 2002; **73**: 363–370.

208. Martin ER, Scott WK, Nance MA, *et al*. Association of single-nucleotide polymorphisms of the tau gene with late-onset Parkinson disease. *JAMA* 2001; **286**: 2245–2250.

209. van der Walt JM, Nicodemus KK, Martin ER, *et al*. Mitochondrial polymorphisms significantly reduce the risk of Parkinson disease. *Am J Hum Genet* 2003; **72**: 804–811.

210. Li YJ, Oliveira SA, Xu P, *et al*. Glutathione S-transferase omega-1 modifies age-at-onset of Alzheimer disease and Parkinson disease. *Hum Mol Genet* 2003; **12**: 3259–3267.

211. van der Walt JM, Noureddine MA, Kittappa R, *et al*. Fibroblast growth factor 20 polymorphisms and haplotypes strongly influence risk of Parkinson disease. *Am J Hum Genet* 2004; **74**: 1121–1127.

212. Healy DG, Abou-Sleiman PM, Ozawa T, *et al*. A functional polymorphism regulating dopamine beta-hydroxylase influences against Parkinson's

disease. *Ann Neurol* 2004; **55**: 443–446.

213. Palmer LJ, Cardon LR. Shaking the tree: mapping complex disease genes with linkage disequilibrium. *Lancet* 2005; **366**: 1223–1234.

214. Wang WY, Barratt BJ, Clayton DG, Todd JA. Genome-wide association studies: theoretical and practical concerns. *Nat Rev Genet* 2005; **6**: 109–118.

215. Hirschhorn JN, Daly MJ. Genome-wide association studies for common diseases and complex traits. *Nat Rev Genet* 2005; **6**: 95–108.

216. Maraganore DM, de Andrade M, Lesnick TG, *et al*. High-resolution whole-genome association study of Parkinson disease. *Am J Hum Genet* 2005; **77**: 685–693.

217. Myers DR. Considerations for genome-wide association studies in Parkinson disease. *Am J Hum Genet* 2006; **78**: 1081–1082.

218. Varilo T, Peltonen L. Isolates and their potential use in complex gene mapping efforts. *Curr Opin Genet Dev* 2004; **14**: 316–323.

219. McInerney-Leo A. Genetic testing in Parkinson's disease. *Mov Disord* 2005; **20**: 908–909.

220. McInerney-Leo A, Hadley DW, Gwinn-Hardy K, Hardy J. Genetic testing in Parkinson's disease. *Mov Disord* 2005; **20**: 1–10.

221. Klein C, Schlossmacher MG. The genetics of Parkinson disease: implications for neurological care. *Nat Clin Pract Neurol* 2006; **2**: 136–146.

222. Klein C. Implications of genetics on the diagnosis and care of patients with Parkinson disease. *Arch Neurol* 2006; **63**: 328–334.

Prion diseases

Simon Mead and John Collinge

Introduction and history

The prion diseases are a closely related group of neurodegenerative conditions that affect both humans and animals. The prototypic disease is scrapie, a naturally occurring disease affecting sheep and goats, which has been recognized in Europe for over 200 years [1] and is present in many countries worldwide. Since the 1980s, a new animal prion disease, bovine spongiform encephalopathy (BSE), has been described in the United Kingdom and is now recognized in most European Union countries, Japan, Canada, and the United States. The human prion diseases have traditionally been classified into Creutzfeldt–Jakob disease (CJD), Gerstmann–Sträussler syndrome (GSS) (also known as Gerstmann–Sträussler–Scheinker disease), and kuru. Although these are rare neurodegenerative disorders, affecting about one to two persons per million worldwide per annum, remarkable attention has recently been focused on these diseases. This is because of the unique biology of the transmissible agent or prion, and also because of the fears that an epidemic of BSE could pose a threat to public health through dietary exposure to infected tissues.

The distinctive feature of prion diseases is their transmissibility, first demonstrated by the transmission of scrapie by inoculation between sheep (and goats) with prolonged incubation periods [2]. Both the animal and human conditions share common histopathological features: the classical triad of spongiform vacuolation (affecting any part of the cerebral gray matter), neuronal loss, and astrocytic proliferation that may be accompanied by amyloid plaques [3]. In 1959, Hadlow drew attention to similarities between kuru and scrapie at the neuropathological, clinical, and epidemiological levels, leading to the suggestion that the human diseases may also be transmissible [4,5]. A landmark in the field was the transmission, by intracerebral inoculation with brain homogenates into chimpanzees, of first kuru and then CJD by Gajdusek and colleagues in 1966 and 1968, respectively [6,7]. The new criterion of transmissibility allowed diagnostic criteria for CJD to be assessed and refined. Atypical cases could be classified as CJD on the basis of their transmissibility.

The nature of the transmissible agent in these diseases has been a subject of heated debate. Progressive enrichment of brain homogenates for infectivity resulted in the isolation of a protease resistant sialoglycoprotein, designated the prion protein (PrP), by Prusiner and co-workers in 1982, in fractions enriched for scrapie infectivity (designated PrP^{Sc} for the scrapie isoform of the protein) [8]. The protease resistant PrP extracted from affected brains was demonstrated, in 1985, to be encoded by a single copy chromosomal gene, rather than by a putative nucleic acid. The normal product of the PrP gene is protease sensitive and designated PrP^{C} (denoting the cellular isoform of the protein). No differences in amino acid sequence between PrP^{Sc} and PrP^{C} have been identified. PrP^{Sc} is known to be derived from PrP^{C} by a posttranslational process [9,10]. The precise mechanisms of this conversion process and subsequent neurotoxicity remain unclear.

Clinical features of human prion diseases

The clinically defined categories: CJD, GSS, and kuru may be divided further into three etiological categories: sporadic, acquired, and inherited.

Sporadic (classical) Creutzfeldt–Jakob disease

Epidemiological studies do not provide any evidence for an association between sheep scrapie and the occurrence of CJD in humans [11]. Sporadic CJD occurs in all countries with a random case distribution and an annual incidence of one to two per million. Classical (sporadic) CJD is a rapidly progressive multifocal dementia, usually with myoclonus. The onset is typically in the 45 to 75 year age group, with peak onset between 60 and 65 years. Clinical progression may occur over weeks, progressing to akinetic mutism and death within two to three months. Approximately 70% of cases die in less than six months. About 10% of cases have a clinical duration of more than two years. Prodromal features, present in about one third of cases, include fatigue, insomnia, depression, weight loss, headaches, general malaise, and ill-defined pain sensations. In addition to mental deterioration and myoclonus, frequent additional neurological features include extrapyramidal signs, cerebellar ataxia, pyramidal signs, and cortical blindness.

Acquired prion disease: iatrogenic and variant Creutzfeldt–Jakob disease

While prion diseases can be transmitted to experimental animals by inoculation, it is important to appreciate that they are not contagious in humans. Documented case-to-case spread has only occurred by cannibalism (kuru) or following accidental inoculation with prions. Such iatrogenic routes include the use of inadequately sterilized intracerebral electrodes, dura mater and corneal grafting, and from the use of human cadaveric pituitary-derived growth hormone or gonadotrophin. Interestingly, cases arising from intracerebral or optic inoculation manifest clinically as classical CJD, with a rapidly progressive dementia, while those resulting from peripheral inoculation present frequently with a progressive cerebellar ataxia initially, reminiscent of kuru. Unsurprisingly, the incubation period in intracerebral cases is short (19–46 months for dura mater grafts) as compared to peripheral cases (mean estimated at about 15 years).

The appearance of a novel acquired human prion disease, variant CJD (vCJD), in the United Kingdom from 1995 onwards, and the experimental evidence that this is caused by the same prion strain as that causing BSE in cattle, raised the possibility that an epidemic of vCJD will occur in the United Kingdom and other countries as a result of dietary or other exposure to BSE prions [12,13]. These concerns, together with the iatrogenic transmission of

preclinical vCJD via blood transfusion [14–16] and potentially via medical and surgical procedures, have led to an intensification of efforts to understand the molecular basis of prion propagation and to develop rational therapeutics.

Variant CJD has a clinical presentation in which behavioral and psychiatric disturbances predominate and in some cases there are marked sensory phenomena (notably dysesthesia or pain in the limbs or face) [17,18]. Initial referral is often to a psychiatrist – the most prominent feature is depression – but anxiety, withdrawal, and behavioral change are also frequent. Other features include delusions, emotional lability, aggression, insomnia, and auditory and visual hallucinations. In most patients, a progressive cerebellar syndrome develops with gait and limb ataxia. Dementia develops later in the clinical course. Myoclonus is seen in most patients and prominent chorea occurs in some cases. The age at onset ranges from teenagers to old age (mean late 20s) and the clinical course is unusually prolonged (median 14 months).

Variant CJD can be diagnosed by detection of characteristic PrP immunostaining and PrP^{Sc} on tonsil biopsy [18,19]. Importantly, PrP^{Sc} is only detectable in tonsil and other lymphoreticular tissues in vCJD, and not other forms of human prion disease, indicating that it has a distinctive pathogenesis. The PrP^{Sc} type detected on Western blot in vCJD tonsil has a characteristic pattern. The neuropathological appearances of vCJD are striking and consistent [20]. While there is widespread spongiform change, gliosis, and neuronal loss, most severe in the basal ganglia and thalamus, the most remarkable feature is the abundant PrP amyloid plaques in cerebral and cerebellar cortex. These consist of kuru-like, florid (surrounded by spongiform vacuoles), and multicentric plaque types. The florid plaques, seen previously only in scrapie, are a particularly unusual but highly consistent feature. There is also abundant pericellular PrP deposition in the cerebral and cerebellar cortex and in the molecular layer of the cerebellum. Some of the features of vCJD are reminiscent of kuru [21], in which behavioral changes and progressive ataxia predominate. In addition, peripheral sensory disturbances are well recognized in the kuru prodrome. Kuru plaques are seen in about 70% of cases and are especially abundant in younger kuru cases. The observation that iatrogenic prion disease related to peripheral exposure to human prions has a more kuru-like than CJD-like clinical picture may well be relevant and would be consistent with a peripheral prion exposure in vCJD. The relatively stereotyped clinical presentation and neuropathology of vCJD contrasts sharply with sporadic CJD. This may be because vCJD is caused by a single prion strain and may also suggest that a relatively homogeneous, genetically susceptible, subgroup of the population with short incubation periods to BSE has been selected to date.

Inherited prion disease

Syndromes and epidemiology

Approximately 10%–15% of human prion disease is inherited and all cases to date have been associated with coding mutations in the prion protein gene (PRNP) of which over 30 distinct types are recognized. The recognition that the familial forms of the human diseases are autosomal dominant inherited conditions, associated with PRNP coding mutations [22,23], as well as being transmissible to laboratory animals by inoculation, strongly supported the contention that the transmissible agent or prion was composed principally of an abnormal isoform of prion protein.

The identification of one of the pathogenic mutations of PRNP in a case with neurodegenerative disease allows diagnosis of an inherited prion disease (IPD) and subclassification according to the mutation [24]. Pathogenic mutations have been described in two groups: (1) point mutations resulting in amino acid substitutions in PrP or production of a stop codon resulting in expression of a truncated PrP; (2) alteration of the number of integral copies of an octapeptide repeat present in a tandem array of five copies in the normal protein (OPRI) (Figure 8.1). Kindreds with inherited prion disease have been described with phenotypes of classical CJD, GSS, and with a range of other neurodegenerative syndromes. Some families show remarkable phenotypic variability, which can encompass both CJD- and GSS-like cases as well as other cases that do not conform to either CJD or GSS phenotypes [25]. Such atypical prion diseases may lack the classical histological features of a spongiform encephalopathy entirely although PrP immunohistochemistry is usually positive [26] (Figure 8.2). Progressive dementia, cerebellar ataxia, pyramidal signs, chorea, myoclonus, extrapyramidal features, pseudobulbar signs, seizures, and amyotrophic features are seen in variable combinations. Core features are shown in Table 8.1.

A number of surveillance reports and screening studies provide useful data about the epidemiology and importance of IPD. Mutation screening of dementia has shown that prion disease is a frequent cause of inherited early onset dementia. Finckh, for example, tested four genes (APP, PSEN1, PSEN2, and PRNP) in 36 patients with familial early onset dementia and found PRNP accounted for four in 12 mutation positive cases [27]. A general epidemiological account of IPD is problematic, however, for a number of reasons. There is considerable geographical variation in the incidence of IPD related to the population genetic effects of drift and migration on ancestral mutations. An accurate incidence of IPD as a proportion of the totality of prion disease is also difficult because of the poor overall ascertainment of prion disease. An autopsy study found that 40% of cases of neuropathological prion disease were undiagnosed while alive [28]. Furthermore, the referral of cases to national CJD surveillance units is likely to be biased toward the phenotype of sporadic CJD rather than more common and slowly progressive neurodegenerative diseases. Despite these issues, a number of units have reviewed the population incidence of IPD, summarized by the EUROCJD group [29]. It remains to be seen if the large populations of South and East Asia will have a similar epidemiology of IPD, but if a generality is to be made in the absence of data from these regions, the most common worldwide PRNP gene mutations are E200K, D178N, P102L, V210I, and 6-OPRI.

Pathogenic missense mutations of PRNP

P102L (c.305C>T)

The P102L mutation, first reported in 1989 in a UK and US family [23], is the archetypal example of the GSS syndrome, which was later described in association with the less frequently occurring F198S, A117V, P105L, G131V, Y145X, H187R, and some D178N mutations. The first case of GSS was described by Gerstmann in 1928 and was followed by a more detailed report on seven other affected members of the same family in 1936 [30]. The classical presentation is a chronic cerebellar ataxia accompanied by pyramidal features, with dementia occurring later. The histological hallmark is the presence of multicentric amyloid plaques. Transmissibility to experimental animals has been demonstrated.

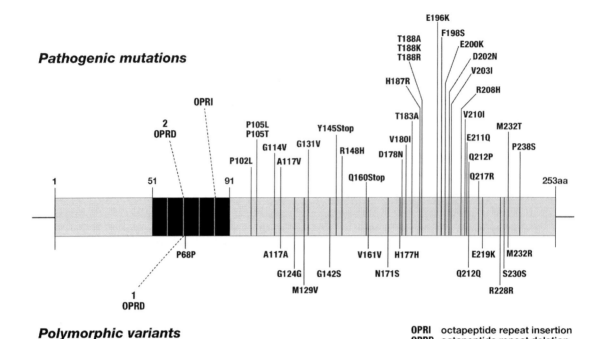

Figure 8.1. Definite or suspected pathogenic mutations are shown above this representation of the prion protein gene. Neutral or prion disease susceptibility/modifying polymorphisms are shown below.

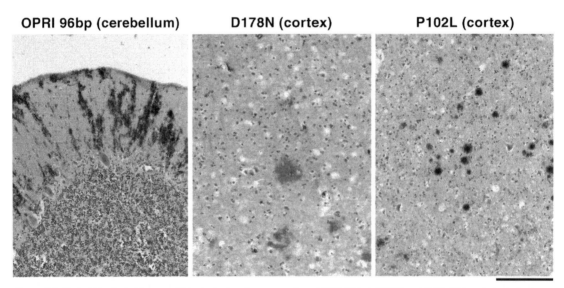

Figure 8.2. Typical histological features of inherited prion disease mutations 4-OPRI (96 bp), D178N, and P102L. Histopathologically, the 4-OPRI mutation shows stripe-like deposits of PrP^{Sc} in the molecular layer of the cerebellum, the D178N mutation shows spongiform change and fluffy deposits of PrP^{Sc}, and the P102L mutation shows multiple unicentric plaques of PrP^{Sc} deposition. Classical Gerstmann–Sträussler syndrome is associated with uni- or multicentric PrP plaques in the cerebellar cortex and cerebral cortex with variable spongiform change and neurofibrillary tangles; fatal familial insomnia is associated with anterior and dorsomedial thalamic atrophy with variable extrathalamic spongiosis and gliosis; and classical familial Creutzfeldt–Jakob disease is associated with cortical neuronal loss, spongiosis, gliosis, and variable PrP deposits. Immunohistochemistry with prion protein antibody ICSM35 is shown. Scale bar is 150 μm. (Images provided by Professor S. Bradner.)

Table 8.1. Typical age of onset, range, and clinical features of inherited prion disease mutations

Mutation	Median onset age (years)	Range (years)	Clinical features	Modification by codon 129 genotype	Transmission
P102L	50	25–70	GSS, heterogeneous	Yes	Yes
P105L	45	38–50	GSS, spastic paraparesis	Not known	Not known
G114V	22	18–27	GSS, neuropsychiatric and extrapyramidal signs prominent	Not known	Not known
A117V	40	20–64	GSS with early cognitive, neuropsychiatric, extrapyramidal features	Yes	No
G131V	42		GSS	Not known	Not known
Y145X	38		Dementia	Not known	No
R148H	72	63–82	CJD	Not known	Not known
Q160X	40	32–48	Dementia	Not known	Not known
D178N	50	20–72	FFI, CJD	Possible	Yes
V180I	74	58–81	CJD	Not known	Not known
T183A	45	37–49	Prominent behavioral abnormalities, one patient with dementia and no additional signs	Not known	Not known
H187R	32	20–53	Early onset with personality disorder in one family	Not known	Not known
T188A	82		CJD	Not known	Not known
T188K	59		CJD	Not known	Not known
E196K	69		CJD	Not known	Not known
F198S	56	40–71	GSS	Yes	Not known
E200K	58	33–78	CJD	Yes	Yes
D202N	73		Dementia	Not known	Not known
V203I	69		CJD	Not known	Not known
R208H	59	58–60	CJD	Not known	Not known
V210I	58	54–68	CJD	Not known	Yes
E211Q	69		CJD	Not known	Not known
Q212P	60		Ataxia, no dementia	Not known	Not known
Q217R	64	62–66	CJD, frontotemporal dementia	Not known	Not known
4-OPRI	62	56–82	CJD	Not known	Not known
5-OPRI	45	26–61	GSS, CJD, variable, some with prominent extrapyramidal signs	Yes	Not known
6-OPRI	34	20–53	GSS, CJD, variable, personality and psychiatric features and extrapyramidal signs	Yes	Yes

Table 8.1. (cont.)

Mutation	Median onset age (years)	Range (years)	Clinical features	Modification by codon 129 genotype	Transmission
7-OPRI	29	23–35	GSS, CJD, variable, personality and psychiatric features	Not known	Yes
8-OPRI	38	21–55	GSS, CJD, variable, personality and psychiatric features	Not known	Yes
9-OPRI	44	34–54	GSS	Not known	Not known
2-OPRD			CJD	Not known	Not known

Modification by codon 129 and transmission to laboratory animals is shown where known. In this table, GSS is used to refer to the clinical combination of a slowly progressive ataxia, spasticity, and dementia.
GSS, Gerstmann–Sträussler syndrome; CJD, Creutzfeldt–Jakob disease; FFI, fatal familial insomnia.

Phenotypic variability is a major feature: median age of onset in 52 reported cases was 50 years (range 25–70 years) and median duration of disease was four years (range 5 months to 17 years) [31–36]. Families with amyotrophic features [37] and patients with a rapidly deteriorating course are seen occasionally. The variable involvement of wild-type PrP in the disease process may contribute to phenotypic heterogeneity [38].

P105L (c.314C>T)

This mutation was originally reported in three Japanese families [39] with a history of spastic paraparesis and dementia, and the clinical duration is about five years. There were no periodic synchronous discharges on EEG. Neuropathological examination showed plaques in the cerebral cortex (but not cerebellum) and neuronal loss, but no spongiosis. Neurofibrillary tangles were variably present. A more recent case series described clinical and pathological heterogeneity, with only half the patients having a spastic paraparesis. The age of onset of eight cases ranged from 38 to 50 years [40]. This mutation has also been seen in the United Kingdom (unpublished).

G114V (c.341G>T)

Reported in a single Uruguayan family with five affected individuals [41], this mutation is associated with a remarkably early age of onset and early mood and psychiatric disturbances (range 18–27 years). Unusually, two living family members in their fifth decade of life carrying the mutation had no signs of disease.

A117V (c.350C>T)

First described in a French family [42] and subsequently in a US family of German origin [43], clinical features of this mutation are presenile dementia with pyramidal signs, parkinsonism, pseudobulbar features, and cerebellar signs. Neuropathologically, PrP immunoreactive plaques are usually present, but spongiosis and tau pathology are variable. This mutation has also been identified in a large family in the United Kingdom [44]. Of 39 reported patients, age of onset ranged from 20 to 64 years.

G131V (c.392G>T)

This mutation was reported in a patient with a nine-year progressive cortical dementia with onset when aged 42 years [45]. Intense PrP deposition was seen at autopsy in the molecular layer of the cerebellum with little spongiform change.

Y145X (c.435T>G)

This mutation was detected in a Japanese patient with a clinical diagnosis of Alzheimer's disease. She developed memory disturbance at the age of 38 years with a duration of illness of 21 years. Neuropathological examination revealed typical Alzheimer-like pathology without spongiform change [46]. Many PrP plaques along with paired helical filaments were seen in the cortex.

R148H (c.443G>A)

Reported in two patients with a sporadic CJD-like phenotype, aged 63 and 82 yeas, this mutation is not definitely pathogenic [47,48]. The same change has been found in a healthy chimpanzee [49].

Q160X (c.478C>T)

This mutation was found in a screen of families with early onset dementia without neurological signs [27]. Two members of one family aged 32 and 48 years at onset segregate for the mutation with dementia. No analysis of brain tissue has been performed.

D178N (c.532G>A)

This mutation was first reported in Finnish families with a CJD-like illness [50]. Subsequently, the same mutation was identified in families with a condition known as fatal familial insomnia (FFI). A large family case series was reported by Medori *et al.* (1992) [51], who described an untreatable insomnia, dysautonomia, and myoclonus. Histopathologically, selective degeneration of the anteroventral and dorsomedial thalamus with variable cortical spongiform change and weak PrP immunocytochemical staining was seen [52].

In 1992, Goldfarb *et al.* [53] established a haplotypic relationship between codon 129 and 178, whereby the mutation on a 129M chromosome leads to FFI, and the mutation on a 129V chromosome leads to familial CJD. However, there are pedigrees that segregate both the FFI and CJD phenotype [54], and it has become increasingly recognized that autonomic and sleep disturbances may accompany other *PRNP* gene mutations, sometimes overtly [55]. Patients with D178N reported to the CJD surveillance unit in Germany were less clinically distinct than the first reported FFI families in that none were clinically diagnosed with FFI owing to an absence of obvious insomnia and no positive family history was obtained in four of nine individuals [56]. Pocchiari *et al.* (1998) noted that of the patients presenting with overt sleep disturbance to a CJD unit, four of nine cases had sporadic CJD, one had a V210I mutation, but none had the D178N mutation [57]. Of 72 case reports, the median age of onset was 50 years (range 20–72 years) and the median duration of disease was 11 months (range 5 months to 4 years).

CJD-like codon 178 patient material has frequently transmitted to experimental animals while the FFI type did not transmit to laboratory primates [58]. However, transmission of FFI to mice has been reported [59,60].

V180I (c.538G>A)

This mutation has now been described in nine elderly Japanese patients without family history [61]. The presentation was similar to sporadic CJD, but overall progression was slower and age of onset later (range 58–81 years). The EEG did not show pseudoperiodic sharp wave activity. Neuropathological examination demonstrated spongiform change, neuronal loss, and astrocytosis.

T183A (c.547A>G)

This mutation was reported in a Brazilian family with nine affected family members. The clinical picture mimicked frontotemporal dementia with a mean onset of 45 years and duration of four years [62]. Parkinsonian features were also present in some patients. Neuropathological examination revealed severe spongiform change and neuronal loss in the deep cortical layers and putamen with little gliosis. PrP immunoreactivity was demonstrated in the putamen and cerebellum. A second occurrence in a patient with dementia and no additional neurological signs has since been described [27].

H187R (c.560A>G)

This mutation has been reported in two families with differing clinical phenotypes. In the first, onset ranged from 37 to 53 years in three patients examined, with limb ataxia, dysarthria, and cognitive decline [63]. More recently, a large family report included many individuals with disease onset in the third decade of life and prominent childhood personality disorder [64] similar to that described in the large UK 6-OPRI pedigree. No distinctive neuropathological features were detected in four brains examined. Tau pathology has been variably observed.

T188A (c.562A>G), T188K (c.563C>A), T188R (c.563C>G)

The T188A mutation has been found in an octogenarian with clinical and autopsy features of CJD [65].

109

The mutation T188K was identified in a 59-year-old patient with a rapidly progressive dementia and dysarthria [27]; prion disease has not been confirmed. The T188R mutation was discovered in a single patient from a screen of those referred to a German CJD surveillance unit [66]; similarly, prion disease has not been confirmed.

E196 K (c.586G>A)

This mutation was seen in a French patient, aged 69 years, with rapidly progressive dementia. Other family members were affected with a similar disease [67]. The autopsy showed features typical of CJD.

F198S (c.593T>C)

This mutation was described in a single large Indiana kindred. Neuropathologically, there were widespread Alzheimer-like neurofibrillary tangles in the cortex and subcortical nuclei in addition to PrP amyloid plaques [68]. There is an apparent codon 129 effect with this mutation, in that individuals heterozygous at codon 129 have a later age of onset than homozygotic individuals.

E200K (c.598G>A)

The typical clinical presentation of this mutation is a rapidly progressive dementia with myoclonus and pyramidal, cerebellar, or extrapyramidal signs. The median age of onset in 112 reported cases (including some summarized data) was 58 years with a median duration of seven months [55,69–75]. Although the age of onset is slightly younger than that for sporadic CJD, Kahana and Zilber (1991) found no unique clinical features that distinguish patients with the E200K mutation from those with sporadic CJD [76]. The neuropathology is also similar to that of sporadic CJD, often with an absence of PrP plaques. However, in E200K patients with 129M homozygosity, a peculiar perpendicular stripe-like PrP deposit has been described in the molecular layer of the cerebellum [77]. Transmission to experimental animals has been demonstrated.

The E200K mutation is the most common cause of IPD worldwide. As the mutation occurs by deamination of a CpG dinucleotide, it is not surprising that haplotype ancestry has shown multiple occurrences in human history [74,78,79]. Multiple ancestral mutations have led to distinct geographical clusters with a high incidence of disease, most notably in Libyan Jews, which had prompted investigators to make an epidemiological link with ingestion of sheep's brain tissue. At least four separate mutational events are responsible for the global distribution of the mutation [78]. Clustering has led to the occurrence of a small number of individuals homozygous for the E200K mutation. These patients have a slightly earlier age of onset at 50 years, but overall, the homozygous and heterozygous phenotypes are similar, confirming the true dominance of this *PRNP* gene mutation [80].

Expressivity of the E200K mutation is highly variable, manifesting in a wide range of age of onset of disease. Examination and genetic testing of unaffected relatives detect asymptomatic mutation carriers in old age, implying that penetrance is incomplete. The codon 129 polymorphism may determine these to a limited extent [75]. The E219K polymorphism (c.655G>A) may also modify the phenotype [79]. Atypical clinical presentations include those with peripheral neuropathy [72,81], supranuclear gaze palsy [82], and sleep disturbance [55]; the pathogenesis of these atypical presentations is not well understood.

D202N (c.604G>A)

Detected in an English patient clinically diagnosed with Alzheimer's disease, this mutation had an onset age of 73 years and duration of six years. No spongiform change was noted but abundant PrP deposition with tau pathology was found in the cerebrum and cerebellum [32].

V203I (c.607G>A)

This mutation was seen in an Italian patient aged 69 years, with brief but fatal illness consisting of diplopia, confusion, hallucinosis, and myoclonus [67]. The autopsy showed features typical of CJD.

R208H (c.623G>A)

This mutation was first reported in a single patient with CJD without details of the family history or phenotype [83]. Capellari *et al.* (2005) subsequently reported a patient with a typical clinical presentation of CJD associated with the R208H mutation. The autopsy showed spongiform degeneration and synaptic PrP deposition [84]. A third report concerned a man with a long history of memory problems and emotional disturbance, who died aged 61 years after a seven-month rapid decline. The autopsy showed kuru-like plaques of PrP deposition and spongiform change [85].

V210I (c.628G>A)

This mutation is the most common cause of inherited prion disease in Italy, cases being concentrated in the Campania and Apulia regions [86]. Presentation is typical of sporadic CJD except that the mean age of onset is slightly younger (about 55 years of age). There are likely to be multiple ancestral occurrences of the mutation as cases have been reported from Africa [87], Japan [88], and China [89].

E211Q (c.631G>C)

This mutation was seen in a patient with cerebellar ataxia and behavioral abnormalities, followed by dementia and myoclonus, with age of onset at 69 years. Other family members were affected [67]. The autopsy showed features typical of CJD.

Q212P (c.635A>G)

Little information is available, but this mutation has been found in a single patient from the United States with a progressive ataxia and onset when aged 60 years. At autopsy, spongiform change, moderate amounts of PrP deposition, degeneration of the corticospinal tracts, and Lewy bodies were detected [32].

Q217R (c.650A>G)

First reported in a single Swedish family, the presentation of this mutation was dementia followed by gait ataxia, dysphagia, and confusion [90]. Prominent neurofibrillary tangles were found at autopsy. This pathological feature was confirmed by a second case [91], clinically diagnosed with frontotemporal dementia.

M232T (c.695T>C)

This mutation was found in a single Polish patient with a GSS-like phenotype [92].

P238S (c.712C>T)

This mutation was discovered in a single patient from a screen of those referred to a German CJD surveillance unit [66]; prion disease has not been confirmed.

1-, 2-, or 3-octapeptide repeat insertional mutations

The addition of a small number of octapeptide repeats in the N-terminal region of PrP may result in a CJD-like illness. As these mutations have not been described to segregate in families and have been found coincidentally or in population screens, it is difficult to distinguish whether they are rare polymorphisms or incompletely penetrant IPD mutations.

The 1-OPRI mutation was initially reported in a single French individual; the patient presented at age 73 years with dizziness followed by visual agnosia, cerebellar ataxia, and intellectual impairment with diffuse periodic activity on EEG. Myoclonus and cortical blindness developed and he progressed to akinetic mutism. The disease duration was four months. The patient's father had died aged 70 years from an undiagnosed neurological disorder. No neuropathological information is available [93]. Subsequently, two further patients with a CJD-like illness, which in one was confirmed at autopsy, have been associated with a 1-OPRI mutation [94].

The 2-OPRI mutation has been reported in a US family [95]; the proband had a CJD-like phenotype both clinically and pathologically, with a typical EEG and an age at onset of 58 years. However, the proband's mother had onset of cognitive decline at age 75 years with a slow progression to a severe dementia over 13 years. The maternal grandfather had a similar late onset (at age 80 years) and slow progressive cognitive decline over 15 years. A second report of a Dutch patient with a distinct 2-OPRI mutation was diagnosed with presenile dementia and ataxia [96]. MRI was atypical of prion disease with extensive white matter signal change.

The 3-OPRI mutation has only recently been detected. It was first found in a screen of healthy Chinese individuals [97]. Subsequently, a different 3-OPRI mutation was reported in a patient with a clinical and pathological phenotype typical of CJD.

A number of reports detail the 4-OPRI mutation, which typically has late onset and short duration with no family history [98]. This mutation was first reported in an individual who died at the age of 63 years of hepatic cirrhosis [99] but with no history of neurological illness. This was the first recorded case of a *PRNP* gene insertional mutation other than in an affected or an at-risk individual.

Five different 4-OPRI mutations have been reported in six affected individuals, each differing in the DNA sequence from the original four-repeat insertion, although all of the mutations encode the same PrP. Laplanche *et al.* (1995) reported a 4-OPRI mutation in an 82-year-old French woman who developed progressive depression and behavioral changes [93]. She progressed over three months to akinetic mutism with pyramidal signs and myoclonus. The EEG showed pseudoperiodic complexes. The duration of illness was four months. There was no known family history of neurological illness.

Another 4-OPRI mutation was seen in a patient with classical clinical and pathological features of CJD, with the exception of the unusual finding of pronounced PrP immunoreactivity in the molecular layer of the cerebellum, typical of OPRI neuropathology [100]. The latter finding supports the pathogenicity of this mutation.

5-, 6-, 7-, 8-, or 9-octapeptide repeat insertional mutations

Insertion of more than four additional octapeptide repeats in the N-terminal region of PrP causes inherited prion disease with an autosomal dominant pattern. The prototypic example is the insertion of an additional six extra octapeptide repeats. This mutation has some historical importance as it was the first described *PRNP* gene mutation in a small UK family [22]. Genealogical work demonstrated a common ancestor of this family and a larger pedigree with over 50 affected individuals [101]. In 2006, this pedigree was updated and now comprises over 86 affected individuals and about 100 individuals at risk of disease affording a detailed analysis of the phenotype and its determinants [102].

Clinical and pathological features of the UK pedigree are highly variable. Cortical dementia, often with apraxia, is the core feature with additional neurological signs including cerebellar ataxia, pyramidal and extrapyramidal signs, myoclonus, chorea, and seizures in declining order of frequency. The age of onset ranges from the third to sixth decade of life, and duration of disease ranges from an aggressive condition mistaken for sporadic CJD to a slowly progressive neurodegenerative disease over more than two decades. The polymorphism at *PRNP* codon 129 accounts for a proportion of this variability. Insertional mutation carriers associated with heterozygosity at

codon 129 have a delayed age of onset by approximately a decade compared with patients homozygous at codon 129 [101], accounting for 41% of the variance in age of onset.

The 6-OPRI mutation has been transmitted to laboratory mice with incubation times comparable with that expected of sporadic CJD [102]. Analysis of PrP^{Sc}-type indicates a molecular heterogeneity within this single pedigree, although given a small sample size, no conclusion can be made about whether this impacts on phenotypic heterogeneity.

The existence of a premorbid personality disorder in prion disease was first reported in this pedigree, characterized by criminality, aggression, delinquency, and hypersexuality [25]. Other clinicians have ascribed psychiatric symptoms in IPD to the early stages of a neurodegenerative disease [41,103], although the abnormalities described by Collinge *et al.* (1992) [25] dated from early childhood in some cases. The presence of personality disorders with such an early onset may indicate a role for the normal function of PrP in the healthy brain that is abrogated by certain mutations.

Four different types of the 5-OPRI mutation have been reported [99,104–106]. The age of onset ranged from 31 to 61 years with marked heterogeneity of clinical duration.

The 7-OPRI mutation has been reported in a US family. Clinical features were mood change, abnormal behavior, confusion, aphasia, cerebellar signs, involuntary movements, rigidity, dementia, and myoclonus. The age at onset was 23–35 years and the clinical duration 10 to over 13 years. The EEG was atypical. Neuropathological examination showed spongiform change, neuronal loss, and gliosis to varying degrees [99]. Experimental transmission has been demonstrated. Another three mutations with a similar phenotype have since been described [107].

The 8-OPRI mutation was first reported in a French family with clinical features including abnormal behavior, cerebellar signs, mutism, pyramidal signs, myoclonus, tremor, intellectual slowing, and seizures; the disease duration ranged from 3 months to 13 years. The EEG findings included diffuse slowing, slow wave burst suppression, and periodic triphasic complexes. Neuropathological examination revealed spongiform change, neuronal loss, gliosis, and multicentric plaques in the cerebellum [99]. Experimental transmission has been reported. Two other families [103,108] with prominent psychological or psychiatric changes are now known.

The 9-OPRI mutation was first reported in a single case from the United Kingdom [109]. The clinical onset was approximately 54 years with falls, axial rigidity, myoclonic jerks, and progressive dementia. Although there was no clear family history of a similar illness, the mother had died at age 53 years with a cerebrovascular event. The maternal grandmother had died at age 79 years with senile dementia. The EEG was atypical. Neuropathological examination showed no spongiform encephalopathy but marked deposition of plaques, which in the cerebellum and the basal ganglia showed immunoreactivity with PrP antisera [110]. In the hippocampus, there were neuritic plaques positive for both β-amyloid protein and tau. Some neurofibrillary tangles were also seen. In some respects, therefore, the pathology resembled Alzheimer's disease. Experimental transmission studies have not been attempted. A second, German family with a 9-OPRI mutation of different sequence has also been reported [111].

The neuropathology of the OPRI mutation has been studied by Vital *et al.* (1998) and King *et al.* (2003) [112,113]. The degree of spongiosis and astrocytosis seen was highly variable between cases. Obvious plaques of PrP deposition in the cerebellum were seen only in those patients with 8- or 9-OPRI mutations. For smaller OPRI mutations, PrP deposition was visualized by immunocytochemistry as elongated deposits in the molecular layer of the cerebellum.

2-octapeptide repeat deletional mutation

A two-repeat deletion has been described in two individuals with CJD [114,115].

Non-pathogenic *PRNP* polymorphisms

The coding sequences of mammalian prion protein genes are highly conserved in a similar way to other structural proteins, presumably by deleterious selection of coding mutations. Despite this conservation, a number of common human coding polymorphisms have been characterized in different populations [116,117], some of which have an important role in disease modification or susceptibility.

M129V (c.385A>G)

Foremost among the polymorphisms of the gene *PRNP* is at codon 129 between methionine and valine [118], which has a strong disease susceptibility and phenotype modifying effect [119–125]. Codon 129

has a susceptibility or modifying effect in all categories of prion disease. Variant CJD demonstrates this effect most dramatically: all genetically tested definite cases have been homozygous for 129M [17,18] (our unpublished observations). A single codon 129 heterozygous patient, who had received blood from a donor subsequently diagnosed with vCJD, was found to have widespread prion protein deposition in the peripheral lymphoreticular system at autopsy, having died of an unrelated cause [14]. It remains to be seen whether individuals of different genotypes will succumb to vCJD, or a similar phenotype of prion disease, in the BSE-exposed UK and other European populations. Sporadic CJD also shows a susceptibility effect at codon 129 with ~90% of patients having either methionine or valine homozygous genotypes [120].

Aside from vCJD, outbreaks of acquired prion disease have been caused by human–human transmission of prions by cadaver derived growth hormone injections, the use of dura mater in neurosurgery, corneal transplantation, and intracerebral electrodes. These outbreaks have remained small owing to the limited exposed group, but patients with a heterozygous genotype at codon 129 are protected. Our largest experience of an acquired human prion disease comes from kuru, a devastating epidemic of prion disease spread by ritualistic cannibalism in the Fore and neighboring linguistic groups of the Eastern Highlands of Papua New Guinea. At its peak in the 1950s, kuru was the leading cause of death in young women in the South Fore. Although precise epidemiological data are not available, both methionine and valine homozygous individuals had a mean age of onset of disease in early adulthood, whereas heterozygous individuals had a delayed onset into middle age [121], some with incubation periods of over 50 years [122]. Such a high disease incidence, coupled with the effect of heterozygosity to delay disease onset through reproductive age, affords the opportunity for strong selection pressure. Surviving elderly women in the present-day South Fore population, who lived through the epidemic, show marked Hardy–Weinberg disequilibrium at the *PRNP* gene with an excess of codon 129 heterozygosity, illustrating the population genetic effect of the kuru epidemic [116,123].

E219K (c.655G>A)

This polymorphism is found in South and East Asia. No cases of sporadic CJD with either one or two 219K alleles have been reported [124], indicating a powerful disease resistance effect of this allele.

G142S (c.424G>A), N171S (c.512A>G), M232R (c.695T>G)

The G142S and N171S polymorphisms have been found in African derived populations [116,125]. Their role in disease susceptibility is unclear.

The M232R polymorphism was first found on the opposite allele to the V180I mutation in a Japanese patient with prion disease [126]; it was further demonstrated in seven Japanese patients with progressive dementia, myoclonus, and periodic synchronous discharges in the EEG (in all except one 84-year-old patient). The duration of illness ranged from 4 to 24 months. However, the recent finding of this change in a screen of 16 healthy Japanese individuals [125] and in a patient with dementia with Lewy bodies [127] suggests that this change is, in fact, a non-pathogenic polymorphism.

1-octapeptide repeat deletion polymorphism

This change is an uncommon (~1%) polymorphism in European populations with no known disease-modifying or susceptibility effect [128].

Genetic counseling and presymptomatic testing

Since a direct gene test has become available, it has been possible to provide an unequivocal diagnosis in patients with inherited forms of the disease. This has also led to the possibility of performing presymptomatic testing of unaffected but at-risk family members, as well as antenatal testing [129]. Because of the effect of *PRNP* codon 129 genotype on the age of onset of disease associated with some mutations, it is possible to determine within a family whether a carrier of a mutation will have an early or late onset of disease. Most of the mutations appear to be fully penetrant; however, experience with some is extremely limited. In families with the V210I, D178N, and E200K mutations, there are examples of elderly unaffected gene carriers who appear to have escaped the disease. Genetic counseling is essential prior to presymptomatic testing and follows a protocol similar to that established for Huntington's

disease. A positive PrP gene analysis has important consequences for other family members, and it is preferable to have discussed these issues with others in the immediate family before testing. Following the identification of a mutation, the wider family should be referred for genetic counseling. It is vital to counsel both those testing positive for mutations and those untested but at risk that they should not be blood or organ donors and they should inform surgeons, including dentists, of their risk status prior to significant procedures as precautions may be necessary to minimize risk of iatrogenic transmission.

The strong genetic susceptibility to acquired and sporadic prion diseases does not justify the use of the polymorphism (M129V or E219K) data for predictive purposes. Patients heterozygous at codon 129 are diagnosed with sporadic CJD, and these patients may be atypical in their clinical presentation. Although all patients with vCJD to date have been homozygous for methionine, our experience with kuru suggests that other genotypes will eventually become affected with longer subclinical phases, with differing clinical, pathological, and molecular phenotypes [122,130].

Therapeutics

All known forms of prion diseases are invariably fatal, following a relentlessly progressive course, and there is no effective therapy. The duration of illness in sporadic patients is very short with a mean duration of three to four months. However, in some of the inherited cases, the duration can be 20 years or more. Symptomatic treatment of various neurological and psychiatric features can be provided and a range of supportive services are likely to be required in the later stages of the disease (see UK National Prion Clinic website for factsheets and specialist advice: http://www.nationalprionclinic.org). While no effective treatment for the human disease is known, several drugs are currently being studied in patients. In the United Kingdom, a clinical trial for evaluation of quinacrine CJD, designated the MRC PRION-1 trial, has been conducted.

Current agents are unlikely to stop prion propagation and may, at best, be expected to delay disease progression. Clearly, advances toward early diagnosis, to allow therapies to be used prior to extensive neuronal loss, will be important. While the challenge of interrupting this aggressive, non-focal, and uniformly fatal neurodegenerative process is daunting, major advances in understanding the basic processes of prion propagation and neurotoxicity are being made. Considerable optimism is provided by the recent finding that onset of clinical disease in established neuroinvasive prion infection in a mouse model can be halted and, indeed, early pathology reversed [131]. A number of approaches to rational therapeutics are being studied in experimental models. Anti-PrP antibodies have been shown to block progression of peripheral prion propagation in mouse models and humanized versions of these antibodies could, in principle, be developed and used for both postexposure prophylaxis and during established clinical disease. In the longer term, the development of drugs that selectively bind PrP^{Sc} or which bind to PrP^{C} to inhibit its conversion might be able to block prion propagation and allow natural clearance mechanisms to eradicate remaining PrP^{Sc} and thus cure prion infection.

References

1. McGowan JP. Scrapie in sheep. *Scottish J Agric* 1922; **5**: 365–375.

2. Cuillé J, Chelle PL. La maladie dite tremblante du mouton est-elle inocuable? *CR Acad Sci* 1936; **203**: 1552–1554.

3. Beck E, Daniel PM. Neuropathology of transmissible spongiform encephalopathies. In Prusiner SB, McKinley MP, eds. *Prions: Novel Infectious Pathogens Causing Scrapie and Creutzfeldt-Jakob Disease*. San Diego, CA, USA: Academic Press, 1987; 331–385.

4. Klatzo I, Gajdusek DC, Zigas V. Pathology of kuru. *Lab Invest* 1959; **8**: 799–847.

5. Hadlow WJ. Scrapie and kuru. *Lancet* 1959; **ii**: 289–290.

6. Gajdusek DC, Gibbs CJ Jr, Alpers MP. Experimental transmission of a kuru-like syndrome to chimpanzees. *Nature* 1966; **209**: 794–796.

7. Gibbs CJ Jr, Gajdusek DC, Asher DM, *et al.* Creutzfeldt-Jakob disease (spongiform encephalopathy): transmission to the chimpanzee. *Science* 1968; **161**: 388–389.

8. Oesch B, Westaway D, Walchli M, *et al.* A cellular gene encodes scrapie PrP 27–30 protein. *Cell* 1985; **40**: 735–746.

9. Borchelt DR, Scott M, Taraboulos A, *et al.* Scrapie and cellular prion proteins differ in their kinetics of synthesis and topology in cultured cells. *J Cell Biol* 1990; **110**: 743–752.

10. Caughey B, Raymond GJ. The scrapie-associated form of PrP is made from a cell surface precursor that is both protease- and phospholipase-sensitive. *J Biol Chem* 1991; **266**: 18217–18223.

11. Brown P, Cathala F, Raubertas RF, *et al.* The epidemiology of Creutzfeldt-Jakob disease: conclusion of a 15-year investigation in France and review of the world literature. *Neurology* 1987; **37**: 895–904.

12. Ghani AC, Ferguson NM, Donnelly CA, *et al.* Epidemiological determinants of the pattern and magnitude of the vCJD epidemic in Great Britain. *Proc R Soc Lond B Biol Sci* 1999; **265**: 2443–2452.

13. Collinge J. Variant Creutzfeldt-Jakob disease. *Lancet* 1999; **354**: 317–323.

14. Peden AH, Head MW, Ritchie DL, *et al.* Preclinical vCJD after blood transfusion in a PRNP codon 129 heterozygous patient. *Lancet* 2004; **364**: 527–529.

15. Llewelyn CA, Hewitt PE, Knight RS, *et al.* Possible transmission of variant Creutzfeldt-Jakob disease by blood transfusion. *Lancet* 2004; **363**: 417–421.

16. Wroe SJ, Pal S, Siddique D, *et al.* Clinical presentation and pre-mortem diagnosis of variant Creutzfeldt–Jakob disease associated with blood transfusion: a case report. *Lancet* 2006; **368**: 2061–2067.

17. Zeidler M, Stewart G, Cousens SN, *et al.* Codon 129 genotype and new variant CJD. *Lancet* 1997; **350**: 668.

18. Hill AF, Butterworth RJ, Joiner S, *et al.* Investigation of variant Creutzfeldt–Jakob disease and other human prion diseases with tonsil biopsy samples. *Lancet* 1999; **353**: 183–189.

19. Hill AF, Zeidler M, Ironside J, Collinge J. Diagnosis of new variant Creutzfeldt-Jakob disease by tonsil biopsy. *Lancet* 1997; **349**: 99–100.

20. Will RG, Ironside JW, Zeidler M, *et al.* A new variant of Creutzfeldt-Jakob disease in the UK. *Lancet* 1996; **347**: 921–925.

21. Alpers MP. Epidemiology and clinical aspects of kuru. In Prusiner SB, McKinley MP, eds. *Prions: Novel Infectious Pathogens Causing Scrapie and Creutzfeldt-Jakob Disease*. San Diego, CA, USA: Academic Press, 1987; 451–465.

22. Owen F, Poulter M, Lofthouse R, *et al.* Insertion in prion protein gene in familial Creutzfeldt-Jakob disease. *Lancet* 1989; **1**: 51–52.

23. Hsiao K, Baker HF, Crow TJ, *et al.* Linkage of a prion protein missense variant to Gerstmann–Straussler syndrome. *Nature* 1989; **338**: 342–345.

24. Collinge J, Harding AE, Owen F, *et al.* Diagnosis of Gerstmann–Straussler syndrome in familial dementia with prion protein gene analysis. *Lancet* 1989; **2**: 15–17.

25. Collinge J, Brown J, Hardy J, *et al.* Inherited prion disease with 144 base pair gene insertion. II: Clinical and pathological features. *Brain* 1992; **115**: 687–710.

26. Collinge J, Owen F, Poulter M, *et al.* Prion dementia without characteristic pathology. *Lancet* 1990; **336**: 7–9.

27. Finckh U, Muller-Thomsen T, Mann U, *et al.* High prevalence of pathogenic mutations in patients with early-onset dementia detected by sequence analyses of four different genes. *Am J Hum Genet* 2000; **66**: 110–117.

28. Bruton CJ, Bruton RK, Gentleman SM, Roberts GW. Diagnosis and incidence of prion (Creutzfeldt–Jakob) disease: a retrospective archival survey with implications for future research. *Neurodegeneration* 1995; **4**: 357–368.

29. Kovacs GG, Puopolo M, Ladogana A, *et al.* Genetic prion disease: the EUROCJD experience. *Hum Genet* 2005; **118**: 166–174.

30. Gerstmann J, Sträussler E, Scheinker I. Über eine eigenartige hereditär-familiäre Erkrankung des Zentralnervensystems. Zugleich ein Beitrag zur Frage des vorzeitigen lakalen Alterns. *Z Neurol* 1936; **154**: 736–762.

31. Young K, Clark HB, Piccardo P, *et al.* Gerstmann–Straussler–Scheinker disease with the *PRNP* P102L mutation and valine at codon 129. *Mol Brain Res* 1997; **44**: 147–150.

32. Piccardo P, Dlouhy SR, Lievens PMJ, *et al.* Phenotypic variability of Gerstmann–Straussler–Scheinker disease is associated with prion protein heterogeneity. *J Neuropathol Exp Neurol* 1998; **57**: 979–988.

33. Barbanti P, Fabbrini G, Salvatore M, *et al.* Polymorphism at codon 129 or codon 219 of *PRNP* and clinical heterogeneity in a previously unreported family with Gerstmann–Straussler–Scheinker disease (PrP-P102L mutation). *Neurology* 1996; **47**: 734–741.

34. Hainfellner JA, Brantner-Inthaler S, Cervenáková L, *et al.* The original Gerstmann–Straussler–Scheinker family of Austria: divergent clinicopathological phenotypes but constant PrP genotype. *Brain Pathol* 1995; **5**: 201–211.

35. Adam J, Crow TJ, Duchen LW, *et al.* Familial cerebral amyloidosis and spongiform encephalopathy. *J Neurol Neurosurg Psychiatry* 1982; **45**: 37–45.

36. Tanaka Y, Minematsu K, Moriyasu H, *et al.* A Japanese family with a variant of Gerstmann–Straussler–Scheinker disease. *J Neurol Neurosurg Psychiatry* 1997; **62**: 454–457.

37. Kretzschmar HA, Kufer P, Riethmuller G, *et al.* Prion protein mutation at codon 102 in an Italian family with Gerstmann–Straussler–Scheinker syndrome. *Neurology* 1992; **42**: 809–810.

38. Wadsworth JD, Joiner S, Linehan JM, *et al.* Phenotypic heterogeneity in inherited prion disease (P102L) is associated with differential propagation of protease-resistant wild-type and mutant prion protein. *Brain* 2006; **129**: 1557–1569.

39. Kitamoto T, Amano N, Terao Y, *et al.* A new inherited prion disease (PrP-P105L mutation) showing spastic paraparesis. *Ann Neurol* 1993; **34**: 808–813.

40. Yamada M, Itoh Y, Inaba A, *et al.* An inherited prion disease with a PrPP105L mutation – clinicopathologic and PrP heterogeneity. *Neurology* 1999; **53**: 181–188.

41. Rodriguez MM, Peoc'h K, Haik S, *et al.* A novel mutation (G114V) in the prion protein gene in a family with inherited prion disease. *Neurology* 2005; **64**: 1455–1457.

42. Doh ura K, Tateishi J, Sasaki H, *et al.* Pro–leu change at position 102 of prion protein is the most common but not the sole mutation related to Gerstmann–Straussler syndrome. *Biochem Biophys Res Commun* 1989; **163**: 974–979.

43. Hsiao KK, Cass C, Schellenberg GD, *et al.* A prion protein variant in a family with the telencephalic form of Gerstmann–Straussler–Scheinker syndrome. *Neurology* 1991; **41**: 681–684.

44. Mallucci GR, Campbell TA, Dickinson A, *et al.* Inherited prion disease with an alanine to valine mutation at codon 117 in the prion protein gene. *Brain* 1999; **122**: 1823–1837.

45. Panegyres PK, Toufexis K, Kakulas BA, *et al.* A new *PRNP* mutation (G131V) associated with Gerstmann–Straussler–Scheinker disease. *Arch Neurol* 2001; **58**: 1899–1902.

46. Kitamoto T, Iizuka R, Tateishi J. An amber mutation of prion protein in Gerstmann–Straussler syndrome with mutant PrP plaques. *Biochem Biophys Res Commun* 1993; **192**: 525–531.

47. Krebs B, Lederer RM, Windl O, *et al.* Creutzfeldt–Jakob disease associated with an R148H mutation of the prion protein gene. *Neurogenetics* 2005; **6**: 97–100.

48. Pastore M, Chin SS, Bell KL, *et al.* Creutzfeldt–Jakob disease (CJD) with a mutation at codon 148 of prion protein gene:

relationship with sporadic CJD. *Am J Pathol* 2005; **167**: 1729–1738.

49. Soldevila M, Andres AM, Blancher A, *et al.* Variation of the prion gene in chimpanzees and its implication for prion diseases. *Neurosci Lett* 2004; **355**: 157–160.

50. Goldfarb LG, Haltia M, Brown P, *et al.* New mutation in scrapie amyloid precursor gene (at codon 178) in Finnish Creutzfeldt–Jakob kindred. *Lancet* 1991; **337**: 425.

51. Medori R, Tritschler HJ, LeBlanc AC, *et al.* Fatal familial insomnia, a prion disease with a mutation in codon 178 of the prion protein gene: study of two kindreds. In Prusiner SB, Collinge J, Powell J, Anderton B, eds. *Prion Diseases of Humans and Animals.* London, UK: Ellis Horwood, 1992; 180–187.

52. Lugaresi E, Medori R, Baruzzi PM, *et al.* Fatal familial insomnia and dysautonomia, with selective degeneration of thalamic nuclei. *N Engl J Med* 1986; **315**: 997–1003.

53. Goldfarb LG, Petersen RB, Tabaton M, *et al.* Fatal familial insomnia and familial Creutzfeldt–Jakob disease: disease phenotype determined by a DNA polymorphism. *Science* 1992; **258**: 806–808.

54. McLean CA, Storey E, Gardner RJM, *et al.* The D178N (cis-129M) "fatal familial insomnia" mutation associated with diverse clinicopathologic phenotypes in an Australian kindred. *Neurology* 1997; **49**: 552–558.

55. Chapman J, Arlazoroff A, Goldfarb LG, *et al.* Fatal insomnia in a case of familial Creutzfeldt–Jakob disease with the codon 200Lys mutation. *Neurology* 1996; **46**: 758–761.

56. Zerr I, Giese A, Windl O, *et al.* Phenotypic variability in fatal familial insomnia (D178N–129M) genotype. *Neurology* 1998; **51**: 1398–1405.

57. Pocchiari M, Ladogana A, Petraroli R, *et al.* Recent Italian FFI cases. *Brain Pathol* 1998; **8**: 564–566.

58. Brown P, Gibbs CJ Jr, Rodgers Johnson P, *et al.* Human spongiform encephalopathy: the National Institutes of Health series of 300 cases of experimentally transmitted disease. *Ann Neurol* 1994; **35**: 513–529.

59. Collinge J, Palmer MS, Sidle KCL, *et al.* Transmission of fatal familial insomnia to laboratory animals. *Lancet* 1995; **346**: 569–570.

60. Tateishi J, Brown P, Kitamoto T, *et al.* First experimental transmission of fatal familial insomnia. *Nature* 1995; **376**: 434–435.

61. Jin K, Shiga Y, Shibuya S, *et al.* Clinical features of Creutzfeldt–Jakob disease with V180I mutation. *Neurology* 2004; **62**: 502–505.

62. Nitrini R, Rosemberg S, Passos Bueno MR, *et al.* Familial spongiform encephalopathy associated with a novel prion protein gene mutation. *Ann Neurol* 1997; **42**: 138–146.

63. Cervenakova L, Buetefisch C, Lee HS, *et al.* Novel PRNP sequence variant associated with familial encephalopathy. *American J Med Genet*, 1999; **88**: 653–656.

64. Hall DA, Leehey MA, Filley CM, *et al.* PRNP H187R mutation associated with neuropsychiatric disorders in childhood and dementia. *Neurology* 2005; **64**: 1304–1306.

65. Collins S, Boyd A, Fletcher A, *et al.* Novel prion protein gene mutation in an octogenarian with Creutzfeldt–Jakob disease. *Arch Neurol* 2000; **57**: 1058–1063.

66. Windl O, Giese A, Schulz-Schaeffer W, *et al.* Molecular genetics of human prion diseases in Germany. *Hum Genet* 1999; **105**: 244–252.

67. Peoc'h K, Manivet P, Beaudry P, *et al.* Identification of three novel mutations (E196K, V203I, E211Q) in the prion protein gene (PRNP) in inherited prion diseases with Creutzfeldt–Jakob disease phenotype. *Hum Mutat* 2000; **15**: 482.

68. Dlouhy SR, Hsiao K, Farlow MR, *et al.* Linkage of the Indiana kindred of Gerstmann–Sträussler-Scheinker disease to the prion protein gene. *Nat Genet* 1992; **1**: 64–67.

69. Bertoni JM, Brown P, Goldfarb LG, *et al.* Familial Creutzfeldt–Jakob disease (codon 200 mutation) with supranuclear palsy. *JAMA* 1992; **268**: 2413–2415.

70. Inoue I, Kitamoto T, Doh-ura K, *et al.* Japanese family with Creutzfeldt–Jakob disease with codon 200 point mutation of the prion protein gene. *Neurology* 1994; **44**: 299–301.

71. Collinge J, Palmer MS, Campbell TA, *et al.* Inherited prion disease (PrP lysine 200) in Britain: two case reports. *BMJ* 1993; **306**: 301–302.

72. Antoine JC, Laplanche JL, Mosnier JF, *et al.* Demyelinating peripheral neuropathy with Creutzfeldt–Jakob disease and mutation at codon 200 of the prion protein gene. *Neurology* 1996; **46**: 1123–1127.

73. Miyakawa T, Inoue K, Iseki E, *et al.* Japanese Creutzfeldt–Jakob disease patients exhibiting high incidence of the E200K PRNP mutation and located in the basin of a river. *Neurol Res* 1998; **20**: 684–688.

74. Goldfarb LG, Brown P, Mitrova E, *et al.* Creutzfeldt–Jacob disease associated with the PRNP codon 200Lys mutation: an analysis of

45 families. *Eur J Epidemiol* 1991; 7: 477–486.

75. Mitrova E, Belay G. Creutzfeldt–Jakob disease with E200K mutation in Slovakia: characterization and development. *Acta Virol* 2002; 46: 31–39.

76. Kahana E, Zilber N. Do Creutzfeldt–Jakob disease patients of Jewish Libyan origin have unique clinical features? *Neurology* 1991; 41: 1390–1392.

77. Jarius C, Kovacs GG, Belay G, et al. Distinctive cerebellar immunoreactivity for the prion protein in familial (E200K) Creutzfeldt–Jakob disease. *Acta Neuropathol* 2003; 105: 449–454.

78. Lee HS, Sambuughin N, Cervenakova L, et al. Ancestral origins and worldwide distribution of the PRNP 200K mutation causing familial Creutzfeldt–Jakob disease. *Am J Hum Genet* 1999; 64: 1063–1070.

79. Seno H, Tashiro H, Ishino H, et al. New haplotype of familial Creutzfeldt–Jakob disease with a codon 200 mutation and a codon 219 polymorphism of the prion protein gene in a Japanese family. *Acta Neuropathol* 2000; 99: 125–130.

80. Simon ES, Kahana E, Chapman J, et al. Creutzfeldt–Jakob disease profile in patients homozygous for the PRNP E200K mutation. *Ann Neurol* 2000; 47: 257–260.

81. Chapman J, Brown P, Goldfarb LG, et al. Clinical heterogeneity and unusual presentations of Creutzfeldt–Jakob disease in Jewish patients with the PRNP codon 200 mutation. *J Neurol Neurosurg Psychiatry* 1993; 56: 1109–1112.

82. Bertoni JM, Label LS, Sackelleres JC, Hicks SP. Supranuclear gaze palsy in familial Creutzfeldt–Jakob disease. *Arch Neurol* 1983; 40: 618–622.

83. Mastrianni JA, Iannicola C, Myers R, Prusiner SB. Identification of a new mutation of the prion protein gene at codon 208 in a patient with Creutzfeldt–Jakob disease. *Neurology* 1995; 45: A201.

84. Capellari S, Cardone F, Notari S, et al. Creutzfeldt–Jakob disease associated with the R208H mutation in the prion protein gene. *Neurology* 2005; 64: 905–907.

85. Basset-Leobon C, Uro-Coste E, Peoc'h K, et al. Familial Creutzfeldt–Jakob disease with an R208H-129V haplotype and kuru plaques. *Arch Neurol* 2006; 63: 449–452.

86. Ladogana A, Puopolo M, Poleggi A, et al. High incidence of genetic human transmissible spongiform encephalopathies in Italy. *Neurology* 2005; 64: 1592–1597.

87. Mouillet-Richard S, Teil C, Lenne M, et al. Mutation at codon 210 (V210I) of the prion protein gene in a North African patient with Creutzfeldt–Jakob disease. *J Neurol Sci* 1999; 168: 141–144.

88. Furukawa H, Kitamoto T, Hashiguchi H, Tateishi J. A Japanese case of Creutzfeldt–Jakob disease with a point mutation in the prion protein gene at codon 210. *J Neurol Sci* 1996; 141: 120–122.

89. Shyu WC, Hsu YD, Kao MC, Tsao WL. Panencephalitic Creutzfeldt–Jakob disease in a Chinese family – unusual presentation with PrP codon 210 mutation and identification by PCR-SSCP. *J Neurol Sci* 1996; 143: 176–180.

90. Hsiao K, Dlouhy SR, Farlow MR, et al. Mutant prion proteins in Gerstmann–Sträussler–Sheinker disease with neurofibrillary tangles. *Nat Genet* 1992; 1: 68–71.

91. Woulfe J, Kertesz A, Frohn I, et al. Gerstmann–Straussler–Scheinker disease with the Q217R mutation mimicking frontotemporal dementia. *Acta Neuropathol* 2005; 110: 317–319.

92. Liberski P, Bratosiewicz J, Barcikowska M, et al. A case of Gerstmann–Straussler–Scheinker disease (GSS) with Met to Thr mutation at codon 232 of the PRNP gene. *Brain Pathol* 2000; 10: 669.

93. Laplanche JL, Delasnerie Laupretre N, Brandel JP, et al. Two novel insertions in the prion protein gene in patients with late-onset dementia. *Hum Mol Genet* 1995; 4: 1109–1111.

94. Pietrini V, Puoti G, Limido L, et al. Creutzfeldt–Jakob disease with a novel extra-repeat insertional mutation in the PRNP gene. *Neurology* 2003; 61: 1288–1291.

95. Goldfarb LG, Brown P, Little BW, et al. A new (two-repeat) octapeptide coding insert mutation in Creutzfeldt–Jakob disease. *Neurology* 1993; 43: 2392–2394.

96. Van Harten B, Van Gool WA, Van Langen IM, et al. A new mutation in the prion protein gene: a patient with dementia and white matter changes. *Neurology* 2000; 55: 1055–1057.

97. Yu SL, Jin L, Sy MS, et al. Polymorphisms of the PRNP gene in Chinese populations and the identification of a novel insertion mutation. *Eur J Hum Genet* 2004; 12: 867–870.

98. Yanagihara C, Yasuda M, Maeda K, et al. Rapidly progressive dementia syndrome associated with a novel four extra repeat mutation in the prion protein gene. *J Neurol Neurosurg Psychiatry* 2002; 72: 788–791.

99. Goldfarb LG, Brown P, McCombie WR, et al. Transmissible familial

Creutzfeldt–Jakob disease associated with five, seven, and eight extra octapeptide coding repeats in the *PRNP* gene. *Proc Natl Acad Sci USA* 1991; **88**: 10926–10930.

100. Campbell TA, Palmer MS, Will RG, *et al.* A prion disease with a novel 96-base pair insertional mutation in the prion protein gene. *Neurology* 1996; **46**: 761–766.

101. Poulter M, Baker HF, Frith CD, *et al.* Inherited prion disease with 144 base pair gene insertion. I: Genealogical and molecular studies. *Brain* 1992; **115**: 675–685.

102. Mead S, Poulter M, Beck J, *et al.* Inherited prion disease with six octapeptide repeat insertional mutation – molecular analysis of phenotypic heterogeneity. *Brain* 2006; **129**: 2297–2317.

103. Laplanche JL, El Hachimi KH, Durieux I, *et al.* Prominent psychiatric features and early onset in an inherited prion disease with a new insertional mutation in the prion protein gene. *Brain* 1999; **122**: 2375–2386.

104. Beck G, Kawano T, Naba I, *et al.* A case with a 120 base pair insertional mutation in the prion protein gene: the first case in Japan. *J Neurol Neurosurg Psychiatry* 2005; **76**: 756–757.

105. Cochran EJ, Bennett DA, Cervenáková L, *et al.* Familial Creutzfeldt–Jakob disease with a five-repeat octapeptide insert mutation. *Neurology* 1996; **47**: 727–733.

106. Skworc KH, Windl O, Schulz-Schaeffer WJ, *et al.* Familial Creutzfeldt–Jakob disease with a novel 120-bp insertion in the prion protein gene. *Ann Neurol* 1999; **46**: 693–700.

107. Lewis V, Collins S, Hill AF, *et al.* Novel prion protein insert mutation associated with prolonged neurodegenerative

illness. *Neurology* 2003; **60**: 1620–1624.

108. Van Gool WA, Hensels GW, Hoogerwaard EM, *et al.* Hypokinesia and presenile dementia in a Dutch family with a novel insertion in the prion protein gene. *Brain* 1995; **118**: 1565–1571.

109. Owen F, Poulter M, Collinge J, *et al.* A dementing illness associated with a novel insertion in the prion protein gene. *Mol Brain Res* 1992; **13**: 155–157.

110. Duchen LW, Poulter M, Harding AE. Dementia associated with a 216 base pair insertion in the prion protein gene. Clinical and neuropathological features. *Brain* 1993; **116**: 555–567.

111. Krasemann S, Zerr I, Weber T, *et al.* Prion disease associated with a novel nine octapeptide repeat insertion in the PRNP gene. *Mol Brain Res* 1995; **34**: 173–176.

112. Vital C, Gray F, Vital A, *et al.* Prion encephalopathy with insertion of octapeptide repeats: the number of repeats determines the type of cerebellar deposits. *Neuropathol Appl Neurobiol* 1998; **24**: 125–130.

113. King A, Doey L, Rossor M, *et al.* Phenotypic variability in the brains of a family with a prion disease characterized by a 144-base pair insertion in the prion protein gene. *Neuropathol Appl Neurobiol* 2003; **29**: 98–105.

114. Beck J, Mead S, Campbell TA, *et al.* Two-octapeptide repeat deletion of prion protein associated with rapidly progressive dementia. *Neurology* 2001; **57**: 354–356.

115. Capellari S, Parchi P, Wolff BD, *et al.* Creutzfeldt–Jakob disease associated with a deletion of two repeats in the prion protein gene. *Neurology* 2002; **59**: 1628–1630.

116. Mead S, Stumpf MP, Whitfield J, *et al.* Balancing selection at the prion protein gene consistent with prehistoric kuru-like epidemics. *Science* 2003; **300**: 640–643.

117. Soldevila M, Calafell F, Andres AM, *et al.* Prion susceptibility and protective alleles exhibit marked geographic differences. *Hum Mutat* 2003; **22**: 104–105.

118. Owen F, Poulter M, Collinge J, Crow TJ. Codon 129 changes in the prion protein gene in Caucasians. *Am J Hum Genet* 1990; **46**: 1215–1216.

119. Collinge J, Palmer MS, Dryden AJ. Genetic predisposition to iatrogenic Creutzfeldt–Jakob disease. *Lancet* 1991; **337**: 1441–1442.

120. Palmer MS, Dryden AJ, Hughes JT, Collinge J. Homozygous prion protein genotype predisposes to sporadic Creutzfeldt–Jakob disease. *Nature* 1991; **352**: 340–342.

121. Cervenakova L, Goldfarb L, Garruto R, *et al.* Phenotype-genotype studies in kuru: implications for new variant Creutzfeldt–Jakob disease. *Proc Natl Acad Sci USA* 1999; **95**: 13239–13241.

122. Collinge J, Whitfield J, McKintosh E, *et al.* Kuru in the 21st century – an acquired human prion disease with very long incubation periods. *Lancet* 2006; **367**: 2068–2074.

123. Lee HS, Brown P, Cervenáková L, *et al.* Increased susceptibility to kuru of carriers of the *PRNP* 129 methionine/methionine genotype. *J Infect Dis* 2001; **183**: 192–196.

124. Shibuya S, Higuchi J, Shin RW, Tateishi J, Kitamoto T. Codon 219 Lys allele of PRNP is not found in sporadic Creutzfeldt–Jakob disease. *Ann Neurol* 1998; **43**: 826–828.

125. Soldevila M, Andres AM, Ramirez-Soriano A, *et al.* The

prion protein gene in humans revisited: lessons from a worldwide resequencing study. *Genome Res* 2006; **16**: 231–239.

126. Kitamoto T, Ohta M, Doh-ura K, *et al.* Novel missense variants of prion protein in Creutzfeldt–Jakob disease or Gerstmann–Straussler syndrome. *Biochem Biophys Res Commun* 1993; **191**: 709–714.

127. Koide T, Ohtake H, Nakajima T, *et al.* A patient with dementia with Lewy bodies and codon 232 mutation of PRNP. *Neurology* 2002; **59**: 1619–1621.

128. Palmer MS, Mahal SP, Campbell TA, *et al.* Deletions in the prion protein gene are not associated with CJD. *Hum Mol Genet* 1993; **2**: 541–544.

129. Collinge J, Poulter M, Davis MB, *et al.* Presymptomatic detection or exclusion of prion protein gene defects in families with inherited prion diseases. *Am J Hum Genet* 1991; **49**: 1351–1354.

130. Wadsworth JD, Asante EA, Desbruslais M, *et al.* Human prion protein with valine 129 prevents expression of variant CJD phenotype. *Science* 2004; **306**: 1793–1796.

131. Mallucci G, Dickinson A, Linehan J, *et al.* Depleting neuronal PrP in prion infection prevents disease and reverses spongiosis. *Science* 2003; **302**: 871–874.

Channelopathies

Michael G. Hanna and Dimitri M. Kullmann

Introduction

In recent years, an increasing number of single-gene neurogenetic disorders have been identified in which the primary genetic defect resides in an ion channel [1]. These disorders have become known as the neurological channelopathies and may be divided into those that affect the peripheral nervous system (principally skeletal muscle) and those that affect the central nervous system (CNS). For many of these single-gene channelopathies, the fusion of advances in the fields of genetics and cellular electrophysiology has provided a detailed understanding of the molecular pathophysiology.

The molecular mechanisms underlying the paroxysmal nature of many common neurological diseases, such as epilepsy and migraine, have always been something of an enigma. It is now clear that certain forms of inherited epilepsy and migraine are caused by mutations in ion channel genes. This has led many to suspect that the genetic contribution to common forms of epilepsy and migraine may reside in ion channel genes, and this is currently an important focus of research in the field.

There are at least 40 separate single-gene neurological channelopathies known at present. It is likely that clinicians in neurology and genetics will encounter neurological channelopathies. In this chapter, we aim to provide a clinicians' guide to the key clinical, genetic, and treatment aspects of the main single-gene neurological channelopathies. We have considered the major skeletal muscle channelopathies followed by the main CNS channelopathies.

Skeletal muscle channelopathies

The skeletal muscle channelopathies (Table 9.1) were the first to be defined at a genetic level. The combination of genetic and cellular electrophysiological research has led to a detailed understanding of the molecular pathophysiology of most of the skeletal

Table 9.1. Skeletal muscle channelopathies – a genetic classification

Gene	Channel	Disease	Inheritance
CACNA1S*	Calcium channel L-type calcium α-subunit	HypoPP MH	AD
SCN4A*	Sodium channel Nav1.4 α-subunit	HyperPP PMC PAM HypoPP	AD
KCNJ2*	Potassium channel Kir2.1	Andersen's syndrome	AD
CLCN-1*	Chloride channel ClC1	Myotonia congenita	AD or AR
RYR1	Ryanodine receptor Ca release channel	Malignant hyperthermia Central core disease	AD

HypoPP, hypokalemic periodic paralysis; MH, malignant hyperthermia; HyperPP, hyperkalemic periodic paralysis; PMC, paramyotonia congenita; PAM, potassium aggravated myotonia; AD, autosomal dominant; AR, autosomal recessive.
* indicates DNA-based diagnosis available in the United Kingdom.

muscle channelopathies. It is now clear that these channelopathies are generally characterized by a disturbance in skeletal muscle excitability. It is helpful to review the key processes of excitation–contraction coupling and action potential generation.

Excitation–contraction coupling in skeletal muscle

The process of excitation–contraction coupling in skeletal muscle is dependent entirely on normally functioning ion channels. For voluntary muscle contraction to occur, the action potential initiated by motor neuron activity has to be transferred to skeletal muscle. This transfer takes place at the specialized neuromuscular junction. As the action potential invades the presynaptic terminal, voltage-gated presynaptic calcium channels open, resulting in a small increase in the calcium concentration in the terminal. This increased calcium initiates release of acetylcholine into the synaptic space, which binds to the postsynaptic acetylcholine receptor – a ligand-gated ion channel. Acetylcholine induced opening of the receptor results in end plate potentials that summate, causing a self-propagating action potential in the sarcolemma. Transmission of this action potential along the T-tubule system (that part of the sarcolemma that invaginates into the muscle fiber) is the prerequisite for calcium induced muscle contraction. The action potential invading the T-tubule leads to an interaction between the T-tubule membrane-located calcium channel (CACNA1S) and the ryanodine receptor (RYR1) located in the membrane of the muscle sarcoplasmic reticulum. This interaction results in opening of the ryanodine receptor, allowing calcium to be released from the sarcoplasmic reticulum into the myoplasm and calcium induced activity of the contractile system.

Skeletal muscle action potential generation

The resting membrane potential of muscle fibers is determined by the high chloride channel conductance of the membrane in the resting state. Muscle fiber membrane excitability depends on normal activation and inactivation properties of ion channels. In response to a depolarizing stimulus, the upstroke of an action potential is caused by the opening of voltage-gated sodium channels (Nav1.4 encoded by the gene *SCN4A*) allowing a rapid inward sodium current to develop. Rapid closure – fast inactivation – of the sodium channel is essential for the initiation of repolarization. Repolarization is promoted further by the opening of delayed rectifier potassium channels that allow efflux of potassium from the muscle fiber. After-potentials (repetitive depolarizations following an action potential) are limited by the high chloride channel conductance present in the resting muscle fiber membrane – mediated by the homodimeric chloride channel [encoded by the gene *CLCN1*].

It is now recognized that the skeletal muscle channelopathies are disorders characterized by altered muscle fiber membrane excitability. Genetic mutations in many of the ion channels involved in excitation–contraction coupling and action potential genesis have been shown to be causative (Table 9.1).

Periodic paralysis

The periodic paralyses (PP) are disorders in which patients experience focal or generalized episodes of muscle weakness of variable duration. Traditionally, they have been characterized on the basis of the serum potassium during an attack. This classification is useful clinically, although a genetic classification has now emerged (see Table 9.1).

Hyperkalemic periodic paralysis

Hyperkalemic periodic paralysis (hyperPP) is an autosomal dominant skeletal muscle channelopathy. Patients typically experience attacks of muscle weakness starting in the first decade of life. Precipitants to attacks vary but may include rest following exercise, cold, potassium ingestion, or stress. Attacks may vary in severity from mild weakness to total paralysis. The duration of attacks is shorter than in hypokalemic periodic paralysis (hypoPP) and is usually less than two hours. Typically, the attack frequency declines with age but patients may develop a fixed myopathy of variable severity. Muscle biopsy in such cases often reveals tubular aggregates and/or a vacuolar change. In humans, unlike in equines, death is extremely rare in hyperPP or hypoPP. Cardiac arrhythmias are also uncommon (see following discussion of Andersen's syndrome).

Hyperkalemic periodic paralysis is caused by "gain of function" point mutations in the muscle sodium channel SCN4A. Sodium channel α-subunit mutations (SCN4A) [2–3] lead to defective fast inactivation of the skeletal muscle sodium channel [4]. The resulting persisting inward sodium current (a gain of function) impairs repolarization and increases membrane excitability. Depending on the degree of increased membrane excitability, a patient may experience myotonia or paralysis. Some genotype/phenotype correlations can be made. For example, the most frequent point mutation, T704M, which causes 60% of cases frequently causes permanent late-onset muscle weakness. Another frequent mutation,

I1592M, is often associated with myotonia as well as paralysis.

Attacks of weakness are associated with high serum potassium and high urinary potassium excretion. However, the serum potassium may remain within the normal range and a supra-normal potassium may rapidly autocorrect; therefore, measurement as early as possible in an attack is important. The creatine kinase may be normal or modestly elevated up to about 300 U/L. Many attacks are brief and do not require treatment. If necessary, acute attacks can be terminated by ingestion of carbohydrate or inhaled salbutamol [5]. Preventative treatment with acetazolamide or a thiazide diuretic may be required [6]. It remains unproven if reducing attack frequency with such agents reduces the likelihood of the subsequent development of myopathy.

Hypokalemic periodic paralysis

Hypokalemic periodic paralysis is the most common form of periodic paralysis with an incidence estimated to be 1 in 100 000. It is inherited in an autosomal dominant manner but *de novo* dominant mutations seem to account for up to one third of cases. The attacks may be brought on by a period of exercise followed by rest or by carbohydrate loading. It is common for attacks to develop in the early hours of the morning from sleep, particularly if a large carbohydrate meal was taken late in the previous evening. Attack duration is much longer then in hyperPP and may be hours to days. Serum potassium is typically low at the onset but may normalize quickly. As in all forms of PP attack, frequency tends to decline with age but a fixed myopathy may develop. Myotonia does not occur in hypoPP.

Point mutations in two separate muscle channel genes may cause hypoPP. The majority of cases harbor one of three point mutations in the L-type calcium channel, CACNA1S, also known as hypoPP type 1 [7]. Far less frequent mutations have been described in the muscle sodium channel SCN4A, also known as hypoPP type 2. Available evidence indicates that hypoPP associated with mutations in either of these channels leads to "loss of function".

Mutations in the L-type calcium channel α_1-subunit (dihydropyridine receptor) (CACNA1S) [8,9] located on chromosome 1q31, account for about 70% of cases of hypoPP [10]. All mutations are arginine substitutions in the voltage sensor (S4) of the channel protein.

It remains unclear how mutations in CACNA1S, which does not have a major role in determining muscle membrane excitability, result in attacks of paralysis. The normal channel has two roles: (1) as a slow voltage-activated calcium channel, and (2) excitation–contraction coupling with the ryanodine receptor. Although the role of this channel in determining membrane excitability is unclear, molecular expression studies of mutated channels have shown enhanced inactivation of the channel [11]. Therefore, it seems that loss of the normal function of the channel is necessary for the attacks of paralysis.

Hypokalemic periodic paralysis associated with CACNA1S mutations exhibits reduced penetrance in females (50%) compared to complete penetrance in males. About half of the women who have the R528H mutation and one third of those with the R1239H mutation are asymptomatic. In contrast, more than 90% of males with a disease-causing mutation are symptomatic. Specific mutations appear to have discrete clinical features (e.g. R528H is common), with later onset and associated myalgias.

Hypokalemic periodic paralysis can also be caused by missense mutations in the voltage sensor of domain 2 of SCN4A [10,12]. Expression studies indicate that the SCN4A mutations associated with hypoPP cause loss of function of the channel. There is some evidence that such hypoPP cases may experience worsening of attacks with prominent myalgia when exposed to acetazolamide. In this setting, an alternative carbonic anhydrase inhibitor, dichlorphenamide, seems to be effective [10]. SCN4A mutations are an uncommon cause of hypoPP in the United Kingdom [13].

Periodic paralysis with cardiac arrhythmias
Andersen's syndrome

Andersen's syndrome is an autosomal dominant potassium-sensitive periodic paralysis associated with ventricular arrhythmias and characteristic facial and skeletal features [14]. The morphological features are often subtle but include low-set ears, hypertelorism, clinodactyly, and syndactyly. Bidirectional ventricular tachycardia is a frequent and potentially serious arrhythmia. From a practical point of view, this disorder should be considered in any case of periodic paralysis with arrhythmia. It is not uncommon that the resting electrocardiograph (EKG) shows bigeminy.

Andersen's syndrome is a channelopathy caused by mutations in a potassium channel termed Kir2.1. This inward rectifying potassium channel Kir2.1 is encoded by the gene *KCNJ2* on chromosome 17q23 [15]. The functional channel is a homotetramer important for cardiac and skeletal muscle membrane hyperpolarization and also has a role in skeletal bone precursor cell migration and fusion during development. Functional expression studies have shown loss of function from a dominant negative effect on wild-type channel subunits, producing a reduced inwardly rectifying potassium current [16]. There is intrafamilial variability and partial manifestation of the phenotype is common. Serum potassium during an attack is most commonly low but may be normal or high. In patients with hypokalemia, oral potassium supplements may improve the weakness. In some families, increasing plasma potassium concentration with acetazolamide improves arrhythmias at the expense of exacerbating weakness [17]. Once the diagnosis is made, detailed cardiac assessment is needed. However, the optimum management to prevent malignant arrhythmias is not certain.

Inherited myotonic disorders

Myotonia is the term given to delayed relaxation of skeletal muscle following voluntary contraction. In most situations, myotonia is most marked following initial muscle contraction and usually abates after repeated muscle activity (the "warm-up phenomenon"). Electophysiologically, myotonia is a disturbance of the normal excitability of the skeletal muscle membrane. There is an abnormally increased excitability of the membrane such that in response to a depolarizing stimulus (i.e. a nerve impulse) rather than a single muscle contraction being initiated, multiple contractions occur, and this results in the delayed relaxation observed clinically. Electromyographic (EMG) and other electrophysiological studies have shown that, in normal muscle, a depolarizing stimulus results in a single action potential; the muscle fiber will contract and then relax. In contrast, in myotonic muscle, after the same stimulus, repetitive action potential firing occurs and the muscle fiber will repeatedly contract thereby delaying relaxation. Patients presenting with isolated pure myotonia are most likely to have myotonia congenita although potassium aggravated myotonia may need to be considered.

Paramyotonia congenita and myotonic dystrophy have specific clinical features that usually make distinction from the pure myotonic disorders straightforward.

Myotonia congenita
Thomsen's disease
Patients with this condition usually present between infancy and adulthood with mild myotonia that may be constant or intermittent. Patients often describe marked muscle stiffness at the onset of activity, but the more they continue the less stiff the muscles become – the so-called warm-up phenomenon. While 90% of cases show myotonia on EMG, only 50% have percussion myotonia on examination. There is usually normal power at rest, although a minority of patients have proximal weakness. Muscle hypertrophy and myalgia may occur. The EMG shows myotonia with a distal predominance, which is present even in early childhood, and the warm-up effect can be observed electrophysiologically.

Thomsen's disease is caused by mutations in a muscle voltage-gated chloride channel (CLCN1) located on chromosome 7q35 [18]. It is transmitted as an autosomal dominant trait with variable penetrance, although 90% of affected individuals are symptomatic. The resting membrane potential in skeletal muscle is mainly dependent upon the chloride channel conductance. Mutations in channel subunits associated with the dominant disease may interfere with dimer formation by exerting a dominant negative effect on wild-type subunits [19]. Because chloride conductance is necessary to stabilize the high resting membrane potential of skeletal muscle, a loss of chloride conductance caused by the mutation results in partial depolarization of the membrane. This creates the electrophysiological condition of increased excitability necessary for myotonia to occur [20].

Becker's disease
The Becker form of myotonia congenita is more severe than Thomsen's disease, with an earlier age of onset. As in Thomsen's disease, there is myotonia with the warm-up phenomenon but patients also have significant muscle hypertrophy, especially in the gluteal muscles. In addition, there may be mild distal muscle weakness. Sudden momentary loss of power with short amounts of exercise is a characteristic feature in many patients. For example, after sitting

for a period, an attempt to stand may precipitate momentary weakness of the quadriceps muscle. The EMG shows frequent myotonic discharges and the warm-up effect can be demonstrated. In contrast to Thomsen's disease, the motor units are frequently mildly myopathic. Becker's disease is also caused by mutations in the muscle chloride channel (CLCN1) [18]; that is, the two forms of myotonia congenita are allelic. However, Becker's disease is inherited in an autosomal recessive manner. There is a male predominance, suggesting reduced penetrance or a milder clinical phenotype in females. Mutations have been found throughout the gene, with point, nonsense, missense mutations, and deletions identified. Most patients are compound heterozygotes.

Molecular expression studies have shown that most recessive mutations result in a loss of function of the chloride channel monomer. Hence, recessive disease, as expected, is a loss of function process.

Many patients with myotonia congenita do not require medication, but those that do usually respond well to mexilitine, in our experience. Other antimyotonic agents can be considered, and include phenytoin, but are less effective [21]. Mexilitene causes use-dependent blockade of sodium channels and stops the production of repetitive runs of action potentials and, hence, reduces muscle stiffness. Ultimately, a specific chloride channel opening agent would be the ideal therapy for these patients but such a drug has not been developed to date. Accurate genetic counseling is important and this relies on the availability of a precise DNA-based diagnosis.

Potassium aggravated myotonias

This is an umbrella term for several rare conditions owing to mutations in the sodium channel, SCN4A. Clinically, patients exhibit pure myotonia of variable severity, which can be particularly sensitive to potassium ingestion. Attacks of severe myotonia may be precipitated by potassium loading with no associated weakness. Various terms have been used to describe these disorders and these are summarized as follows.

Myotonia fluctuant

This involves mild myotonia that varies in severity from day to day with no weakness or cold sensitivity. Stiffness typically develops during rest following a period of exercise and lasts for approximately one

hour. It is exacerbated by potassium and depolarizing agents (e.g. suxamethonium) and may interfere with respiration. The EMG shows myotonia that increases after exercise [22].

Myotonia permanens

These patients experience severe continuous myotonia that may interfere with respiration. There is often marked muscle hypertrophy, especially in the neck and shoulders [22].

Acetazolamide responsive myotonia congenita

This condition is characterized by muscle hypertrophy, myotonia, and myalgia, aggravated by potassium loading and improved by acetazolamide [8].

Paramyotonia congenita

Paradoxical myotonia is stiffness (myotonia) that appears during exercise and worsens with continued activity. The EMG at rest often shows some myotonia although it is less prominent than in the other myotonias previously described. Low temperature often precipitates symptoms in these patients and cooling produces repetitive spontaneous motor unit discharges with a decrement in the muscle action potential amplitude.

Paramyotonia congenita (PMC) is caused by mutations in the voltage-gated skeletal muscle sodium channel α-subunit (SCN4A) [9] on chromosome 17q35 and PMC, therefore, is allelic with hyperPP. Paramyotonia congenita is inherited as a highly penetrant autosomal dominant trait. Mutations have been found throughout the gene, although exon 24 appears to be a hotspot for mutations [23]. Paramyotonia congenita associated point mutations are gain of function. However, the resulting impairment of fast inactivation is less than that associated with mutations associated with hyperPP. Mexiletene is an effective symptomatic treatment for PMC [24].

Myotonia in myotonic dystrophy type 1 and type 2

Myotonic dystrophy is one of the most common genetic muscle disorders in adult neuromuscular practice. It is a multisystem disorder of variable severity ranging from severe, often lethal congenital myotonic dystrophy to minimal myopathy myotonia with cataracts only. Common clinical features include distal muscle myopathy, myotonia, subcapsular catar-acts, cardiac conduction defects, and endocrinopathy. Two types of myotonic dystrophy are now recognized on clinical grounds: DM1 and DM2 (also known as proximal myotonic myopathy, PROMM). Clinically, useful distinguishing features of DM2 include the proximal distribution of the muscle weakness and the prominence of pain, also usually in a proximal distri-bution. DM1 is caused by an unstable CTG repeat in the 3′ untranslated region of the myotonic dystrophy protein kinase gene (*DMPK* on chromosme 19). DM2 associates with a CCTG repeat in the zinc finger protein gene *ZNF9*. Recently, it has been demonstrated that reduced expression of the chloride channel at the muscle fiber membrane is the basis of the myotonia in both DM1 and DM2. The reduced expression seems to be at the level of processing of the primary RNA transcript of the chloride channel gene [25].

In myotonic dystrophy patients where myotonia requires treatment, similar strategies are employed as previously outlined for myotonia congenita. How-ever, close attention to potential cardiac arrhythmias is essential.

Malignant hyperthermia

Malignant hyperthermia syndrome

Malignant hyperthermia syndrome (MHS) is an important cause of death during anesthesia, with an estimated incidence of between 1 in 7000 and 1 in 50 000 of anesthetics given. Malignant hyperthermia syndrome is a skeletal muscle channelopathy caused by dysfunction of the muscle ryanodine receptor. In response to certain anesthetic agents (including volatile agents and depolarizing muscle relaxants), a pathological increase in myoplasmic calcium concentration occurs. This results in hyperthermia, rhabdomyolysis, muscle rigidity, metabolic acidosis, hyperkalemia, and hypoxia. Without prompt treat-ment with dantrolene, mortality can be as high as 70% [26]. Susceptibility tests (mainly the in vitro contraction test [IVCT]) may be diagnostic and can be applied to family members after an affected indi-vidual has been identified. The IVCT test requires a large fresh muscle biopsy, after which either the halothane or the caffeine contracture test may be performed.

Disordered muscle calcium regulation is now known to underlie the pathophysiology of MHS.

A trigger (such as anesthesia) leads to excessive activation of the ryanodine receptor calcium release channel and, thus, calcium is released from sarco-plasmic reticulum stores. Calcium reuptake from the cytoplasm may also be impaired. The increased cyto-plasmic calcium leads to the clinical features [27]. Dantrolene inhibits release of calcium from the sar-coplasmic reticulum [28], and early administration has reduced the mortality rate from 70% to approxi-mately 10%. Mutations in the ryanodine receptor (RYR1) on chromosome 19q13 [29] are found in 50% of MH families and 20% of all MH patients. Over 30 mutations have been identified; most are missense and 50% lie between exons 39 and 46 [30,31]. However, there is genetic heterogeneity [32], with at least five dominantly inherited suscepti-bility loci identified. These include: (1) the sodium channel α_1-subunit (SCN4A) [33], allelic with hyperPP; (2) the skeletal muscle voltage-dependent L-type calcium channel (dihydropyridine receptor) α_2/δ-subunit (CACNL2A) [34]; (3) the L-type calcium chan-nel (dihydropyridine receptor) α_1-subunit (CACNA1S) [35,36], allelic with hypoPP; and (4) unknown genes located on chromosome 3q13.1 (MHS 4) [37] and chromosome 5p (MHS 6) [38].

Central core disease

This is a congenital myopathy with susceptibility to MH. The clinical features include a nonprogressive myopathy with facial and proximal weakness and hypotonia. Occasionally, muscle cramps following exercise are seen. More than a quarter of patients with central core disease (CCD [MHS 1]) have a tendency to MH; however, about 40% of cases at risk for MH are asymptomatic. In such cases, adequate precau-tions prior to anesthesia are not possible. Central core disease is characterized pathologically by the presence of a central core lesion throughout the length of type I muscle fibers. Missense mutations in the skeletal muscle ryanodine receptor gene (RYR1) have been identified in some families with CCD [39]. There are also several other primary muscle disorders with an associated susceptibility to an MH-like reaction. These include myotonia congenita, periodic paralysis, myotonic dystrophy type I, Duchenne and Becker muscular dystrophy, mitochondrial disorders, carni-tine palmitoyl transferase deficiency, and Brody's myopathy. Caution in relation to anesthesia, there-fore, is advised in all these groups.

Congenital myasthenic syndromes

There are some very rare congenital myasthenic syndromes associated with defects in the key processes that underlie efficient neuromuscular junction transmission. The most common defects are mutations in the subunits of the postsynaptic acetylcholine receptor. These myasthenic syndromes may be considered to be genetic ligand-gated channelopathies and are reviewed by Engel *et al.* (2003) [40].

Neuronal channelopathies (Table 9.2)

Ion channels and neuronal function

Ion channels are at least as important for neuronal signaling as they are for muscle contraction. However, although sodium channels play a very similar role in both cell types, the resting membrane potential of neurons is set principally by potassium rather than by chloride channels. Correspondingly, membrane repolarization in neurons is mediated mainly by an outward potassium flux controlled by voltage-sensitive potassium channels. Another difference from muscle cells is that individual neurons express a very large number of different ion channels, both ligand-gated and voltage-gated. Reflecting the heterogeneity among distinct neuronal types, the repertoire of channels expressed (encoded by many genes, most of which may be alternatively spliced) is highly variable. Distinct ion channels are also expressed in different parts of the neuron; namely, the soma, the axon initial segment (where the action potential is normally initiated), nodal and paranodal segments of myelinated axons, presynaptic varicosities and terminals, and synaptic and extrasynaptic areas of dendrites and dendritic spines.

The impact of ion channel mutations for CNS disease is rapidly expanding. Although most of the inherited neuronal channelopathies are dominantly inherited, this may simply reflect the relative difficulty of recognizing rare recessively inherited disorders and elucidating their cause. Interestingly, many of the disorders are characterized by paroxysms of abnormal brain function against a background of normal development and function. (How a life-long abnormality of ion channels can cause only intermittent symptoms is a major puzzle. Indeed, a partial explanation is only available for hyperPP, where muscle depolarization exacerbates extracellular potassium accumulation.)

Neuronal channelopathies can be classified by syndrome or by gene, both of which are problematic.

Table 9.2. Neuronal channelopathes – a genetic classification

Gene	Channel	Disease	Inheritance
GLRA1*	Glycine receptor α1 subunit	Hyperekplexia	AD/AR
CACN1A*	Calcium channel CaV2.1 α1 subunit	EA2 FHM SCA6	AD
KCNA1*	Potassium channel Kv1.1	EA1	AD
KCNQ2/KCNQ3*	Potassium channel	BFNC	AD
CHRNA4/CHRNB2*	Nicotinic ACh receptor α4 and β2 subunits	ADNFLE	AD
SCN1A*	Sodium channel NaV1.1	GEFS+ SMEI FHM	AD Sporadic AD
SCN2A*	Sodium channel NaV1.2	GEFS+	AD
SCN1B*	Sodium channel β1 subunit	GEFS+	AD
CLCN2*	Chloride channel	IGE	AD

EA1, episodic ataxia type 1; EA2, episodic ataxia type 2; FHM, familial hemiplegic migraine; SCA6, spinocerebellar ataxia type 6; BFNC, benign familial neonatal convulsions; ADNFLE, autosomal dominant nocturnal frontal lobe epilepsy; GEFS+, generalized epilepsy with febrile seizures plus; SMEI, severe myoclonic epilepsy of infancy; IGE, idiopathic generalized epilepsy; AD, autosomal dominant; AR, autosomal recessive.

Some ion channel genes are known to be affected in very few patients, perhaps as few as one family, and the list of such genes continues to grow. As for a syndromic classification, some presentations are highly nonspecific, for instance idiopathic epilepsy, for which a monogenic cause accounts for only a minuscule proportion of patients. Rather than providing a comprehensive list of mutations that have been reported, we will concentrate on some of the more unusual syndromes that may raise the suspicion of causation by an ion channel mutation: hyperekplexia, episodic ataxia, hemiplegic migraine, erythromelalgia, and nocturnal frontal lobe epilepsy. These diagnoses by no means make a genetic cause, let alone an inherited channelopathy, inevitable. Rather, in the context of a positive family history, they raise the possibility of a mutation in one of a small number of genes. We will also discuss the confusing relationship between ion channel mutations and epilepsy.

Hereditary hyperekplexia

Hereditary hyperekplexia can present in the neonatal period with stiffness and cyanotic attacks, but more characteristically, patients exhibit a dramatically exaggerated startle response to unexpected noises and other stimuli, with stereotypic posturing of the upper limbs and contraction of facial and neck muscles, sometimes leading to falls. The severity of the response usually slowly abates with age, and the disorder can respond to clonazepam.

Hyperekplexia can exhibit either dominant or recessive inheritance. Some patients have been shown to exhibit compound heterozygosity (inheritance of two presumably recessive alleles from asymptomatic parents). The most commonly affected gene is GLRA1 [41], which encodes the α1 subunit of glycine receptors. The α1 subunit assembles with β subunits to form the adult form of glycine receptors, which are widely expressed in the spinal cord and brainstem, where, together with GABA$_A$ receptors, they mediate fast inhibitory neurotransmission. Hyperekplexia associated mutations are loss of function, although they have highly variable effects on channel trafficking, ligand binding, and transduction of binding to channel opening. Recessively inherited mutations are frequently unable to form a functional channel at all, implying that one wild-type allele alone is sufficient to subserve normal inhibitory signaling.

Some kindreds with hyperekplexia do not have GLRA1 gene mutations, but instead have mutations of other genes involved in glycinergic signaling or in targeting glycine receptors to synapses [42]. These are rare, however.

Episodic ataxia

Two forms of episodic ataxia caused by ion channel mutations are recognized, both of which are inherited in an autosomal dominant manner. In episodic ataxia type 1 (EA1), patients have brief attacks (seconds to minutes) of incoordination, dominated by gait ataxia and often triggered by sudden movements and stress. In between attacks, patients typically have neuromyotonia or myokymia, manifesting as muscle stiffness, twitching, and small amplitude involuntary movements of the fingers. Epilepsy is over-represented among patients with EA1 [43], and the severity of the ataxia and neuromyotonia vary among kindreds, as does the response to treatment with carbamazepine or acetazolamide.

Episodic ataxia type 1 is caused by mutations of the voltage-gated potassium channel gene KCNA1 [44]. This gene encodes a pore-forming subunit Kv1.1, which assembles in a tetramer to form a delayed rectifier-type channel; that is, a channel that opens relatively slowly upon membrane depolarization, thereby allowing potassium ions to flow out of the neuron. Kv1.1 coassembles with other members of the Kv1 family, as well as cytoplasmic auxiliary subunits, and depending on the exact composition of the heteromeric assembly, the channel's biophysical properties can be quite variable. It is expressed widely in the CNS as well as in motor axons, where it contributes to repolarizing the membrane after action potentials.

Episodic ataxia type 1 associated mutations are loss of function, and have variable deleterious effects on channel assembly, trafficking, and kinetics [45,46]. This gives rise to the prediction that, following membrane depolarization, neurons that normally express Kv1.1 should have impaired repolarization. Thus, there is an analogy between the presumed mechanism of neuromyotonia in EA1, arising from spontaneous motor axon activity, and of repetitive muscle fiber action potentials in myotonia congenita. A mutant mouse expressing a human EA1 mutation provides support for the hypothesis that ataxia arises in an analogous way from excessive release of GABA from inhibitory synaptic terminals in the cerebellum [47]. Why ataxia in EA1 patients should be paroxysmal, however, is quite mysterious. Interestingly, when comparing different mutations, there is some correlation between the severity of the clinical syndrome and the degree to which potassium channel function is reduced, with the most severe mutations associated with a dominant negative effect on coexpressed wild-type channel subunits [48].

Episodic ataxia type 2 (EA2) differs from EA1 in that the paroxysms are generally longer lasting (hours) and dominated by dysarthria, diplopia, and gait ataxia. Patients often have nausea and dysphoric symptoms during attacks, which are sometimes diagnosed as basilar migraine. In addition, patients generally have evidence of a mild but slowly progressive cerebellar disorder, with prominent interictal nystagmus. Attacks are frequently precipitated by stress and can be prevented or alleviated by acetazolamide.

Episodic ataxia type 2 is caused by mutations of the calcium channel gene *CACNA1A*, which encodes the α_1 pore-forming subunit of CaV2.1, also known as the P/Q-type channel [49]. This channel is abundantly expressed in cerebellar granule and Purkinje cells. It is also present presynaptically at most synapses in the brain and at the neuromuscular junction, where it mediates a large fraction of the calcium influx that triggers neurotransmitter exocytosis. Episodic ataxia type 2 associated mutations are loss of function. The degree of reduction of calcium channel flux can be partial as shown for some missense mutations, or complete as expected to occur for premature stop codons or splice site mutations. Why a reduction in calcium channel function should lead to a paroxysmal and progressive cerebellar disorder is not clear, but inspection of some spontaneous inbred mouse strains that have mutations of the gene *CACNA1A* suggests that the expression of several other calcium channels is altered, possibly as an indirect developmental consequence. Whether this also occurs in humans with EA2 is not known.

Familial hemiplegic migraine

Episodic ataxia type 2 is only one of several allelic disorders caused by mutations of the gene *CACNA1A*. Familial hemiplegic migraine (FHM) is an especially severe form of migraine with aura, where the aura can cause reversible hemiparesis, transmitted in an autosomal dominant manner. One of the two genes linked to FHM is *CACNA1A*, although in contrast to EA2, all the mutations are missense [49]. Distinct mutations

are associated with different degrees of severity, and many cause an additional mild progressive cerebellar ataxia [50]. Other variable features include reversible coma and a myasthenic syndrome.

Whether FHM mutations are loss or gain of function is controversial. Although most of them reduce the maximal calcium current mediated by CaV2.1 relative to wild-type when expressed in vitro, it has been argued that the current passing through a single channel might be increased [51]. However, alterations of expression of other calcium channels may also occur, and this might have different consequences in cerebellar neurons and transmitter release sites [52]. A mutant mouse strain expressing a human FHM mutation shows a lowered threshold for cortical spreading depression [53], which is presumed to be the substrate of the aura, but the mechanisms linking altered calcium channel function to the neuronal depolarization and ion shifts underlying spreading depression are unclear.

A second gene linked to FHM, *ATP1A2*, encodes a sodium–potassium pump [54]. Although this is not, strictly speaking, an ion channel, it is also intimately involved in maintaining the transmembrane ion gradients that underlie resting potentials and action potentials. The mutations of this gene are also loss of function, and so can be expected to lead to depolarization and impaired ion homeostasis in the brain, possibly explaining a lowered threshold for cortical spreading depression and aura.

A third gene, *SCN1A*, encodes a sodium channel [55]. Surprisingly, mutations of the same gene have been identified in both sporadic and inherited epilepsy (see following discussion).

Although there are other FHM loci, the genes responsible have yet to be identified. Patients with sporadic hemiplegic migraine are infrequently found to have *CACNA1A* gene mutations. It is too early to determine whether genetic insights into the causation of FHM will lead to new therapies. Although EA2 clearly responds to acetazolamide, this drug has a much less marked success rate in FHM. Flunarizine has been found to be successful in the treatment of migraine, and it has been speculated that this reflects its action on calcium channels.

Spinocerebellar ataxia type 6

A third allelic disorder linked to *CACNA1A* gene mutations is spinocerebellar ataxia type 6 (SCA6) [56]. Patients exhibit a relatively pure, slowly progressive, cerebellar degeneration. This is a relatively common cause of autosomal dominant cerebellar ataxia in Japan, and is usually a result of an expanded trinucleotide repeat encoding a polyglutamine sequence in the C-terminus of the channel. It is uncertain whether it causes cerebellar degeneration because of an effect on channel function or because of a direct toxic effect of the peptide.

Hereditary erythromelalgia

Patients with erythromelalgia (also known as erythermalgia) experience burning pain of the extremities associated with redness, precipitated or worsened by cold. Rarely, the disorder is transmitted in an autosomal dominant manner, and is caused by missense mutations of the sodium channel NaV1.7, encoded by the gene *SCN9A* [57]. This channel is expressed in small diameter neurons in the dorsal root ganglia. The mutations that have been studied are gain of function; that is, the channel opens more readily at intermediate levels of membrane depolarization, possibly leading to hyperexcitability or spontaneous firing of unmyelinated sensory axons [58]. Some patients respond to sodium channel blocking drugs such as mexilitine or lignocaine.

Epilepsy

Many studies indicate a strong genetic contribution to the risk of developing idiopathic generalized epilepsy, as well as febrile seizures. However, Mendelian patterns of inheritance are extremely rare in families with multiple affected individuals. This has led to the view that idiopathic (and possibly cryptogenic) epilepsy is a polygenic disorder (or "quantitative trait"), arising when several common gene variants, each of which has a weak contribution to the disease, occur together in an individual. Ion channel genes are prominent candidate quantitative trait loci, a view that was vindicated when the first Mendelian epilepsies were elucidated.

Autosomal dominant nocturnal frontal lobe epilepsy

Autosomal dominant nocturnal frontal lobe epilepsy (ADNFLE) is an uncommon epilepsy, which is characterized by convulsive seizures frequently arising from sleep or while waking. Consciousness is commonly preserved, and patients sometimes have violent thrashing movements of the lower limbs. Because the interictal EEG is often normal, and the ictal electrographic changes overlooked, the disease is sometimes misdiagnosed as a parasomnia or functional disorder. Two loci for ADNFLE have been shown to harbor the genes encoding the nicotinic acetylcholine receptor subunits α4 and β2. Autosomal dominant nocturnal frontal lobe epilepsy is caused by missense mutations of either of the genes encoding these subunits, *CHRNA4* and *CHRNB2*, respectively [54,59]. The subunits coassemble to form an abundant type of nicotinic receptor expressed in the CNS. Nicotinic receptors mediate rapid cholinergic neurotransmission and are candidate targets of tobacco derived nicotine. Their physiological role is uncertain, as is the mechanism by which missense mutations cause frontal lobe epilepsy, not least because distinct mutations appear to have highly variable and inconsistent effects on ligand binding, opening kinetics, and ion permeability. Patients generally respond to carbamazepine and other anti-epileptic drugs acting on sodium channels (e.g. phenytoin, lamotrigine). It has been suggested that mutant nicotinic receptors themselves might also be targets of carbamazepine, but this remains to be confirmed.

Benign familial neonatal convulsions

Benign familial neonatal convulsions (BFNC) are manifested by brief seizures that resolve by six weeks of age, although they can persist in a small proportion of patients. Again, two loci harbor two closely related ion channel genes, in this case *KCNQ2* and *KCNQ3*, which encode potassium channel subunits. These subunits coassemble to form a heteromeric channel that is a major target of muscarinic (G protein-coupled) cholinergic neurotransmission. Benign familial neonatal convulsions is caused by missense mutations, which are loss of function [60–62]. A simple hypothesis to explain the hyperexcitability of brain circuits underlying BFNC is that the potassium conductance mediated by KCNQ2–KCNQ3 heteromers is smaller than normal. However, why the seizures should resolve spontaneously is unclear, as is the precipitating event for seizures in the first place. Because the condition remits spontaneously, drug treatment is generally not indicated.

Generalized epilepsy with febrile seizures plus

This is perhaps the most confusing area in the neurological channelopathies. The term generalized epilepsy with febrile seizures plus (GEFS+) was coined to describe an autosomal dominant form of epilepsy, in which affected individuals suffer from febrile seizures in childhood, and/or febrile seizures persisting beyond childhood, or afebrile seizures [63]. GEFS+ is not a syndrome in the conventional sense, because individuals carrying a given mutation within a kindred can be highly variable, ranging from asymptomatic (implying incomplete penetrance) to severe epileptic encephalopathy. Several genes have been linked to this familial syndrome: *SCN1B*, *SCN1A*, *SCN2A*, and *GBRG2*.

The gene *SCN1B* encodes the β1 sodium channel subunit. This coassembles with either of two α pore-forming subunits, NaV1.1 and NaV1.2, which are encoded by *SCN1A* and *SCN2A*, respectively. Heterozygous missense mutations of all three genes have been identified in distinct GEFS+ families [64–66]. The mechanism by which these sodium channel mutations causes epilepsy is controversial. The first mutation identified disrupts a cysteine bond in the β1 subunit, and prevents the normal functions of β1, among which is an acceleration of fast inactivation. Thus, the GEFS+ mutation of *SCN1B* causes sodium channels to close more slowly than normal [64]. This is effectively a gain of sodium current, reminiscent of the effect of hyperPP mutations of *SCN4A*. Although some mutations of *SCN1A* have been shown to interfere with fast inactivation [67], there is also evidence for loss of function effects on activation kinetics [68]. If the net effect is loss of function, this is unexpected because it would be anticipated to have a similar effect to many anti-epileptic drugs that act on sodium channels (e.g. phenytoin, carbamazepine, lamotrigine). Therefore, it may be necessary to invoke some indirect effects of the mutation, akin to what has been speculated to occur in the CACNA1A-linked disorders above.

The gene *GBRG2* encodes the γ2 subunit of GABA_A receptors. This subunit contributes to targeting GABA_A receptors to inhibitory synapses, and also modulates the sensitivity to GABA and benzodiazepine drugs. The mutations associated with GEFS+ are loss of function; that is, they are predicted to impair GABAergic transmission [69–71].

Why a single ion channel mutation should give rise to such a pleomorphic seizure disorder is not known. However, a likely explanation is that, on its own, the mutation is sufficient to destabilize brain circuits to such an extent that spontaneous synchronous firing of neurons (i.e. the electrographic component of a seizure) occurs spontaneously. However, where in the brain these paroxysms arise, and which circuits they involve, is also influenced by other factors, most plausibly subtle functional variants in other genes that affect neuronal signaling.

It is too early to tell whether the insights into the causation of GEFS+ will lead to new therapies. Reflecting the heterogeneity of the syndrome, affected patients range from benign seizure disorders not requiring treatment to severe refractory epilepsy.

Severe myoclonic epilepsy of infancy

Severe myoclonic epilepsy of infancy (SMEI), or the Dravet syndrome, is a severe pediatric epilepsy that is associated with frequent episodes of status epilepticus and cognitive and motor regression. Affected children generally do not survive to adulthood. It usually arises in the absence of a family history. Several studies have shown that *de novo* heterozygous mutations of the gene *SCN1A*, mainly premature stop codons and splice site mutations predicted to give rise to nonfunctional proteins, occur in a large proportion of children with SMEI [72,73]. This fact alone provides further support to the view that loss of sodium channel function can give rise to epilepsy, although the mechanisms by which this happens are unknown.

Conclusions

The previously described list of ion channels, now known to be involved in monogenic disorders, is not complete. Among others are the CNS chloride channel gene *CLCN2* (associated with idiopathic generalized epilepsy [74]), the GABA_A receptor subunit gene *GBRA1* (associated with juvenile myoclonic epilepsy [75]), and the calcium-gated potassium channel gene *KCNMA1* (causing generalized epilepsy associated with paroxysmal dyskinesia [76]). Recently, it has become apparent that mutations of some ion channel genes do not cosegregate with the disease but may instead be susceptibility factors; for instance, the calcium channel gene *CACNA1H* (associated with sporadic childhood absence epilepsy [77]). Inherited variability in the coding sequence of the *GABRD* gene, encoding the δ subunit of GABA_A receptors, has also been suggested to act as a susceptibility factor for generalized epilepsy [78]. It remains to be determined whether a small number of ion channel genes harbor susceptibility factors accounting for a large part of the population risk of developing idiopathic epilepsy and other paroxysmal neurological diseases. An alternative view is that each ion channel gene individually contributes to only a relatively small part of the heritability of these disorders. Nevertheless, because there are several hundred ion channel genes expressed in neurons and muscle, this family of genes as a whole remains the best candidate group to account for the population risk. By extension, genes encoding proteins involved in the trafficking and modulation of ion channel function are also strong candidates. Indeed, two genes that have been implicated in monogenic epilepsy have recently been reported to modulate the function of calcium and potassium channels [79,80].

A further fertile area of research is the role of inherited variability of ion channels in the drug treatment of neurological disease. This is hinted at by the recent observation that a common polymorphism in the sodium channel gene *SCN1A* (the same gene involved in GEFS+, SMEI, and FHM) associates with the dosage of carbamazepine or phenytoin prescribed to patients with epilepsy [81]. Because NaV1.1, encoded by *SCN1A*, is a target of these drugs and the polymorphism affects the splicing of this gene, this genetic association points to a direct mechanism linking inherited variability of ion channels to the treatment of epilepsy.

Acknowledgments

We thank Dr TD Graves for help in preparing this manuscript. Our research is supported by the Medical Research Council, the Wellcome Trust, the National Institutes of Health USA, and the Guarantors of Brain. Our clinical channelopathy service is supported by the Department of Health Specialist commissioning (NSCAG) UK.

References

1. Kullmann DM, Hanna MG. Neurological disorders caused by inherited ion-channel mutations. *Lancet Neurol* 2002; **1**: 157–166.

2. Ptacek LJ, George AL Jr, Griggs RC, *et al.* Identification of a mutation in the gene causing hyperkalemic periodic paralysis. *Cell* 1991; **67**: 1021–1027.

3. Bendahhou S, Cummins TR, Tawil R, *et al.* Activation and inactivation of the voltage-gated sodium channel: role of segment S5 revealed by a novel hyperkalaemic periodic paralysis mutation. *J Neurosci* 1999; **19**: 4762–4771.

4. Hayward LJ, Sandoval GM, Cannon SC. Defective slow inactivation of sodium channels contributes to familial periodic paralysis. *Neurology* 1999; **52**: 1447–1453.

5. Hanna MG, Stewart J, Schapira AH, *et al.* Salbutamol treatment in a patient with hyperkalaemic periodic paralysis due to a mutation in the skeletal muscle sodium channel gene (SCN4A). *J Neurol Neurosurg Psychiatry* 1998; **65**: 248–250.

6. Hoskins B, Vroom FQ, Jarrell MA. Hyperkalemic periodic paralysis. Effects of potassium, exercise, glucose, and acetazolamide on blood chemistry. *Arch Neurol* 1975; **32**: 519–523.

7. Ptacek LJ, Tawil R, Griggs RC, *et al.* Dihydropyridine receptor mutations cause hypokalemic periodic paralysis. *Cell* 1994; **77**: 863–868.

8. Ptacek LJ, Tawil R, Griggs RC, *et al.* Sodium channel mutations in acetazolamide-responsive myotonia congenita, paramyotonia congenita, and hyperkalemic periodic paralysis. *Neurology* 1994; **44**: 1500–1503.

9. Ptacek LJ, George AL Jr, Barchi RL, *et al.* Mutations in an S4 segment of the adult skeletal muscle sodium channel cause paramyotonia congenita. *Neuron* 1992; **8**: 891–897.

10. Sternberg D, Maisonobe T, Jurkat-Rott K, *et al.* Hypokalaemic periodic paralysis type 2 caused by mutations at codon 672 in the muscle sodium channel gene SCN4A. *Brain* 2001; **124**: 1091–1099.

11. Jurkat-Rott K, Lehmann-Horn F, Elbaz A, *et al.* A calcium channel mutation causing hypokalemic periodic paralysis. *Hum Mol Genet* 1994; **3**: 1415–1419.

12. Bulman DE, Scoggan KA, van Oene MD, *et al.* A novel sodium channel mutation in a family with hypokalemic periodic paralysis. *Neurology* 1999; **53**: 1932–1936.

13. Davies NP, Eunson LH, Samuel M, Hanna MG. Sodium channel gene mutations in hypokalemic periodic paralysis: an uncommon cause in the UK. *Neurology* 2001; **57**: 1323–1325.

14. Sansone V, Griggs RC, Meola G, *et al.* Andersen's syndrome: a distinct periodic paralysis. *Ann Neurol* 1997; **42**: 305–312.

15. Plaster NM, Tawil R, Tristani-Firouzi M, *et al.* Mutations in Kir2.1 cause the developmental and episodic electrical phenotypes of Andersen's syndrome. *Cell* 2001; **105**: 511–519.

16. Tristani-Firouzi M, Jensen JL, Donaldson MR, *et al.* Functional and clinical characterization of KCNJ2 mutations associated with LQT7 (Andersen syndrome). *J Clin Invest* 2002; **110**: 381–388.

17. Junker J, Haverkamp W, Schulze-Bahr E, *et al.*

Amiodarone and acetazolamide for the treatment of genetically confirmed severe Andersen syndrome. *Neurology* 2002; **59**: 466.

18. Koch MC, Steinmeyer K, Lorenz C, *et al.* The skeletal muscle chloride channel in dominant and recessive human myotonia. *Science* 1992; **257**: 797–800.

19. Kubisch C, Schmidt-Rose T, Fontaine B, *et al.* CLC-1 chloride channel mutations in myotonia congenita: variable penetrance of mutations shifting the voltage dependence. *Hum Mol Genet* 1998; 7: 1753–1760.

20. Wu FF, Ryan A, Devaney J, *et al.* Novel CLCN1 mutations with unique clinical and electrophysiological consequences. *Brain* 2002; **125**: 2392–2407.

21. Ceccarelli M, Rossi B, Siciliano G, *et al.* Clinical and electrophysiological reports in a case of early onset myotonia congenita (Thomsen's disease) successfully treated with mexiletine. *Acta Paediatr* 1992; **81**: 453–455.

22. Ricker K, Moxley RT 3rd, Heine R, Lehmann-Horn F. Myotonia fluctuans. A third type of muscle sodium channel disease. *Arch Neurol* 1994; **51**: 1095–1102.

23. Davies NP, Eunson LH, Gregory RP, *et al.* Clinical, electrophysiological, and molecular genetic studies in a new family with paramyotonia congenita. *J Neurol Neurosurg Psychiatry* 2000; **68**: 504–507.

24. Weckbecker K, Wurz A, Mohammadi B, *et al.* Different effects of mexiletine on two mutant sodium channels causing paramyotonia congenita and hyperkalemic periodic paralysis. *Neuromuscul Disord* 2000; **10**: 31–39.

25. Charlet-B N, Saykur RS, Singh G, *et al.* Loss of the muscle-specific chloride channel in type 1 myotonic dystrophy due to misregulated alternative splicing. *Mol Cell* 2002; **10**: 45–53.

26. Hogan K. The anesthetic myopathies and malignant hyperthermias. *Curr Opin Neurol* 1998; **11**: 469–476.

27. Jurkat-Rott K, McCarthy T, Lehmann-Horn F. Genetics and pathogenesis of malignant hyperthermia. *Muscle Nerve* 2000; **23**: 4–17.

28. Zhao F, Li P, Chen SR, *et al.* Dantrolene inhibition of ryanodine receptor Ca2+ release channels. Molecular mechanism and isoform selectivity. *J Biol Chem* 2001; **276**: 13810–13816.

29. MacLennan DH, Otsu K, Fujii J, *et al.* The role of the skeletal muscle ryanodine receptor gene in malignant hyperthermia. *Symp Soc Exp Biol* 1992; **46**: 189–201.

30. Quane KA, Keating KE, Manning BM, *et al.* Detection of a novel common mutation in the ryanodine receptor gene in malignant hyperthermia: implications for diagnosis and heterogeneity studies. *Hum Mol Genet* 1994; **3**: 471–476.

31. Manning BM, Quane KA, Ording H, *et al.* Identification of novel mutations in the ryanodine-receptor gene (RYR1) in malignant hyperthermia: genotype-phenotype correlation. *Am J Hum Genet* 1998; **62**: 599–609.

32. Robinson RL, Curran JL, Ellis FR, *et al.* Multiple interacting gene products may influence susceptibility to malignant hyperthermia. *Ann Hum Genet* 2000; **64**: 307–320.

33. Moslehi R, Langlois S, Yam I, Friedman JM. Linkage of malignant hyperthermia and hyperkalemic periodic paralysis to the adult skeletal muscle sodium channel (SCN4A) gene in a large pedigree. *Am J Med Genet* 1998; **76**: 21–27.

34. Iles DE, Lehmann-Horn F, Scherer SW, *et al.* Localization of the gene encoding the alpha 2/delta-subunits of the L-type voltage-dependent calcium channel to chromosome 7q and analysis of the segregation of flanking markers in malignant hyperthermia susceptible families. *Hum Mol Genet* 1994; **3**: 969–975.

35. Monnier N, Procaccio V, Stieglitz P, Lunardi J. Malignant-hyperthermia susceptibility is associated with a mutation of the alpha 1-subunit of the human dihydropyridine-sensitive L-type voltage-dependent calcium-channel receptor in skeletal muscle. *Am J Hum Genet* 1997; **60**: 1316–1325.

36. Stewart SL, Hogan K, Rosenberg H, Fletcher JE. Identification of the Arg1086His mutation in the alpha subunit of the voltage-dependent calcium channel (CACNA1S) in a North American family with malignant hyperthermia. *Clin Genet* 2001; **59**: 178–184.

37. Sudbrak R, Procaccio V, Klausnitzer M, *et al.* Mapping of a further malignant hyperthermia susceptibility locus to chromosome 3q13.1. *Am J Hum Genet* 1995; **56**: 684–691.

38. Robinson RL, Monnier N, Wolz W, *et al.* A genome wide search for susceptibility loci in three European malignant hyperthermia pedigrees. *Hum Mol Genet* 1997; **6**: 953–961.

39. Monnier N, Romero NB, Lerale J, *et al.* An autosomal dominant congenital myopathy with cores and rods is associated with a neomutation in the RYR1 gene encoding the skeletal muscle ryanodine receptor. *Hum Mol Genet* 2000; **9**: 2599–2608.

40. Engel AG, Ohno K, Sine SM. Congenital myasthenic syndromes: progress over the past decade. *Muscle Nerve* 2003; **27**: 4–25.

41. Shiang R, Ryan SG, Zhu YZ, *et al.* Mutations in the alpha 1

subunit of the inhibitory glycine receptor cause the dominant neurologic disorder, hyperekplexia. *Nat Genet* 1993; **5**: 351–358.

42. Harvey RJ, Topf M, Harvey K, Rees MI. The genetics of hyperekplexia: more than startle! *Trends Genet* 2008; **24**: 439–447.

43. Zuberi SM, Eunson LH, Spauschus A, *et al.* A novel mutation in the human voltage-gated potassium channel gene (Kv1.1) associates with episodic ataxia type 1 and sometimes with partial epilepsy. *Brain* 1999; **122**: 817–825.

44. Browne DL, Gancher ST, Nutt JG, *et al.* Episodic ataxia/myokymia syndrome is associated with point mutations in the human potassium channel gene, KCNA1. *Nat Genet* 1994; **8**: 136–140.

45. Adelman JP, Bond CT, Pessia M, Maylie J. Episodic ataxia results from voltage-dependent potassium channels with altered functions. *Neuron* 1995; **15**: 1449–1454.

46. Rea R, Spauschus A, Eunson L, *et al.* Variable K+ channel subunit dysfunction in inherited mutations of KCNA1. *J Physiol* 2002; **538**: 5–23.

47. Herson PS, Virk M, Rustay NR, *et al.* A mouse model of episodic ataxia type-1. *Nat Neurosci* 2003; **6**: 378–383.

48. Eunson LH, Rea R, Zuberi SM, *et al.* Clinical, genetic, and expression studies of mutations in the potassium channel gene KCNA1 reveal new phenotypic variability. *Ann Neurol* 2000; **48**: 647–656.

49. Ophoff RA, Terwindt GM, Vergouwe MN, *et al.* Familial hemiplegic migraine and episodic ataxia type-2 are caused by mutations in the Ca2+ channel gene CACNL1A4. *Cell* 1996; **87**: 543–552.

50. Ducros A, Denier C, Joutel A, *et al.* The clinical spectrum of familial hemiplegic migraine associated with mutations in a neuronal calcium channel. *N Engl J Med* 2001; **345**: 17–24.

51. Tottene A, Fellin T, Pagnutti S, *et al.* Familial hemiplegic migraine mutations increase Ca(2+) influx through single human CaV2.1 channels and decrease maximal CaV2.1 current density in neurons. *Proc Natl Acad Sci USA* 2002; **99**: 13284–13289.

52. Cao YQ, Piedras-Renteria ES, Smith GB, *et al.* Presynaptic Ca2+ channels compete for channel type-preferring slots in altered neurotransmission arising from Ca2+ channelopathy. *Neuron* 2004; **43**: 387–400.

53. van den Maagdenberg AM, Pietrobon D, Pizzorusso T, *et al.* A CACNA1A knockin migraine mouse model with increased susceptibility to cortical spreading depression. *Neuron* 2004; **41**: 701–710.

54. De Fusco M, Becchetti A, Patrignani A, *et al.* The nicotinic receptor beta 2 subunit is mutant in nocturnal frontal lobe epilepsy. *Nat Genet* 2000; **26**: 275–276.

55. Dichgans M, Freilinger T, Eckstein G, *et al.* Mutation in the neuronal voltage-gated sodium channel SCN1A in familial hemiplegic migraine. *Lancet* 2005; **366**: 371–377.

56. Zhuchenko O, Bailey J, Bonnen P, *et al.* Autosomal dominant cerebellar ataxia (SCA6) associated with small polyglutamine expansions in the alpha 1A-voltage-dependent calcium channel. *Nat Genet* 1997; **15**: 62–69.

57. Yang Y, Wang Y, Li S, *et al.* Mutations in SCN9A, encoding a sodium channel alpha subunit, in patients with primary erythermalgia. *J Med Genet* 2004; **41**: 171–174.

58. Cummins TR, Dib-Hajj SD, Waxman SG. Electrophysiological properties of mutant Nav1.7 sodium channels in a painful inherited neuropathy. *J Neurosci* 2004; **24**: 8232–8236.

59. Steinlein OK, Mulley JC, Propping P, *et al.* A missense mutation in the neuronal nicotinic acetylcholine receptor alpha 4 subunit is associated with autosomal dominant nocturnal frontal lobe epilepsy. *Nat Genet* 1995; **11**: 201–203.

60. Biervert C, Schroeder BC, Kubisch C, *et al.* A potassium channel mutation in neonatal human epilepsy. *Science* 1998; **279**: 403–406.

61. Charlier C, Singh NA, Ryan SG, *et al.* A pore mutation in a novel KQT-like potassium channel gene in an idiopathic epilepsy family. *Nat Genet* 1998; **18**: 53–55.

62. Singh NA, Charlier C, Stauffer D, *et al.* A novel potassium channel gene, KCNQ2, is mutated in an inherited epilepsy of newborns. *Nat Genet* 1998; **18**: 25–29.

63. Scheffer IE, Berkovic SF. Generalized epilepsy with febrile seizures plus. A genetic disorder with heterogeneous clinical phenotypes. *Brain* 1997; **120**: 479–490.

64. Wallace RH, Wang DW, Singh R, *et al.* Febrile seizures and generalized epilepsy associated with a mutation in the Na$^+$-channel beta1 subunit gene SCN1B. *Nat Genet* 1998; **19**: 366–370.

65. Escayg A, MacDonald BT, Meisler MH, *et al.* Mutations of SCN1A, encoding a neuronal sodium channel, in two families with GEFS+2. *Nat Genet* 2000; **24**: 343–345.

66. Sugawara T, Tsurubuchi Y, Agarwala KL, *et al.* A missense mutation of the Na$^+$ channel alpha II subunit gene Na(v)1.2 in a patient with febrile and afebrile seizures causes channel dysfunction. *Proc Natl Acad Sci USA* 2001; **98**: 6384–6389.

67. Lossin C, Wang DW, Rhodes TH, *et al.* Molecular basis of an inherited epilepsy. *Neuron* 2002; **34**: 877–884.

68. Alekov AK, Rahman MM, Mitrovic N, *et al.* Enhanced inactivation and acceleration of activation of the sodium channel associated with epilepsy in man. *Eur J Neurosci* 2001; **13**: 2171–2176.

69. Baulac S, Huberfeld G, Gourfinkel-An I, *et al.* First genetic evidence of GABA(A) receptor dysfunction in epilepsy: a mutation in the gamma2-subunit gene. *Nat Genet* 2001; **28**: 46–48.

70. Wallace RH, Marini C, Petrou S, *et al.* Mutant GABA(A) receptor gamma2-subunit in childhood absence epilepsy and febrile seizures. *Nat Genet* 2001; **28**: 49–52.

71. Bianchi MT, Song L, Zhang H, Macdonald RL. Two different mechanisms of disinhibition produced by GABAA receptor mutations linked to epilepsy in humans. *J Neurosci* 2002; **22**: 5321–5327.

72. Claes L, Del-Favero J, Ceulemans B, *et al.* De novo mutations in the sodium-channel gene SCN1A cause severe myoclonic epilepsy of infancy. *Am J Hum Genet* 2001; **68**: 1327–1332.

73. Sugawara T, Mazaki-Miyazaki E, Fukushima K, *et al.* Frequent mutations of SCN1A in severe myoclonic epilepsy in infancy. *Neurology* 2002; **58**: 1122–1124.

74. Haug K, Warnstedt M, Alekov AK, *et al.* Mutations in CLCN2 encoding a voltage-gated chloride channel are associated with idiopathic generalized epilepsies. *Nat Genet* 2003; **33**: 527–532.

75. Cossette P, Liu L, Brisebois K, *et al.* Mutation of GABRA1 in an autosomal dominant form of juvenile myoclonic epilepsy. *Nat Genet* 2002; **31**: 184–189.

76. Du W, Bautista JF, Yang H, *et al.* Calcium-sensitive potassium channelopathy in human epilepsy and paroxysmal movement disorder. *Nat Genet* 2005; **37**: 733–738.

77. Chen Y, Lu J, Pan H, *et al.* Association between genetic variation of CACNA1H and childhood absence epilepsy. *Ann Neurol* 2003; **54**: 239–243.

78. Dibbens LM, Feng HJ, Richards MC, *et al.* GABRD encoding a protein for extra- or peri-synaptic GABAA receptors is a susceptibility locus for generalized epilepsies. *Hum Mol Genet* 2004; **13**: 1315–1319.

79. Schulte U, Thumfart JO, Klocker N, *et al.* The epilepsy-linked Lgi1 protein assembles into presynaptic Kv1 channels and inhibits inactivation by Kvbeta1. *Neuron* 2006; **49**: 697–706.

80. Suzuki T, Delgado-Escueta AV, Aguan K, *et al.* Mutations in EFHC1 cause juvenile myoclonic epilepsy. *Nat Genet* 2004; **36**: 842–849.

81. Tate SK, Depondt C, Sisodiya SM, *et al.* Genetic predictors of the maximum doses patients receive during clinical use of the anti-epileptic drugs carbamazepine and phenytoin. *Proc Natl Acad Sci USA* 2005; **102**: 5507–5512.

Chapter 10

Amyotrophic lateral sclerosis and other disorders of the lower motor neuron

Christopher E. Shaw, Jemeen Sreedharan, Caroline A. Vance, and Ammar Al-Chalabi

Introduction

In this chapter, we will critically review the epidemiology, clinical phenotype, and genetic basis of the heritable forms of amyotrophic lateral sclerosis (ALS) and other disorders of the lower motor neuron (LMN) including Kennedy's disease (spinobulbar muscular atrophy), the spinal muscular atrophies (SMA), and hereditary motor neuropathies (HMN). The identification of mutations in ALS genes in both sporadic (SALS) and familial ALS (FALS) has blurred any distinction between inherited and acquired ALS. The discovery that the TAR DNA binding protein (TDP-43) forms cytoplasmic inclusions within motor neurons and glia in ~90% of ALS cases and that mutations in the gene (*TARDBP*) segregate with disease confirms its pathogenicity. The discovery of mutations in other RNA processing genes, survival motor neuron 1 (SMN1) in SMA, and fused in sarcoma (FUS) and heat shock proteins in HMN have provided new insights into the pathogenesis of the motor neuropathies.

Definition of amyotrophic lateral sclerosis

Amyotrophic lateral sclerosis is also known as Lou Gehrig's disease in the United States and motor neuron disease in the United Kingdom. Amyotrophic lateral sclerosis was originally thought to be a degenerative muscular condition until Charcot published clinicopathological studies, in 1869, emphasizing the involvement of both upper motor neurons (UMNs) and LMNs with sparing of the sensory and autonomic pathways. He used the words amyotrophic (muscle wasting), lateral (corticospinal tracts), and sclerosis (scarring) to describe the principal features. The features that distinguish ALS from other disorders affecting the motor system are rapid progression (survival of approximately 3–5 years), a combination of UMN and LMN signs, and in many cases, mild cognitive impairment (an under-recognized feature). When LMNs degenerate, the muscles they innervate fasciculate, waste, and become profoundly weak. Upper motor neurons reside in the precentral gyrus of the cerebral cortex, and when they degenerate, there is a loss of inhibitory input to the LMNs resulting in muscle spasticity, brisk reflexes, and an extensor plantar response. Motor neurons controlling eye movements, and bladder and bowel sphincters are relatively spared as are sensory and autonomic pathways. The El Escorial Diagnostic Criteria describe a hierarchy of diagnostic certainty based on the number of regions clinically affected and supplemented by neurophysiological tests confirming muscle denervation [1]. These criteria are useful in clinical trials but should not be used clinically as they may add to diagnostic delay.

Most people with ALS have a combination of UMN and LMN signs, but ALS variants include primary lateral sclerosis (PLS) where UMN features predominate, and progressive muscular atrophy (PMA) where LMN features predominate in the early course of the disease. These conditions are usually more slowly progressive, but over time signs of both UMN and LMN degeneration develop. In 25% of patients, symptoms begin with slurred speech or difficulty swallowing (bulbar-onset disease) owing to degeneration of motor neurons in the brainstem. This is characterized by wasting and weakness of the tongue and pharyngeal muscles, and is often combined with poor elevation of the soft palate and an exaggerated gag reflex or jaw jerk. The LMN variant has been named progressive bulbar palsy and the UMN variant pseudobulbar palsy. Pathological studies demonstrate that ubiquitinated TDP-43 positive inclusions are present in the LMNs in the vast majority of patients and confirm that all of these phenotypes fall within the general rubric of ALS [2,3].

Overlap between amyotrophic lateral sclerosis and frontotemporal lobar dementia

The frontotemporal lobar dementias (FTD) are a heterogeneous group of disorders of the frontal and anterior temporal lobes. Frontotemporal lobar dementia is characterized by altered behavior and language deficits. Patients may present with semantic dementia (word meaning is lost) or progressive non-fluent aphasia (difficulties in word finding) [4]. Behavioral changes include socially inappropriate behavior and increased impulsivity. The relative preservation of memory distinguishes FTD from Alzheimer's disease. Interestingly, about 5% of ALS cases may also fulfill diagnostic criteria for FTD, and detailed psychometric testing reveals subtle cognitive deficits in 30% of people with ALS [5]. Pathologically, the FTDs are defined by protein accumulating in cytoplasmic inclusions. Approximately 40% of cases have microtubule associated protein tau (deposited in Pick bodies or neurofibrillary tangles), about 50% have TDP-43 and about 5% have FUS deposited in globular and granular inclusions. Phenotypic overlap between FTD and ALS is recognized increasingly, and the observation that both disorders are TDP-43 proteinopathies provides a molecular link.

Making the diagnosis of amyotrophic lateral sclerosis

Amyotrophic lateral sclerosis is uncommon and the diagnosis can be difficult. A general practitioner may encounter only one case in a working lifetime and may not recognize the earliest symptoms or signs. There is no simple test for ALS and neurologists often delay making a diagnosis until they are absolutely certain. This can lead to prolonged uncertainty for the patient and their families, many of whom are aware of this possibility through the internet. We favor an early and honest discussion of this possibility. A range of investigations (imaging, laboratory-based, and neurophysiological) can be used to exclude potentially treatable conditions that may mimic ALS (Table 10.1). Nerve conduction studies and electromyography are essential to confirm evidence of acute LMN loss in ALS and to exclude myopathy. Muscle biopsy is only helpful if the presentation is atypical or the phenotype suggests inclusion body myositis. Other rare ALS

Table 10.1. Conditions that mimic amyotrophic lateral sclerosis

Condition	Diagnostic screening tests	Clinical phenotype
Structural myelo-radiculopathy (stenosis, osteophytes, syrinx)	MRI	Pain and paresthesiae
Kennedy's disease	Androgen receptor mutation	Very slow progression, gynecomastia, testicular atrophy, hand tremor
Multifocal motor neuropathy	Anti-GM1 ganglioside antibodies, nerve conduction studies	Weakness greater than wasting
Inflammatory myelo-radiculopathy (multiple sclerosis, sarcoidosis)	MRI, lumbar puncture, auto-antibodies, chest X-ray	Sphincter disturbance, paresthesiae
Infectious myelo-radiculopathy (HIV, HTLV1, Lyme disease)	MRI, lumbar puncture, antibodies and polymerase chain reaction to detect infectious agents	Sphincter disturbance, paresthesiae
Adult-onset spinal muscular atrophy	Survival motor neuron 1 gene deletion	Slow progression
Myopathies (inclusion body myositis)	Creatine kinase, muscle biopsy	Weakness of forearm flexors and quadriceps
Diabetic amyotrophy	Glucose, glycosylated hemoglobin	Sensory involvement

mimics have been reported (e.g. hexosaminidase A deficiency), but it is not clinically useful to screen for these in typical ALS cases.

Epidemiology

The incidence of adult-onset classical ALS is 1–2 per 100 000 person–years and the point prevalence is 5–13 per 100 000 [6]. Three populations have a much higher prevalence of ALS, raising the possibility of a strong genetic founder effect. Amyotrophic lateral sclerosis is relatively common in the Chamorro people of Guam and the Marianas Islands (Guamanian Parkinson dementia complex, PDC), the Japanese on the Kii peninsula of Honshu Island, and the Auyu and Jakai peoples of southern West New Guinea. In all three regions, ALS is associated with parkinsonism and FTD, and the pathology demonstrates paired helical tau filaments similar to those in Alzheimer's disease. Genetic studies in affected kindreds have so far been negative [7]. The incidence of Guamanian PDC declined sharply after World War II implying an environmental etiology, while the incidence on the Kii Peninsula is stable and often familial implying a genetic etiology [8].

Familial amyotrophic lateral sclerosis

While the person with sporadic ALS (and their doctors) may not realize the significance of their earliest symptoms, this is not the case in FALS kindreds. Often they have lived with a heavy psychological burden knowing that every muscle cramp, twitch, stiffness, or weakness may herald the onset of ALS. About 1 in 10 affected individuals have a family history of ALS or FTD, typically with autosomal dominant inheritance with age-dependent and incomplete penetrance. In some of these kindreds, penetrance is >90% and the lifetime risk for ALS approaches 50%, while in others it is as low as 20%. Evidence that the disease is familial may only come to light after exhaustive exploration of the extended kindred. Ancestral death following a rapidly progressive gait disturbance, dysarthria, or dysphagia is highly suggestive of ALS, and a history of dementia may also be relevant. Although males are more commonly affected than females in SALS with a ratio of 3:2, the gender ratio in FALS is 1:1 [9]. Apart from a few notable exceptions (described as follows), the clinical presentation of most patients with FALS is identical to that of sporadic disease. The classification of the

Table 10.2. Classification of familial amyotrophic lateral sclerosis disorders

Designation	Locus	Inheritance	Phenotype	Protein
ALS1	21q22	AD	Classical ALS	SOD1
ALS2	2q33	AR	Juvenile PLS	alsin
ALS3	(18q21)	AD	Classical ALS	?
ALS4	9q34	AD	Juvenile HSP+	senataxin
ALS5	15q15	AR	Juvenile ALS	spatacsin
ALS6	16q12	AD	Classical ALS	FUS
ALS7	20ptel	AD	Classical ALS	?
ALS8	20q13	AD	PMA, ?ALS	VAPB
ALS9	14q11	AD/sporadic	Classical ALS	angiogenin
ALS10	1p36	AD	Classical ALS	TDP-43
ALS11	6q21	AD	Classical ALS	FIG4
ALS/FTD1	9q21	AD	Classical ALS+/−FTD	C90RF72
ALS/FTD2	9p13	AD	Classical ALS+/−FTD	?

ALS, amyotrophic lateral sclerosis; FTD, frontotemporal lobar dementia; AD, autosomal dominant; AR, autosomal recessive; PLS, primary lateral sclerosis; HSP, hereditary spastic paraplegia; PMA, progressive muscular atrophy.

different forms of FALS, current as of July 2010, is given in Table 10.2. The most common gene defect in FALS is in *SOD1*, which accounts for about 20% of all dominant kindreds. FUS and TDP-43 mutations are detected in about 1% and 4% of FALS, respectively. The other genes and loci are only very rarely associated with FALS, and in some cases, cause a phenotype very different from that of typical ALS.

Amyotrophic lateral sclerosis 1: Cu/Zn superoxide dismutase

The first successful genome-wide linkage study on FALS described linkage to chromosome 21q21 [10]. Mutations were subsequently identified in the gene encoding Cu/Zn superoxide dismutase (*SOD1*) [11]. Over 140 mutations in *SOD1* have been identified in 20% of FALS and 3%–7% of SALS cases [12,13]. These are listed on the ALSOD website at http:// alsod.iop.kcl.ac.uk/Als. The vast majority are missense mutations, with a smaller number of nonsense mutations, insertions, and deletions. Most mutations are inherited in an autosomal dominant manner, but the D90A mutation appears to be recessive in Scandinavia where homozygotes develop ALS [14]. A few affected D90A heterozygotes have been reported from a few dominant kindreds and occasional sporadic cases. Haplotype studies of markers around the SOD1 locus point to a single ancient founder for all D90A cases, suggesting that it is a very low penetrant mutation and that two copies of the mutant gene are usually required for disease to be manifested [15].

Genotype–phenotype correlation for mutant SOD1

Most SOD1 mutations cause a mixed or predominantly LMN phenotype, and no cases have been reported with a PLS phenotype or significant dementia. Except for a few variants, nearly all SOD1 mutations are associated with a poor prognosis. The most common mutation in the United States, A4V, is particularly aggressive with survival sometimes measured in months, while homozygous D90A patients have a slower progression with an average survival of 14 years [16]. The I113T mutation has a very low penetrance and is the most frequent mutation found in sporadic ALS cases [13,17]. Apart from these exceptions, there is a relatively poor correlation between the position of a mutation within the gene, survival, or disease penetrance.

Disease mechanisms in mutant SOD1

SOD1 exists as a homodimer acting to remove potentially harmful superoxide radicals. It is ubiquitously expressed at high levels in most tissues including the brain, but it is not known why mutations should be selectively toxic to motor neurons. Mice knocked out for SOD1 are healthy, hence mutations do not cause disease through a loss of function. Mice transgenically expressing many different mutant forms of SOD1 all develop progressive paralysis and die prematurely, indicating that mutant SOD1 gains a toxic property, probably owing to protein misfolding and aggregation [18]. Misfolded proteins place stress on the endoplasmic reticulum, can sequester protective chaperones, and overwhelm the ubiquitin proteasome system, which is responsible for protein recycling. The failure of molecular chaperones to clear mutant SOD1 leads to its aggregation, which has an impact on a variety of subcellular organelles and homeostatic functions (reviewed in [19]). Changes in the shape and function of mitochondria, which may impair neuronal energy sources and contribute to oxidative stress, are an early feature in mutant SOD1 mice. Aggregates of SOD1 affect the transport of many cargoes within axons (including mitochondria), and retraction of motor neurons forming the neuromuscular junction are an early feature of disease. Studies in transgenic mice where mutant SOD1 has been deleted from specific cell populations have shown that mutant SOD1 contributes to disease through several cell types. Damage to astrocyte glutamate transporters combined with increased permeability of neuronal glutamate receptors may contribute to excitotoxicity of motor neurons. It is likely that many of these pathogenic mechanisms contribute to motor neuron dysfunction and death. Protein aggregation is a feature of most adult-onset neurodegenerative diseases, including Alzheimer's, Huntington, and Parkinson's disease, and many of the same homeostatic pathways are disturbed; thus, therapies aimed at ameliorating protein aggregation and enhancing its clearance may be more widely applicable.

Amyotrophic lateral sclerosis 2: *alsin*

Amyotrophic lateral sclerosis 2 is a very rare autosomal recessive disorder characterized by a slowly ascending spasticity that begins in infancy or early childhood and progresses over many decades. Mutations in the gene *alsin* were subsequently detected, but only 13 mutations have been reported to date and there is no genetic association with ALS [20–22]. Most mutations cause protein truncation and a loss of alsin function, which affects neurite outgrowth [23].

Amyotrophic lateral sclerosis 3: locus at chromosome 18q21

A large European kindred with classical adult-onset ALS was reported to show linkage to chromosome 18q21 [24]; however, this family was subsequently shown to have FUS mutations (Teepu Sidduque, personal communication).

Amyotrophic lateral sclerosis 4: *SETX*/senataxin

An 11-generation Caucasian American family with an autosomal dominant, juvenile-onset, slowly progressive motor neuron disorder was linked to chromosome 9q34 [25]. Heterozygous point mutations were eventually detected in the gene *SETX* (encoding senataxin) in this and two other kindreds [26]. Onset is before the age of 25 years, with distal limb weakness and amyotrophy, and UMN signs in the limbs. Bulbar muscles and cognition are spared and the life expectancy is normal. Interestingly, homozygous nonsense and compound heterozygous missense mutations in *SETX* cause ataxia-oculomotor-apraxia type 2 (AOA2) [27]. Senataxin contains a DNA/RNA helicase domain with homology to the gene *IGHMBP2*, which encodes for an RNA processing protein. Mutation of *IGHMBP2* is seen in autosomal recessive infantile-onset spinal muscular atrophy and respiratory distress type 1 (SMARD1) [28].

Amyotrophic lateral sclerosis 5: *SPG11* (spatacsin)

Several kindreds from Tunisia and Germany with autosomal recessive juvenile ALS (ARJALS) were linked to chromosome 15q15.1–21.1 [29]. They develop progressive gait disturbance, presenting with mixed UMN and LMN features between eight and 18 years of age. They develop dysarthria after three to four years and survive between 10 and 25 years from symptom onset. The phenotype is closer to classical adult-onset ALS and ultimately fatal. Although the causative gene in these ALS5 kindreds has not been published, a recent candidate gene approach in a separate cohort of 25 families with ARJALS identified 12 mutations in the *SPG11* gene (encoding spatacsin). This gene is present within the ALS5 locus.

Amyotrophic lateral sclerosis 6: *FUS/TLS*

In 2003, four families of European ancestry with typical autosomal dominant ALS were independently linked to chromosome 16q12 [30–32]. The causative mutations have recently been found in the *FUS* gene, which codes for FUS [33,34]. *FUS* mutations have been found in various ALS cohorts around the world in sporadic as well as familial cases and account for about 5% of FALS. Most mutations are dominant, suggesting a toxic gain of function, or a dominant negative effect. A consanguineous family demonstrates recessive inheritance of a *FUS* mutation, suggesting the coinheritance of a protective factor [33]. Mutant FUS isoforms demonstrate an increased propensity to accumulate within the cytoplasm in vitro, and cytoplasmic FUS inclusions are seen in postmortem spinal cord specimens [33,34]. Interestingly, these inclusions are negative for ubiquitin and TDP-43. This suggests that different mechanistic pathways may occur in ALS6 cases compared to sporadic ALS.

FUS is similar to TDP-43 (see following discussion) in that it contains glycine-rich domains and an RNA binding domain, and it is also able to bind DNA. FUS is implicated in tumorigenesis as a component of fusion genes that result in the creation of aberrant transcription factors [35]. FUS has important roles in gene transcription and is implicated in various components of the transcriptional machinery, including RNA polymerase II, nuclear factor κB, and non-coding RNAs [36–38]. Critical roles in DNA repair have also been ascribed to FUS [38]. Both FUS and TDP-43 are components of the Drosha complex, suggesting a role in microRNA and ribosomal biogenesis [39]. As with TDP-43, FUS is a predominantly nuclear protein but can shuttle between the nucleus and cytoplasm. FUS may have roles in RNA transport and synaptic plasticity, RNA maturation, and splicing [38,40].

Amyotrophic lateral sclerosis 7 linked to chromosome 20p13

Linkage to chromosome 20p13 with a peak LOD score of 3.64 was described in a North American kindred with typical ALS [32]. Recombination defined only a 1 Mb region, but no gene mutation has been reported to date.

Amyotrophic lateral sclerosis 8: VAPB

In 2004, a four-generation Brazilian family of Portuguese ancestry with a LMN disorder was linked to chromosome 20q13 [41]. The P56S missense mutation was subsequently identified in the VAMP/synaptobrevin associated membrane protein B (VAPB) in this and six other Brazilian kindreds who share a common founder [42,43]. VAPB localizes to the endoplasmic reticulum and Golgi apparatus and is involved in intracellular trafficking of vesicles [43]. The mutation causes striking intracellular aggregates of VAPB, but the disease mechanism is unknown [43].

Amyotrophic lateral sclerosis 9: *ANG*/angiogenin

A synonymous exonic single nucleotide polymorphism (SNP) (rs11701) in the gene encoding angiogenenin (*ANG*) was associated with susceptibility to ALS in the Irish population [44]. To date, 17 missense mutations in the *ANG* gene have been reported in ALS cases but two of these mutations have also been found in controls [45–53]. These mutations are predominantly in Celtic populations (Irish and Scottish), and segregation with disease has not yet been demonstrated in familial kindreds. Several ANG mutations demonstrate impaired angiogenic properties, possibly because of impaired nuclear localization and reduced ribonuclease activity [49]. The K17I mutation has also been found in a kindred with familial ALS-FTD [46], but the disease also cosegregates with a TARDBP mutation (Leonard van den Berg, personal communication). Previously, TDP-43 positive inclusions have been identified at postmortem in a patient with a K17I mutation [54].

Amyotrophic lateral sclerosis 10: *TARBDP*/TDP-43

The most frequent neuropathological hallmark of ALS is the accumulation of ubiquitinated inclusions in surviving motor neurons in the brainstem and spinal cord. The major protein aggregate is a detergent resistant fragment of the TAR DNA binding protein (TDP-43). These inclusions are present in ~30% of FTD and ~95% of ALS cases [55]. Linkage to chromosome 1p36, which contains the *TARDBP* gene locus (encoding TDP-43), was demonstrated in a large British ALS kindred, and the M337V mutation was shown to segregate with disease [56]. Over 30 other missense mutations and a truncation mutation have now been reported in FALS and SALS, and all but one reside in the C-terminal domain [57]. TDP-43 is a DNA and RNA binding protein that is involved in regulating gene transcription and RNA processing (see section on ALS6, FUS).

Amyotrophic lateral sclerosis 11: FIG4

Heterozygous mutations in the lipid phosphatase FIG4 have been shown to cause approximately 2% of ALS and PLS in patients of European ancestry [58].

Other familial amyotrophic lateral sclerosis related genes
Dynactin

A family with a slowly progressive LMN disorder with stridor and dysphonia was linked to chromosome 2p13 and the G59S mutation identified in the p150 subunit of dynactin, *DCTN1* [59]. Mutations in the gene *DCTN1* were subsequently found in one patient with apparently sporadic ALS, one with FALS, and in a single pedigree in two affected and two unaffected individuals [60]. A further missense mutation has also been described in an autosomal dominant kindred with ALS-FTD [61]. The detection of DCTN1 mutations in ALS cases is of great interest, but it is not proof of pathogenicity.

DAO

A single family with typical ALS was recently linked to a dominant mutation in D-amino acid oxidase (DAO) [62]. Confirmation of its pathogenic role awaits the identification of other kindreds carrying this mutation or other mutations in FALS kindreds.

OPTN

Mutations in the gene *OPTN*, encoding optineurin, are associated with autosomal recessive and dominant ALS. OPTN mutations were found in a handful of Japanese ALS cases [63]. Two different homozygous mutations, both predicted to cause premature termination, were found in consanguineous families. A further missense mutation was found in autosomal dominant kindreds. The pathogenicity of the homozygous mutations is likely to be because of a loss of function as a result of nonsense mediated decay of mRNA transcripts. The dominant missense mutation may act through an as yet unknown toxic gain of function. Initial pathological analysis of an individual with a dominant OPTN mutation identified typical TDP-43 inclusions as seen in SALS. Interestingly, these inclusions were also positive for optineurin. Furthermore, they found optineurin to be a component of inclusions in SALS and in mutant SOD1 associated ALS, suggesting that optineurin may have a broader role in ALS pathogenesis.

Although its functions remain unclear, optineurin is a ubiquitously expressed, cytoplasmic, and perinuclear protein. It associates with the Golgi apparatus and is implicated in vesicle transport, apoptosis, and transcription. Further genetic and pathological studies are needed to determine the wider role of optineurin in ALS pathogenesis. Notably, OPTN mutations are a cause of primary open angle glaucoma [64]. It will be interesting to elucidate how OPTN mutations can cause neurodegeneration in such seemingly disparate locations as the retina and the motor pathways.

Amyotrophic lateral sclerosis– frontotemporal lobe dementia 1 and 2 linked to chromosomes 9q21 and 9p13

Five families with autosomal dominant classical ALS and FTD were linked to a region on chromosome 9q21–q22 (ALS-FTD1) [65]. Very recently, two groups have identified a non-coding hexanucleotide repeat (C90RF72). This appears to account for a very significant proportion of both familial and spastic ALS and FTD cases [65a,65b]. Genome-wide scans in two unrelated families with FTD/ALS were linked to overlapping loci on chromosome 9p13 (ALS–FTD2) [66,67]. Several other families have since been linked to this locus, but no causative mutation has been identified [68–70].

Other genetic disorders of the lower motor neuron that can mimic amyotrophic lateral sclerosis
Kennedy's disease

Kennedy's disease or spinobulbar muscular atrophy (SBMA) is commonly mistaken for ALS and should be tested for in any patient with a slowly progressive course, prominent chin and tongue fasciculations, tremor of the outstretched hands, gynecomastia, and testicular atrophy. Nerve conduction studies commonly show a subclinical sensory neuropathy. Inheritance is X-linked recessive and female carriers are almost always asymptomatic. The gene defect is an expanded CAG nucleotide repeat sequence in the androgen receptor gene and a test is widely available.

Spinal muscular atrophy

Autosomal recessive SMA usually presents in infancy or childhood with a regression in motor milestones (e.g. sitting, walking) and 95% of cases are a result of a deletion of the SMN1 gene. A minority of patients can present in early adulthood with a slowly progressive, purely LMN syndrome characterized by wasting, weakness, and absent reflexes. The muscles affected in SMA tend to be proximal with sparing of distal strength and the muscles controlling speech and swallowing.

Genetic counseling

In our experience, genetic counseling has become a significant component of the discussion that follows an initial diagnosis. Many people with SALS seek genetic counseling once they become aware that ALS can be genetic and are better informed about gene testing. The lifetime risk of ALS occurring in the siblings and children of an individual affected by sporadic disease is greater than the general population risk (~1 in 500–1000) because the newly diagnosed individual might have developed a spontaneous mutation and FALS has an age-dependent and variable penetrance. Thus, mutation carriers in previous generations may not have lived long enough to develop disease. The risk is slightly higher if the index case is adopted or has little knowledge of their family history. We usually quote a figure of ~1%–5% although it is very difficult to derive an accurate statistic. We do not recommend SOD1 gene testing in sporadic ALS because the likelihood of detecting a mutation is only ~2%–7% [13,71,72]. Because SOD1 mutations are only detected in 20% of familial cases [11], the absence of a mutation does not substantially decrease the possibility that it is familial. Thus, in our opinion, SOD1 gene testing in SALS can provide either bad news, or false reassurance.

If there is convincing evidence of a first or second degree relative having ALS, the diagnosis is very likely to be familial because the chance of two individuals in the same kindreds independently developing ALS by chance is between 1 in 250 000 and 1 000 000. The diagnosis of FALS must be relayed very sensitively and additional information in the form of information leaflets and counseling immediately made available to all those who wish to obtain further advice. The effects of this diagnosis may be likened to throwing a large rock into a still pond as the ripples of implied risk spread out through the family, creating a great deal of anxiety. If the disease is multigenerational and the phenotype classical ALS, it is very likely to be autosomal dominant and a result of a single gene mutation causing disease in the heterozygous state (to date, no X-linked kindreds have been published). Even if the affected members are all siblings or cousins in the same generation, the inheritance pattern is still likely to be autosomal dominant as most autosomal recessive kindreds have an onset in childhood or adolescence and a single affected generation is likely to reflect reduced penetrance. The risk of inheriting the mutated gene is 50%, but in families with reduced penetrance one can counsel that the risk of developing ALS may be considerably lower. This is certainly true for individuals heterozygous for the I113T and D90A mutations (see following section). Even in families where the age of disease onset appears to be fairly consistent, the variable penetrance does not imply that older at-risk members have a greatly reduced risk as there is no upper age limit when disease can manifest.

Gene testing

In the first instance, gene testing should always be discussed with and offered to the affected index case. Although there is no direct benefit to that person, it will inform and influence the counseling and gene testing offered to other members of the family. If pathogenic mutations are identified through a diagnostic test, other unaffected members can undergo predictive testing for the same mutation, should they wish. The decision to undergo diagnostic or predictive testing is intensely personal and there is no right decision. The genetic counselor should take an entirely neutral position and help the individual to make the decision that is right for him/her. Diagnostic testing for an affected individual can be done on the first visit following diagnosis, but predictive gene testing in an unaffected at-risk person usually

involves two initial counseling sessions followed by a three-month cooling off period before formal consent is obtained and blood is drawn for the gene test. The counselor makes a fixed follow-up appointment and will not review the test result until the day of the appointment. This facilitates neutral communication in the interim. The issue of familiality and gene testing can be very divisive within families and the person being tested should be given the option of sharing or restricting news of the results with other family members. Someone wishing to have a predictive gene test must be made aware that if he/she is shown to harbor a high-risk mutation, there may be consequences in terms of employment, life assurance, and ability to raise a mortgage. No one can be forced to have a gene test by another individual or organization, but once someone has voluntarily undergone gene testing, he/she may be obligated to disclose the result to his/her employer and other financial agencies. We usually advise people to explore their options and make the necessary arrangements before they undergo gene testing.

Conclusions

Familial ALS is heterogeneous and overlaps with the sporadic form of the disease. The importance of taking an extensive and detailed family history cannot be overstated. Many individuals thought to have sporadic disease subsequently turn out to be familial and the reassurance regarding recurrence risk to their children has been false. If familial disease is suspected, every effort should be made to track down an accurate history and medical records of the other affected individuals to be as certain as possible of the historical diagnosis. Death certificates are notoriously unreliable and corroborating medical record evidence should be sought. Equally important is the phenotype of any relatives with dementia. Symptoms of behavioral or personality change and language deficits early in the course of dementia should raise the suspicion of FTD rather than Alzheimer's disease.

The implications of gene screening should always be discussed in detail with the family prior to testing. Consent and DNA from an affected individual should be obtained before predictive testing in at-risk individuals is considered. The penetrance of different SOD1 mutations in particular varies greatly and must be taken into consideration when ascribing risk to a particular gene carrier. The burden of anxiety on ALS families is huge and they require long-term counseling and support.

A major paradigm shift began in 2006 with identification of TDP-43 as the hallmark protein of ALS and FTD. This was soon followed by the identification of TDP-43 and FUS mutations in ALS and then by the characterization of atypical FTD, which demonstrates FUS inclusions [73]. These discoveries have intensified investigation of the role of RNA-processing in neurodegeneration. These pathological overlaps between ALS and FTD are complemented by growing evidence that a significant number of kindreds with individuals with ALS and/or FTD are linked to chromosome 9p21. More work is needed to explore the clinical and biological links between these two disorders.

For 15 years, mutant SOD1 provided the only genetic model of ALS. However, gene discovery in ALS has accelerated in the past two years and will become even more fruitful with the application of new DNA capture and sequencing technologies. When more ALS genes are identified, we will be in a position to offer mass screening of the population to determine who is at risk. By mapping out common pathogenic pathways, we will be able to develop sensible therapeutic strategies that might arrest or even reverse the disease process.

References

1. Brooks BR, Miller RG, Swash M, Munsat TL. El Escorial revisited: revised criteria for the diagnosis of amyotrophic lateral sclerosis. *Amyotroph Lateral Scler Other Motor Neuron Disord* 2000; **1**: 293–299.

2. Dickson DW, Josephs KA, Amador-Ortiz C. TDP-43 in differential diagnosis of motor neuron disorders. *Acta Neuropathol* 2007; **114**: 71–79.

3. Kim WK, Liu X, Sandner J, et al. Study of 962 patients indicates progressive muscular atrophy is a form of ALS. *Neurology* 2009; **73**: 1686–1692.

4. Hodges JR, Millar B. The classification, genetics and neuropathology of frontotemporal dementia. Introduction to the special topic papers: Part I. *Neurocase* 2001; 7: 31–35.

5. Abrahams S, Goldstein LH, Al-Chalabi A, et al. Relation between cognitive dysfunction and pseudobulbar palsy in amyotrophic lateral sclerosis. *J Neurol Neurosurg Psychiatry* 1997; **62**: 464–472.

6. Kurland LT, Mulder DW. Age-specific incidence rates for motor neuron disease [letter]. *J Neurol Neurosurg Psychiatry* 1987; **50**: 115–116.

7. Morris HR, Steele JC, Crook R, et al. Genome-wide analysis of the parkinsonism-dementia complex of Guam. *Arch Neurol* 2004; **61**: 1889–1897.

8. Kuzuhara S, Kokubo Y. Atypical parkinsonism of Japan: amyotrophic lateral sclerosis-parkinsonism-dementia complex of the Kii peninsula of Japan (Muro disease): an update. *Mov Disord* 2005; **20**: S108–S113.

9. Strong MJ, Hudson AJ, Alvord WG. Familial amyotrophic lateral sclerosis, 1850–1989: a statistical analysis of the world literature. *Can J Neurol Sci* 1991; **18**: 45–58.

10. Siddique T, Figlewicz DA, Pericak-Vance MA, et al. Linkage of a gene causing familial amyotrophic lateral sclerosis to chromosome 21 and evidence of genetic-locus heterogeneity [published errata appear in *N Engl J Med* 1991; **325**: 71 and 1991; **325**: 524] [see comments]. *N Engl J Med* 1991; **324**: 1381–1384.

11. Rosen DR. Mutations in Cu/Zn superoxide dismutase gene are associated with familial amyotrophic lateral sclerosis. *Nature* 1993; **364**: 362.

12. Rosen DR. Mutations in Cu/Zn superoxide dismutase gene are associated with familial amyotrophic lateral sclerosis. *Nature* 1993; **362**: 59–62.

13. Shaw CE, Enayat ZE, Chioza BA, et al. Mutations in all five exons of SOD-1 may cause ALS. *Ann Neurol* 1998; **43**: 390–394.

14. Andersen PM, Nilsson P, Ala-Hurula V, et al. Amyotrophic lateral sclerosis associated with homozygosity for an Asp90Ala mutation in CuZn-superoxide dismutase. *Nat Genet* 1995; **10**: 61–66.

15. Parton MJ, Broom W, Andersen PM, et al. D90A-SOD1 mediated amyotrophic lateral sclerosis: a single founder for all cases with evidence for a Cis-acting disease modifier in the recessive haplotype. *Hum Mutat* 2002; **20**: 473.

16. Andersen PM, Nilsson P, Keranen ML, et al. Phenotypic heterogeneity in motor neuron disease patients with CuZn-superoxide dismutase mutations in Scandinavia. *Brain* 1997; **120**: 1723–1737.

17. Hayward C, Swingler RJ, Simpson SA, Brock DJ. A specific superoxide dismutase mutation is on the same genetic background in sporadic and familial cases of amyotrophic

lateral sclerosis [letter]. *Am J Hum Genet* 1996; **59**: 1165–1167.

18. Cleveland DW, Liu J. Oxidation versus aggregation – how do SOD1 mutants cause ALS? *Nat Med* 2000; **6**: 1320–1321.

19. Bento-Abreu A, Van Damme P, Van Den Bosch L, Robberecht W. The neurobiology of amyotrophic lateral sclerosis. *Eur J Neurosci* 2010; **31**: 2247–2265.

20. Al-Chalabi A, Hansen VK, Simpson CL, *et al.* Variants in the ALS2 gene are not associated with sporadic amyotrophic lateral sclerosis. *Neurogenetics* 2003; **4**: 221–222.

21. Hadano S, Yanagisawa Y, Skaug J, *et al.* Cloning and characterization of three novel genes, ALS2CR1, ALS2CR2, and ALS2CR3, in the juvenile amyotrophic lateral sclerosis (ALS2) critical region at chromosome 2q33-q34: candidate genes for ALS2. *Genomics* 2001; **71**: 200–213.

22. Yang Y, Hentati A, Deng HX, *et al.* The gene encoding alsin, a protein with three guanine-nucleotide exchange factor domains, is mutated in a form of recessive amyotrophic lateral sclerosis. *Nat Genet* 2001; **29**: 160–165.

23. Tudor EL, Perkinton MS, Schmidt A, *et al.* ALS2/Alsin regulates Rac-PAK signaling and neurite outgrowth. *J Biol Chem* 2005; **280**: 34735–34740.

24. Hand CK, Khoris J, Salachas F, *et al.* A novel locus for familial amyotrophic lateral sclerosis, on chromosome 18q. *Am J Hum Genet* 2002; **70**: 251–256.

25. Chance PF, Rabin BA, Ryan SG, *et al.* Linkage of the gene for an autosomal dominant form of juvenile amyotrophic lateral sclerosis to chromosome 9q34. *Am J Hum Genet* 1998; **62**: 633–640.

26. Chen YZ, Bennett CL, Huynh HM, *et al.* DNA/RNA helicase gene mutations in a form of juvenile amyotrophic lateral sclerosis (ALS4). *Am J Hum Genet* 2004; **74**: 1128–1135.

27. Moreira MC, Klur S, Watanabe M, *et al.* Senataxin, the ortholog of a yeast RNA helicase, is mutant in ataxia-ocular apraxia 2. *Nat Genet* 2004; **36**: 225–227.

28. Grohmann K, Schuelke M, Diers A, *et al.* Mutations in the gene encoding immunoglobulin mu-binding protein 2 cause spinal muscular atrophy with respiratory distress type 1. *Nat Genet* 2001; **29**: 75–77.

29. Hentati A, Ouahchi K, Pericak-Vance MA, *et al.* Linkage of a commoner form of recessive amyotrophic lateral sclerosis to chromosome 15q15-q22 markers. *Neurogenetics* 1998; **2**: 55–60.

30. Abalkhail H, Mitchell J, Habgood J, Orrell R, De Belleroche J. A New familial amyotrophic lateral sclerosis locus on chromosome 16q12.1–16q12.2. *Am J Hum Genet* 2003; **73**: 383–389.

31. Ruddy DM, Parton MJ, Al-Chalabi A, *et al.* Two families with familial amyotrophic lateral sclerosis are linked to a novel locus on chromosome 16q. *Am J Hum Genet* 2003; **73**: 390–396.

32. Sapp PC, Hosler BA, McKenna-Yasek D, *et al.* Identification of two novel loci for dominantly inherited familial amyotrophic lateral sclerosis. *Am J Hum Genet* 2003; **73**: 397–403.

33. Kwiatkowski TJ Jr, Bosco DA, Leclerc AL, *et al.* Mutations in the FUS/TLS gene on chromosome 16 cause familial amyotrophic lateral sclerosis. *Science* 2009; **323**: 1205–1208.

34. Vance C, Rogelj B, Hortobagyi T, *et al.* Mutations in FUS, an RNA processing protein, cause familial amyotrophic lateral sclerosis type 6. *Science* 2009; **323**: 1208–1211.

35. Crozat A, Aman P, Mandahl N, Ron D. Fusion of CHOP to a novel RNA-binding protein in human myxoid liposarcoma. *Nature* 1993; **363**: 640–644.

36. Law WJ, Cann KL, Hicks GG. TLS, EWS and TAF15: a model for transcriptional integration of gene expression. *Brief Funct Genomic Proteomic* 2006; **5**: 8–14.

37. Yang S, Warraich ST, Nicholson GA, Blair IP. Fused in sarcoma/translocated in liposarcoma: a multifunctional DNA/RNA binding protein. *Int J Biochem Cell Biol* 2010; **42**: 1408–1411.

38. Kovar H. Dr. Jekyll and Mr. Hyde: The two faces of the FUS/EWS/TAF15 protein family. *Sarcoma* 2011; **2011**: 837474.

39. Ling SC, Albuquerque CP, Han JS, *et al.* ALS-associated mutations in TDP-43 increase its stability and promote TDP-43 complexes with FUS/TLS. *Proc Natl Acad Sci USA* 2010; **107**: 13318–13323.

40. Belly A, Moreau-Gachelin F, Sadoul R, Goldberg Y. Delocalization of the multifunctional RNA splicing factor TLS/FUS in hippocampal neurones: exclusion from the nucleus and accumulation in dendritic granules and spine heads. *Neurosci Lett* 2005; **379**: 152–157.

41. Nishimura AL, Mitne-Neto M, Silva HC, *et al.* A novel locus for late onset amyotrophic lateral sclerosis/motor neurone disease variant at 20q13. *J Med Genet* 2004; **41**: 315–320.

42. Nishimura AL, Al-Chalabi A, Zatz M. A common founder for amyotrophic lateral sclerosis type 8 (ALS8) in the Brazilian population. *Hum Genet* 2005; **118**: 499–500.

43. Nishimura AL, Mitne-Neto M, Silva HC, et al. A mutation in the vesicle-trafficking protein VAPB causes late-onset spinal muscular atrophy and amyotrophic lateral sclerosis. *Am J Hum Genet* 2004; **75**: 822–831.

44. Greenway MJ, Alexander MD, Ennis S, et al. A novel candidate region for ALS on chromosome 14q11.2. *Neurology* 2004; **63**: 1936–1938.

45. Fernandez-Santiago R, Hoenig S, Lichtner P, et al. Identification of novel angiogenin (ANG) gene missense variants in German patients with amyotrophic lateral sclerosis. *J Neurol* 2009; **256**: 1337–1342.

46. van Es MA, Diekstra FP, Veldink JH, et al. A case of ALS-FTD in a large FALS pedigree with a K17I ANG mutation. *Neurology* 2009; **72**: 287–288.

47. Paubel A, Violette J, Amy M, et al. Mutations of the ANG gene in French patients with sporadic amyotrophic lateral sclerosis. *Arch Neurol* 2008; **65**: 1333–1336.

48. Gellera C, Colombrita C, Ticozzi N, et al. Identification of new ANG gene mutations in a large cohort of Italian patients with amyotrophic lateral sclerosis. *Neurogenetics* 2008; **9**: 33–40.

49. Crabtree B, Thiyagarajan N, Prior SH, et al. Characterization of human angiogenin variants implicated in amyotrophic lateral sclerosis. *Biochemistry* 2007; **46**: 11810–11818.

50. Wu D, Yu W, Kishikawa H, et al. Angiogenin loss-of-function mutations in amyotrophic lateral sclerosis. *Ann Neurol* 2007; **62**: 609–617.

51. Conforti FL, Sprovieri T, Mazzei R, et al. A novel angiogenin gene mutation in a sporadic patient with amyotrophic lateral sclerosis from southern Italy. *Neuromuscul Disord* 2008; **18**: 68–70.

52. Corrado L, Battistini S, Penco S, et al. Variations in the coding and regulatory sequences of the angiogenin (ANG) gene are not associated to ALS (amyotrophic lateral sclerosis) in the Italian population. *J Neurol Sci* 2007; **258**: 123–127.

53. Greenway MJ, Andersen PM, Russ C, et al. ANG mutations segregate with familial and 'sporadic' amyotrophic lateral sclerosis. *Nat Genet* 2006; **38**: 411–413.

54. Seilhean D, Cazeneuve C, Thuries V, et al. Accumulation of TDP-43 and alpha-actin in an amyotrophic lateral sclerosis patient with the K17I ANG mutation. *Acta Neuropathol* 2009; **118**: 561–573.

55. Neumann M, Sampathu DM, Kwong LK, et al. Ubiquitinated TDP-43 in frontotemporal lobar degeneration and amyotrophic lateral sclerosis. *Science* 2006; **314**: 130–133.

56. Sreedharan J, Blair IP, Tripathi VB, et al. TDP-43 mutations in familial and sporadic amyotrophic lateral sclerosis. *Science* 2008; **319**: 1668–1672.

57. Lagier-Tourenne C, Cleveland DW. Rethinking ALS: the FUS about TDP-43. *Cell* 2009; **136**: 1001–1004.

58. Chow CY, Landers JE, Bergren SK, et al. Deleterious variants of FIG4, a phosphoinositide phosphatase, in patients with ALS. *Am J Hum Genet* 2009; **84**: 85–88.

59. Puls I, Jonnakuty C, LaMonte BH, et al. Mutant dynactin in motor neuron disease. *Nat Genet* 2003; **33**: 455–456.

60. Munch C, Sedlmeier R, Meyer T, et al. Point mutations of the p150 subunit of dynactin (DCTN1) gene in ALS. *Neurology* 2004; **63**: 724–726.

61. Munch C, Rosenbohm A, Sperfeld AD, et al. Heterozygous R1101K mutation of the DCTN1 gene in a family with ALS and FTD. *Ann Neurol* 2005; **58**: 777–780.

62. Mitchell J, Paul P, Chen HJ, et al. Familial amyotrophic lateral sclerosis is associated with a mutation in D-amino acid oxidase. *Proc Natl Acad Sci USA* 2010; **107**: 7556–7561.

63. Maruyama H, Morino H, Ito H, et al. Mutations of optineurin in amyotrophic lateral sclerosis. *Nature* 2010; **465**: 223–226.

64. Rezaie T, Child A, Hitchings R, et al. Adult-onset primary open-angle glaucoma caused by mutations in optineurin. *Science* 2002; **295**: 1077–1079.

65. Hosler BA, Siddique T, Sapp PC, et al. Linkage of familial amyotrophic lateral sclerosis with frontotemporal dementia to chromosome 9q21-q22. *JAMA* 2000; **284**: 1664–1669.

65a. Renton AE, Majounie E, Waite A, et al. A hexanucleotide repeat expansion in C9ORF72 as the cause of chromosome 9p21 linked ALS-FTD. *Neuron* 2011; **72**: 257–268.

65b. Dejesus-Hernandez M, Mackenzie IR, Boeve BF, et al. Expanded GGGGCC hexanucleotide repeat in noncoding region of C9ORF72. *Neuron* 2011; **72**: 245–256.

66. Morita M, Al-Chalabi A, Andersen PM, et al. A locus on chromosome 9p confers susceptibility to ALS and frontotemporal dementia. *Neurology* 2006; **66**: 839–844.

67. Vance C, Al-Chalabi A, Ruddy D, et al. Familial amyotrophic lateral sclerosis with frontotemporal dementia is linked to a locus on chromosome 9p13.2–21.3. *Brain* 2006; **129**: 868–876.

68. Le Ber I, Camuzat A, Berger E, et al. Chromosome 9p-linked families with frontotemporal

dementia associated with motor neuron disease. *Neurology* 2009; **72**: 1669–1676.

69. Momeni P, Schymick J, Jain S, *et al.* Analysis of IFT74 as a candidate gene for chromosome 9p-linked ALS-FTD. *BMC Neurol* 2006; **6**: 44.

70. Valdmanis PN, Dupre N, Bouchard JP, *et al.* Three families with amyotrophic lateral sclerosis and frontotemporal dementia with evidence of linkage to chromosome 9p. *Arch Neurol* 2007; **64**: 240–245.

71. Jackson M, Al-Chalabi A, Enayat ZE, *et al.* Copper/zinc superoxide dismutase 1 and sporadic amyotrophic lateral sclerosis: analysis of 155 cases and identification of a novel insertion mutation. *Ann Neurol* 1997; **42**: 803–807.

72. Jones CT, Swingler RJ, Simpson SA, Brock DJ. Superoxide dismutase mutations in an unselected cohort of Scottish amyotrophic lateral sclerosis patients. *J Med Genet* 1995; **32**: 290–292.

73. Neumann M, Rademakers R, Roeber S, *et al.* A new subtype of frontotemporal lobar degeneration with FUS pathology. *Brain* 2009; **132**: 2922–2931.

147

The muscular dystrophies

Kate Bushby and Una-Marie Sheerin

Introduction

As the gene and protein abnormalities underlying the muscular dystrophies have been elucidated over the last 20 years, diagnostic strategies have adapted to target these defects directly in the majority of cases. This has led to a very high level of precision being achievable for diagnosis and carrier testing. In order to apply these sophisticated diagnostic tools, it is necessary to appreciate the heterogeneity of this group of diseases and their areas of overlap and distinction. It is also useful to understand the frequency and, therefore, prior probability of encountering any of these diseases in a particular population group

(Table 11.1), and the pitfalls and limitations of the available analyses.

All muscular dystrophies are genetic, and the mode of inheritance may be X-linked, autosomal dominant, or autosomal recessive. As the mode of inheritance is of such fundamental importance in the diagnostic process and, of course, to genetic counseling, this is the initial subdivision on which the classification in this chapter will be based. Other divisions are variable and may be based on either the age at onset (e.g. the congenital muscular dystrophies) or the pattern of muscle involvement (e.g. the limb-girdle muscular dystrophies and facioscapulohumeral muscular dystrophy). While

Table 11.1. The relative frequencies of different inherited muscular dystrophies and other muscle disorders in a clinic population of approximately 1000 patients in the northeast of England [117]

Condition	% of Northern region clinic population	First line diagnostic test
Myotonic dystrophy	28%	DNA test for expansion in DMPK(DM1), ZNF9 (DM2)
Dystrophinopathy	20%	DNA test (MLPA) for deletions/duplications
Facioscapulohumeral muscular dystrophy	10%	DNA test for D4Z4 deletion on chromosome 4q35
Spinal muscular atrophy	4%	DNA test for SMN deletions/gene conversion events
Limb-girdle muscular dystrophy	4.5%	Common C826A mutation for LGMD2I, consider lamin A/C mutation testing otherwise likely to require muscle biopsy to select further genetic testing (see Table 11.3)
Bethlem myopathy	<3%	Collagen VI immunolabeling of cultured fibroblasts
Congenital muscular dystrophies	<3%	Muscle biopsy for laminin alpha 2, alpha dystroglycan, and collagen VI will direct genetic testing (see Table 11.3)
Congenital myopathies	<3%	Muscle biopsy for structural features to direct genetic testing
Myofibrillar myopathies	<2%	Muscle biopsy for structural features to direct genetic testing
Emery–Dreifuss muscular dystrophy	<2%	Emerin and lamin A/C mutation analysis: muscle biopsy for emerin positivity
Distal myopathies	<2%	Muscle biopsy for structural features to direct genetic testing

generic tests such as measurement of the serum creatine kinase (CK) level (elevated in most but not all types of muscular dystrophy), electromyography to exclude neurogenic or myotonic processes, and muscle biopsy to exclude metabolic or inflammatory disease are useful in indicating that the primary pathology might be a muscular dystrophy rather than another disorder, none of them can confirm the diagnosis of a particular type of muscular dystrophy when used in isolation. Specific immunoanalysis of muscle biopsies may be very informative in directing genetic analysis in some cases, but the gold standard for diagnosis in the majority of the muscular dystrophies, and certainly for genetic and prognostic counseling, has become the application of specific DNA-based tests. In many cases, this has removed the need for more invasive investigations such as EMG or muscle biopsy and introduced the possibility of applying relatively simple and widely available genetic testing for conditions such as myotonic dystrophy, facioscapulohumeral muscular dystrophy, and the dystrophinopathies (Table 11.1).

Specificity of diagnosis has led to an improved understanding of the natural history of these diseases, the recognition of particular complications, and thereby the need for specific measures for surveillance and proactive management. Although gene-based treatments for muscular dystrophies have not yet impacted on clinical practice, there have been many developments in management that have improved life expectancy and quality of life for affected patients. Together with the provision of precise genetic counseling information, this enhanced prognostic information is a major impetus to achieving a precise diagnosis [1].

X-linked muscular dystrophies

Two important groups of muscular dystrophies belong to this category. The dystrophinopathies, including Duchenne and Becker muscular dystrophy, are among the most common in all populations. X-linked Emery–Dreifuss muscular dystrophy is rare, but carries important implications for diagnosis in terms of the need for monitoring and treatment of the frequent cardiac arrhythmias that complicate this condition.

The dystrophinopathies

This group of disorders comprises at least four clinically recognized entities, all of which are a result of mutations in the *dystrophin* gene on the X chromosome at Xp21. Three of these disorders are muscular dystrophies, and the fourth is a cardiomyopathy phenotype, highlighting the importance of the dystrophin protein in cardiac as well as skeletal muscle.

Duchenne muscular dystrophy

Duchenne muscular dystrophy (DMD) occurs in approximately 1 in 3500 male live births. The mean age of diagnosis is about 4.5 years, although many boys present with delayed motor milestones much earlier [2]. Approximately half of all boys walk later than 18 months of age, but a frequent concomitant delay in speech development may suggest that the problem is not physical, leading to a delay in diagnosis [3]. Affected boys cannot run and very few can jump with two feet together. There is frequent calf hypertrophy, and sometimes hypertrophy of other muscle groups as well. Untreated, the disease is inexorably progressive, with increasing muscle weakness leading to the inability to walk independently by the age of 13 years, and complications of cardiomyopathy and respiratory failure causing death by a mean age of 19 years. Attention to key areas of management has led to a progressive increase in life expectancy [4,5]. The use of corticosteroids to improve muscle strength has become the mainstay of management during the ambulant phase [6–11], while use of cardioprotective drugs and, in particular, the timely initiation of nocturnal/non-invasive ventilation has improved life expectancy into the late twenties and beyond [4,6,12–14].

Becker muscular dystrophy

Although Becker muscular dystrophy (BMD) was initially described as a distinct clinical entity, it is now known that this disorder represents the milder end of the dystrophinopathy spectrum. The defining feature, as distinct from DMD, is the persistence of independent walking beyond the age of 16 years, while an intermediate form of the condition is recognized to describe the boys who have a milder form of DMD and walk independently until between 13 and 16 years. This rather arbitrary yardstick is simply a clinically obvious marker of milder disease. Patients with BMD may present in early childhood, but frequently this is delayed and the mean age at diagnosis is 11 years, with the mean age of loss of independent ambulation being 40 years [15–18]. Occasionally, much milder cases have been described, and some patients may be detected with hyperCKemia or present with cramps and myalgia. Presentation is with proximal muscle weakness, such as difficulty running and climbing stairs. Calf hypertrophy may be pronounced. Muscle cramping especially after exercise can be problematic, and myoglobinuria may be seen. Respiratory impairment is typically late, following wheelchair confinement, but cardiomyopathy is a significant risk and may be out of proportion to the physical disability. Proactive treatment of cardiomyopathy, in some cases even cardiac transplantation, is indicated [6,19].

Manifesting carriers of Duchenne and Becker muscular dystrophy

Figures for the proportion of female carriers of DMD/BMD who show some clinical manifestation of disease depend on the type of clinical problems included as significant. Many carriers of DMD/BMD show some slight elevation of CK levels, and this used to be the mainstay of carrier testing; however, per se this is not enough to suggest the diagnosis of manifesting carrier. Approximately 8%–10% of carriers could be regarded as falling into this group, by manifesting problems with muscle strength, a behavioral/learning phenotype similar to DMD, or cardiomyopathy. While for the majority of manifesting carriers problems are relatively minor and supervene in adult life, a small proportion has severe disease comparable to the clinical course in an affected male patient. In a known family with DMD/BMD, the diagnosis of manifesting carrier may be relatively straightforward; it may be more problematic in a situation where the manifesting carrier has no prior history of these disorders. In some manifesting carriers, a chromosomal abnormality such as Turner syndrome or an X-chromosome translocation may be present to explain the manifestation of symptoms in a female. For the majority of cases, however, no such chromosomal cause can be detected and the reason for the disease is presumed to be the result of uneven lyonization in skeletal muscle, which may be difficult to demonstrate in individual cases [20–26].

X-linked dilated cardiomyopathy

A number of cases of dystrophinopathy have been reported where pathology relates exclusively to the cardiovascular system, with no involvement of the skeletal musculature. These cases have a dilated cardiomyopathy (DCM) and will present not to the neurologist but to the cardiologist. Dystrophinopathy accounts for a relatively small number of cases of DCM, but the diagnosis should be considered in the presence of an X-linked family history. These cases are likely to result from the presence of unusual mutations where the skeletal muscle isoform of dystrophin is unaffected by the mutation [27–30].

Investigation of suspected dystrophinopathy

The clinical assessment of a young boy with suspected DMD should include asking him to run, climb stairs, and jump – the inability to perform these kinds of tasks is much more discriminating than formal muscle assessment. A Gower's maneuver (the necessity to turn onto the front and climb up the thighs) is present in all affected children, but is not specific to DMD. A degree of learning difficulty is also common in affected children. This may be severe in some cases, and a higher incidence of autistic spectrum disorders is also seen in this group [31,32].

The key initial laboratory investigation is the measurement of the serum CK level, which is grossly elevated (typically over 20 times the upper limit of normal, but frequently much more than this), although this is not specific to DMD. In BMD, physical examination will show proximal muscle weakness and frequently calf hypertrophy. Creatine kinase levels are elevated typically to over 10 times the upper limit of normal, and manifesting carriers of DMD/BMD would also be expected to have an elevation of CK, although this can be very variable. A clue to the diagnosis of the manifesting carrier state may be the presence of significant asymmetry of muscle involvement, reflecting the patchy nature of the distribution of pathology. There may be few clues to the diagnosis in cases of isolated cardiomyopathy as, by definition, muscle strength is normal and there may be no elevation of the serum CK. Specific investigation in all cases is mandatory to allow distinction from other types of muscular dystrophy, and since the identification of the dystrophin gene and protein in 1987, this has relied increasingly on the direct demonstration of abnormal gene and/or protein. Protein analysis can be performed by immunolabeling and immunoblotting of muscle biopsy samples, which in addition to providing a clear demonstration of the effect on the abnormal protein, can add some useful prognostic information in the majority of cases [18,33–36]. However, advances in genetic analysis have been rapid, and now a clear and precise diagnosis can frequently be reached rapidly, without the need for invasive testing. Genetic analysis in the huge dystrophin gene (which has 79 exons and remains the largest human gene identified) is aided by the presence of a common mutation type and two mutation hotspots. In the vast majority of cases (up to 80% of cases of BMD and 70% of DMD), the causative mutation is a deletion of multiple exons. Approximately 6%–11% of cases are a result of duplications of multiple exons and the rest are small missense or nonsense mutations. In most laboratories, a standard PCR-based multiplex analysis, concentrating on the mutation hotspots (thereby missing a proportion of mutations, as well as frequently not being able to define the deletion endpoints), is being replaced by a multiplex ligation-dependent probe amplification (MLPA) approach, which allows the detection of deletions and duplications across all exons of the dystrophin gene as well as the full detection of the endpoints of a deletion [37–39]. The detection of the deletion or duplication endpoints is important because the effect of the mutation on the reading frame of the gene is the main determinant of the phenotype, so that the majority of patients with DMD have a mutation that disrupts the reading frame of the gene and, consequently, no or very little protein can be produced, while BMD is usually associated with inframe mutations allowing the production of a protein that is semi-functional. The structure of dystrophin at the protein level allows a degree of redundancy, especially in the central rod domain, so that even large deletions may be compatible with mild disease as long as the reading frame is maintained. Following MLPA analysis of all of dystrophin's exons, at least 70% of mutations in dystrophin would be expected to be found. For the remaining patients, point mutation analysis is mandatory to identify the underlying cause of disease, not only to confirm the diagnosis but also to allow carrier testing of other family members. Using advanced sequencing methodology, it should be possible to identify up to 95% of dystrophin mutations [40,41], although this may be a time-consuming process.

In practice, although there remain arguments for continued muscle biopsies to assess protein production, a practical way to approach the diagnosis of dystrophinopathy is to analyze the gene by MLPA for deletions and duplications, and if this is negative, to organize a muscle biopsy while point mutation analysis is ongoing. Muscle biopsy analysis can provide a reliable assessment of the dystrophin protein status in most cases, especially if immunoblotting is performed as well as immunolabeling, and also provides material that may be needed for analysis if dystrophinopathy is excluded; for example, to advance the diagnosis of one of the forms of limb-girdle muscular dystrophy.

Genetic counseling for dystrophinopathy

Following the identification of a patient with dystrophinopathy, there are frequently many family members who are at risk of being carriers of the disorder. However, the situation is complicated by the high rate of new mutations in the dystrophin gene, so that for the mother of a newly diagnosed case of DMD with no prior family history, there is an equal chance that she is not a carrier, that she has inherited the mutation, and that she is a carrier of a new mutation. Previous methods for trying to determine carrier status in mothers and other maternally related relatives of an index case relied on Bayesian analysis and CK testing to determine the probability of being a carrier, supplemented in later years by haplotyping in the dystrophin gene. This has been almost completely supplanted now by the availability of direct DNA testing. Unfortunately, for the mother of an affected child, even if the familial mutation is somatically absent, there remains a risk of having another affected child owing to the frequent occurrence of germline mosaicism (a risk of up to 20% with transmission of the at-risk chromosome) [42–45]. There is some evidence that the risk depends on the position of the deletion in the dystrophin gene, with proximal deletions associated with a higher risk of germline mosaicism (up to 30%) compared with distally placed deletions (4%) [46,47].

In some situations, for example where there are no samples from affected individuals or obligate carriers, it can be more complex to establish carrier status as the mutation in the family may be hard to establish and, therefore, impossible to exclude. However, even in the absence of a sample from an affected boy,

MLPA and sequencing can dramatically reduce the risk of a woman's carrier status.

Carriers of dystrophin mutations, or where there is a risk of recurrence because of germline mosaicism, frequently seek prenatal or preimplantation diagnosis to avoid the birth of affected children. Many genetic departments maintain registers of women at risk of being carriers of DMD or BMD so that testing for carrier status can be initiated when potential carriers reach adulthood. Current recommendations recognize the risk of cardiac involvement in even asymptomatic DMD and BMD carriers by suggesting that known carriers should be screened by echocardiogram and electrocardiography at diagnosis and on a five-yearly basis with early intervention for any cardiomyopathy [6,48]. However, this risk does not appear to be particularly high before the late teens or indeed later adulthood, so that the practice, common in clinical genetics, of testing for carrier status when a girl reaches the late teens, does not need to be altered for this indication.

X-linked Emery–Dreifuss muscular dystrophy

Despite the fact that the X-linked form of Emery–Dreifuss muscular dystrophy (XL-EDMD) (caused by mutations in the EMD gene encoding the protein emerin) was the subject of the first classical descriptions of this disorder, it is now recognized through the availability of specific testing that the autosomal dominant form caused by mutations in the lamin A/C gene (*LMNA*) is more common than XL-EDMD, and that the range of diseases associated with lamin A/C mutations is much more variable than the rather stereotypic disorder typically seen with emerinopathy. Both emerin and lamin A/C are components of the nuclear lamina [49–55].

The clinical features of classical EDMD are highly distinctive. Muscle weakness and wasting tends to be focused in a humeroperoneal distribution, and may often be relatively mild and nonprogressive. Far more prominent, and which in time may be more disabling, is the presence of typical joint contractures. These are frequently subtle in early childhood but progress with age, involving the elbows and the Achilles tendons almost universally, and frequently also the paraspinal muscles. This phenotype can be seen with both XL-EDMD and autosomal dominant (AD)-EDMD and overlaps with Bethlem myopathy, the other major

myopathic cause of a contractural phenotype but where the muscle weakness is typically more proximal in distribution. In addition, calpainopathy (LGMD2A) can sometimes present with a contractural phenotype.

The crucial management issue for patients with EDMD is the almost invariable cardiac involvement, for which the risk rises steadily with increasing age. The cardiac involvement in XL-EDMD is generally rather more benign and more easily managed than in AD-EDMD, where there is a significant risk of cardiomyopathy and ventricular arrhythmias. Current recommendations in XL-EDMD are for regular assessment for the development of arrhythmia and early intervention with a pacemaker [6].

Clinical examination usually provides a major clue to the diagnosis of EDMD. Serum CK levels are often mildly elevated, up to around 6 times the upper limit of normal, and rarely higher. The diagnosis of XL-EDMD can be suggested on muscle biopsy where, in the majority of cases, there is absence of emerin staining in skeletal muscle [50]. Analysis of skin may also be informative. The finding of mutations (mainly nucleotide substitutions or small deletions) by sequence analysis of the EDMD gene confirms the diagnosis and allows for carrier testing and prenatal diagnosis if requested. As compared to DMD, there is apparently a much lower frequency of manifesting carriers with EDMD, although a small proportion of female carriers may develop cardiac abnormalities, so that screening with EKG is appropriate.

Autosomal recessive muscular dystrophies

The autosomal recessive muscular dystrophies fall into two main groups – the congenital muscular dystrophies and the autosomal recessive forms of limb-girdle muscular dystrophy. For many forms of these heterogeneous diseases, specific genetic or protein-based testing can be very successful in defining a precise diagnosis. As with all autosomal recessive diseases, these conditions are present at a higher prevalence in communities with a high rate of consanguinity, and some founder mutations also occur in specific communities.

The congenital muscular dystrophies

As the name suggests, the congenital muscular dystrophies (CMD) typically present in the first year of life with muscle weakness and hypotonia [56–58]. Four major diagnostic categories are now recognized: (1) laminin alpha-2-deficient CMD (MDC1A); (2) the forms of CMD associated with abnormal glycosylation of alpha dystroglycan (owing to mutations in genes with established or putative glycosyl transferase activity such as *fukutin*, *FKRP*, *LARGE*, *POMT1*, *POMT2*, and *POMGNT1*), which are frequently also associated with brain and/or eye abnormalities; (3) disorders leading to prominent contractures such as Ullrich congenital muscular dystrophy, UCMD, owing to lack of the extracellular matrix protein collagen VI, and rigid spine muscular dystrophy (RSMD), which is genetically heterogeneous with one gene so far identified (*SEPN1*); and (4) primary or secondary alpha 7 integrin deficiency [57,59–64]. Indeed, for all of these groups of diseases, the full spectrum of underlying genetic causes has not yet been defined, and there remains a proportion of affected children in whom a clear diagnosis cannot be achieved. The route to establishing a precise diagnosis in a suspected case of CMD depends on assessment of the clinical findings, the serum CK level, and the results of muscle biopsy (see Table 11.2). In the assessment of a child with suspected CMD, spinal muscular atrophy (SMA), myotonic dystrophy, and Prader–Willi syndrome all need to be considered among the differential diagnoses, and can be easily excluded by the relevant DNA testing. Congenital myopathies and myasthenias may require muscle biopsy and neurophysiological investigation to confirm the diagnosis. Other differential diagnoses may need to be considered in the presence of particular additional features; for example, with congenital cataracts, the differential diagnosis of Marinesco Sjogren syndrome owing to SIL1 mutations needs to be excluded [65].

Clinical and imaging assessment will be useful to determine the presence of any eye or brain involvement. MDC1A is associated with asymptomatic cerebral white matter lesions, which are typically present after six months of age, and there is a higher incidence of epilepsy. By contrast, brain involvement in the alpha dystroglycanopathies tends to be represented by neuronal migration defects, and these children may have learning difficulties, which are severe in some cases. Eye abnormalities may or may not be present in these patients and can range from very subtle problems such as myopia to major structural eye abnormalities. These disorders have

classically been described as muscle–eye–brain disease and Walker–Warburg syndrome. With the identification of the gene defects underlying these syndromes, it is now clear that the phenotypic spectrum associated with mutations in these genes can overlap and indeed be very broad, including even milder late onset limb-girdle dystrophy-like phenotypes, where eye and brain involvement may be mild or absent.

The serum CK level is always high (>10 times the upper limit of normal) in MDC1A and in the alpha dystroglycanopathies. In UCMD, the serum CK is typically around four times the upper limit of normal, while for RSMD, the serum CK is usually normal.

There may be specific clinical features that may help to indicate the likely diagnosis. Muscle hypertrophy is frequently seen in patients with alpha dystroglycanopathies. Children with UCMD tend to have a marked distal joint laxity associated with more proximal contractures. They often have a prominent kyphosis, and typically prominent calcanei. They may have rough skin, with abnormal scarring (atrophic and keloid scarring may both be seen). Rigid SMD may be rather milder than the other types of CMD, with children usually walking independently. Typically, these children develop a specific scoliosis and respiratory failure while still ambulant. *SEPN1* gene mutations have been described in a number of diseases now felt to overlap and share these characteristics, including multicore myopathy and Mallory body myopathy [66–69].

Specific immunolabeling of a muscle biopsy sample will usually allow a distinction to be made between these groups. In MDC1A, there is a loss of laminin alpha 2 and a secondary upregulation of laminin gamma 5. This should direct the search for the causative mutations in the *laminin alpha 2* gene. In the alpha dystroglycanopathies, there is a secondary loss of alpha dystroglycan, and frequently also a secondary loss of laminin alpha 2, which is most likely to be partial. With this pattern of abnormality, the gene defect may lie in *fukutin*, *FKRP*, *POMT1*, *POMT2*, or *POMGNT1*. Further genes for proteins involved in the glycosylation of dystroglycan are likely to be identified in the future. The epidemiology of these conditions is still being elucidated, and it is possible that specific genes are more likely to be involved in specific populations, such as the common founder mutation in the gene *fukutin* in Japan. In most cases

Table 11.2. The key clues to diagnosis in the congenital muscular dystrophies

Type of congenital muscular dystrophy	Typical clinical features	Level of creatine kinase elevation	Findings on muscle immunoanalysis	Gene(s) involved
MDC1A	Severe weakness and progressive contractures. White matter changes on brain MRI after six months of age. Respiratory failure frequent in childhood	>10x normal	Loss of laminin alpha 2, upregulated laminin gamma 5. Milder cases may have partial reduction	*Laminin alpha 2* (LAMA2)
Dystroglycanopathies	Severe weakness, may be some muscle hypertrophy, variable presence of structural brain and eye abnormalities. Respiratory failure in childhood, may be cardiomyopathy	>10x normal	Loss or reduction in alpha dystroglycan, variably reduced laminin alpha 2	*Fukutin, FKRP, LARGE, POMT1, POMT2, POMGNT1* (other genes to be identified)
Ullrich congenital muscular dystrophy	Distal laxity with proximal contractures, kyphosis, and prominent calcanei. Frequent skin abnormalities. May achieve ambulation. Later spinal rigidity, respiratory failure in childhood	Usually ~4x normal, may be upper limit of normal	Loss or reduction of collagen VI immunolabeling in muscle and cultured fibroblasts	*COL6A1, COL6A2,* and *COL6A3*. Note some new dominant mutations reported
Rigid spine muscular dystrophy	Usually achieve independent ambulation, development of characteristic spinal rigidity and scoliosis, respiratory failure while still ambulant	Normal	Normal. May be structural abnormalities on biopsy including multi-/minicores or Mallory bodies	*SEPN1* (other genes to be identified)

It is noteworthy that mutations in some of these genes may also give a milder range of phenotypes, from an LGMD (limb-girdle muscular dystrophy) phenotype for laminin alpha 2 and the dystroglycanopathies and Bethlem myopathy for mutations in collagen VI.

of UCMD, there is loss of collagen VI from the extracellular matrix of the muscle fibers. This reflects the presence of mutations in one of the genes encoding the chains of collagen VI – *COL6A1, COL6A2,* and *COL6A3*. In a proportion of patients with UCMD, rather than the disease being inherited in an autosomal recessive manner, the disease is the result of a new dominant mutation in one or other of the three genes. As this clearly has very different implications for genetic counseling, demonstration of the causative mutation and, in particular, its segregation in the family is necessary to provide the correct advice. As yet, all of the other types of CMD appear to be inherited in a strictly autosomal recessive manner. Rigid SMD1, owing to *SEPN1* gene mutations, may have a variable muscle biopsy pattern, with some cases

showing characteristic core-like structures and others having a more dystrophic pattern. Immunolabeling with antibodies to the various proteins involved in other types of CMD is normal.

From the previous discussion, it follows that the main discriminatory tools in determining the type of CMD are the level of CK elevation followed by muscle biopsy, with particular attention to the labeling patterns for laminin alpha 2, alpha dystroglycan, and collagen VI, after which directed mutation analysis should be possible to allow precise carrier testing, if required, and prenatal diagnosis.

Management implications for children with CMD are broadly similar throughout the group – the provision of suitable aids and appliances to improve posture and mobility; physical therapy to try and delay the development of contractures and scoliosis, which may also require orthopedic input; attention to feeding problems, which may lead to undernourishment and require gastrostomy feeding; and respiratory impairment, which may lead to the requirement for home nocturnal ventilation, even in the first decade of life. Cardiac involvement may be important in the alpha dystroglycanopathies. These interventions have a demonstrable effect on improving length and quality of life in these patients [70,71].

The autosomal recessive limb-girdle muscular dystrophies

This is another highly heterogeneous group of conditions, sharing the characteristic feature of muscle weakness, most usually in the pelvic and shoulder girdle musculature, with onset at any age from childhood to adult life [72,73]. In all populations, limb-girdle muscular dystrophies (LGMD) are less common than dystrophinopathy (Table 11.1), which should always be excluded as a first line before embarking on investigations for LGMD. The relative frequency of the different types of LGMD varies from population to population, with LGMD2I common in Northern Europe while LGMD2A and 2B are more common in Southern European populations. Knowledge of the prevalence of the different types of LGMD in different populations can help to direct a diagnostic strategy – for example, in Northern Europe a common *FKRP* gene mutation is seen in the majority of cases of LGMD2I and may be used as a diagnostic screen before embarking on muscle biopsy. The key features of the different types of LGMD, the investigations that may be most useful in achieving a precise diagnosis, and the management implications of the particular conditions are outlined in Table 11.3. As with CMD, assessment of the clinical history and examination, knowledge of the serum CK levels, and use of a range of antibodies on the muscle biopsy specimens can help to direct mutation testing in the various autosomal recessive LGMD genes. Specific diagnosis thereafter can allow precise carrier testing and prenatal diagnosis and also direct management, as the implications of the different diagnoses do vary with regard to the need for cardiac and respiratory surveillance in particular [72].

The autosomal dominant muscular dystrophies

The group of disorders discussed here comprises a relatively common form of MD, facioscapulohumeral MD, a probably underdiagnosed entity, Bethlem myopathy, and the autosomal dominant forms of LGMD. Myotonic dystrophy, which is one of the most common types of MD and a highly multisystem disorder with significant genetic counseling and management issues, is discussed previously. The autosomal dominant types of MD share several features that are crucial for genetic counseling; namely, frequently highly variable phenotypes within or between different families, the high incidence of new dominant mutations, and the need to address the issue of presymptomatic testing with sensitivity. Many also have very important implications for management of the affected patient.

Facioscapulohumeral muscular dystrophy

Facioscapulohumeral muscular dystrophy (FSHD), an autosomal dominant muscle disease, is one of the most frequent MDs for which molecular genetic testing has become the diagnostic tool of choice. The clinical phenotype associated with FSHD, although variable, is usually very characteristic, and in most cases the diagnosis is readily confirmed by DNA analysis. The majority of patients show a typical pattern of muscle weakness that is often asymmetrical, with upper and lower facial weakness so that patients often report sleeping with their eyes open and being unable to whistle, scapular weakness, a prominent lumbar lordosis, and foot drop. The clinical spectrum of FSHD can, however, sometimes include prominent pelvic-girdle weakness and, in some individuals, only minimal facial muscle involvement, leading to confusion in diagnosis. It can present in an early onset or infantile form, where facial and scapular weakness is usually extreme and progression of muscle weakness may be very rapid. In this infantile form, there is a frequent association with hearing loss and retinal telangiectasia, associated signs that can also be found but are rarely symptomatic in less severely affected cases [74–77]. Early onset cases may be misdiagnosed as Moebius syndrome, and the presence of deafness may distract from the correct diagnosis. Early onset cases are frequently associated with larger than average deletions demonstrable at the

Table 11.3. The autosomal recessive types of limb-girdle muscular dystrophy

Type of limb-girdle muscular dystrophy	Typical clinical features	Level of creatine kinase	Muscle immunoanalysis	Gene involved
LGMD2A	May present with toe walking, scapular winging. Some patients have contractures, often atrophic. Late respiratory failure. One of the more frequent causes of autosomal recessive LGMD in most populations	>10x normal	Muscle immunolabeling normal, but immunoblotting shows reduction in calpain 3 in ~80% cases	*Calpain 3*
LGMD2B	Frequent inability to walk on tip-toe. About 10% may present with calf pain and swelling. Usually calf wasting, biceps wasting. Shoulder girdle weakness usually later than proximal/distal lower limb weakness. More frequent in Southern than Northern Europe	>40x normal	Reduced or absent dysferlin. May be secondary loss of calpain 3 and caveolin 3	*Dysferlin*
LGMD2C-F	May present in Duchenne-/Becker-like way. May be muscle hypertrophy, scapular winging. Cardiac and respiratory complications frequent and surveillance indicated. Higher frequency in populations with high rate of consanguinity	>10x normal	Reduction in components of dystrophin associated complex with usually predominant reduction in sarcoglycans	*Alpha, beta, gamma, delta sarcoglycan.* Founder mutations in some populations
LGMD2G	May be distal weakness. Very rare, reported only in Brazil	<10x normal		*Telethonin*
LGMD2H	Few reported families have proximal weakness	<10x normal		*TRIM32*
LGMD2I	Clinically may resemble Duchenne/Becker MD with frequent muscle hypertrophy. Cardiomyopathy common. Respiratory failure (diaphragmatic) may occur when still ambulant	>10x normal	Reduced alpha dystroglycan on immunolabeling, may be reduction in laminin alpha 2 on immunoblotting	*FKRP* Common mutation (C826A) in Northern European populations
LGMD2J	History of distal weakness in heterozygotes. Seen in homozygous form only in Finland where the mutation is at high frequency	>10x normal	May be secondary loss of calpain 3	*Titin*
LGMD2K	May present early with global delay. May be mental retardation, microcephaly. Upper limb weakness may be worse than lower limb weakness	>10x normal	Reduced alpha dystroglycan	*POMT1* Other glycosyl transferases now also implicated in LGMD phenotypes

DNA level, and are often *de novo*. A recent review of infantile FSHD suggested that, in known families, the risk of having a child with infantile disease was actually relatively low [78]. Presentation in the first five years of life is seen in only about 5% of all gene carriers, with penetrance rising to 21% for ages 5–9 years, 58% for 10–14 years, 86% for 15–19 years, and 95% for ages 20 years and over, whereas non-penetrance is estimated at <2% after the age of 50 years. However, these figures have not been revisited in the light of molecular diagnosis, which has revealed a higher than previously suspected rate of non-penetrant cases.

There is a gender difference in the severity of the disease, with the mean age of onset slightly lower and rate of progression faster in males, and a higher proportion of females than males among asymptomatic cases [79].

DNA testing for FSHD relies on the demonstration of a deletion on chromosome 4q35, which is found in >95% of affected individuals who typically show a DNA fragment size of <30 kb, and in unaffected individuals where a DNA fragment of >40 kb is detected using a double-digest system and a DNA probe known as p13E–11 [79,80]. This test is robust provided appropriate safeguards are taken – there is an important gray area in allele size, between 33 and 40 kb, where it can be hard to designate affected status absolutely. The region deleted on chromosome 4q35 is highly homologous to a region on chromosome 10q26, and although a double or triple digest system (ECOR1/BIn1 and Xap1) usually distinguishes fragments of chromosome 4 and 10 in origin, the degree of homology between the two regions is such that up to 20% of the population will have exchanged material between the two chromosomes. This can lead to potential difficulties in interpretation of the test results unless additional analysis, such as pulsed field gel electrophoresis or dosage to delineate the chromosome 4 and 10 fragments, is carried out. Two allelic variants of the 4q subtelomere (4qA and 4qB) exist, which are almost equally common in the Caucasian population but, uniquely, 4qA is associated with FSHD [80,81]. Therefore, further distinction of pathogenic versus non-pathogenic repeat arrays relies on the identification of these polymorphic variants (so-called allele A fragments) and also methylation status, as the presence of a D4Z4 deletion leads to hypomethylation of the site, with a correlation again with allele size – the shortest alleles

being the most subject to hypomethylation. Providing these potential pitfalls in diagnosis are taken into account, this analysis has taken an important place in the diagnostic setting, with a role in clinical diagnosis, presymptomatic testing, and prenatal diagnosis where this is sought. A statistical correlation appears to exist between fragment size and severity especially in sporadic cases, with the smallest fragments (and therefore the largest deletions) detected in the youngest-onset and most severe cases, which often tend to be *de novo* cases or children of an unaffected carrier parent with somatic mosaicism. Offspring of a mildly affected mosaic FSHD patient generally will develop a more severe phenotype than expected on the basis of the phenotype of the FSHD parent. In patients with somatic mosaicism, a relationship between the severity of the disease and the combination of the residual repeat size and the proportion of cells carrying the disease allele seems to exist [79]. These correlations have been extended to predict a severe course in patients with the largest deletions. Fragment size does not, however, account for all of the variability seen in the disease, and within families, where all affected individuals have the same fragment size, a huge range of severity may be seen. This intrafamilial variability, at least in part, may be explained by the occurrence of somatic mosaicism [82]. The counseling of a family must include the lack of certainty about likely progression of the disease – while a gene carrier can be identified through the use of DNA testing, this carries with it no prediction as to the likely course of the disease. This is, therefore, a critical point for discussion in families planning presymptomatic or prenatal diagnosis.

The ability to diagnose FSHD specifically has led to the recognition of a high rate of new mutations and of the existence of non-penetrant cases. Previously, it could be hard to decide whether a minor degree of facial or shoulder girdle weakness in a parent of an affected child was significant, and the occurrence of two or more affected children in families without a clearly affected parent led to the suggestion that there might be an autosomal recessive form of the disease. When apparently *de novo* cases are reappraised in the light of molecular genetic testing, the deletion is found in a non-penetrant parent in approximately 19% of cases. It can now be demonstrated directly that the proportion of new mutations ranges between 9.6% and 33%. Even if the deletion is not found in lymphocyte DNA from the parents, owing to the high frequency of somatic mosaicism, siblings of an isolated case probably have a risk in the region of 10% of being affected as well [81].

Management of patients with FSHD depends on the severity of the case and the predominant symptoms. Screening for deafness and retinal telangiectasia, at least in the most severe cases, is probably worthwhile. Extreme lumbar lordosis is often a major problem for the severe infantile cases [78]. In older patients, pain may be a particular problem, which may require the use of pain-killers and graded exercise to try to overcome it [83,84]. Foot drop may respond to splinting, and scapular winging may respond well to scapular fixation [78]. Rarely, patients with FSHD require support for swallowing or respiratory problems. Cardiac involvement is very unusual and most likely not a primary complication of the disease.

Bethlem myopathy

Bethlem myopathy is an autosomal dominant disorder characterized by the combination of a relatively mild proximal myopathy and variable contractures, which leads to diagnostic confusion with EDMD [63,85,86]. It is, in itself, a genetically heterogeneous disorder, with mutations in the three genes COL6A1, COL6A2, and COL6A3 having been described in association with a Bethlem myopathy phenotype [63,64,87–93].

Bethlem myopathy may present at any age. It may be recognizable from birth, with affected children sometimes presenting with torticollis and contractures. Prenatal onset of muscle weakness with diminished fetal movements has been suggested in some families, and affected infants are often hypotonic with delayed motor milestones. Proximal muscle weakness from childhood onward tends to be only slowly progressive and there may be long periods of time when the condition does not progress at all. Other patients may be asymptomatic in childhood and present with mild muscle weakness and contractures in adult life. However, considerable disability may be seen in some patients in late adult life, with more than two thirds of patients over the age of 50 years requiring aids for outdoor ambulation, and some reports of respiratory failure secondary to diaphragmatic paralysis. The major hallmark of this condition is the development of contractures especially of the fingers, wrists, elbows, and ankles, and these, in addition to

weakness, contribute to disability [85,94,95]. The contractures can be quite dynamic in nature during childhood, and hypermobility of distal interphalangeal joints can be present together with long finger flexion contractures (although this is less marked than in the allelic condition UCMD: see previous section). Skin features typically seen in connective tissue disorders, such as keloid formation and "cigarette paper" scarring as well as follicular hyperkeratosis, can also be present in patients with Bethlem myopathy. Clinically, the condition may show overlap with autosomal dominant forms of LGMD because of the proximal muscle weakness, especially as the full spectrum of the disease, such as the characteristic contractures, may not be seen in every patient. The presence of the contractures may cause confusion with EDMD, particularly if a rigid spine is present. Exclusion of these diagnoses is crucial because of the critical need for cardiac surveillance and treatment. In Bethlem myopathy, there is no evidence of any primary cardiac involvement.

Currently, the diagnosis of Bethlem myopathy relies on the detection of a mutation in any of three collagen genes, COL6A1, COL6A2, and COL6A3. As yet, it is impossible to draw clear conclusions on genotype–phenotype correlations. However, specific mutations tend to be strictly associated with a particular phenotype, and site-specific effects impairing particular steps in the complex intracellular and extracellular assembly process of collagen VI are likely to explain the degree of negative effect of individual mutations [64]. It follows that for a patient with Bethlem myopathy, there is not a risk of having a child with UCMD unless the affected person by chance has a partner who is a UCMD carrier. However, in counseling the patient with Bethlem myopathy about their risk of having an affected child, it is important to bear in mind the variability that may be associated with the phenotype.

Unlike the complete or partial absence of collagen VI immunolabeling on muscle biopsies and dermal fibroblast cultures, which is very useful in UCMD patients, the immunohistochemical findings in Bethlem patients appear less clear cut as yet, although immunolabeling of cultured fibroblasts holds promise in detecting the frequently subtle collagen VI changes [96]. A secondary deficiency of the basal lamina component laminin β1 has been demonstrated in muscle biopsies of adult patients with Bethlem myopathy [97]. Despite the fact that this secondary protein reduction may be seen in a variety of other primary muscle conditions, it may act as a pointer toward the diagnosis in patients with a suggestive phenotype.

Management of Bethlem myopathy is focused on the physiotherapeutic and, if necessary, orthopedic management of the progressive contractures. Monitoring for the development of respiratory impairment by measurement of forced vital capacity in sitting and lying (thereby detecting any diaphragmatic involvement) is necessary, and some patients may develop nocturnal respiratory insufficiency requiring ventilatory support. Cardiac involvement does not appear to be a part of the Bethlem myopathy phenotype.

The autosomal dominant forms of limb-girdle muscular dystrophy and associated diseases

The group of disorders that has come to be recognized in the autosomal dominant LGMD classification includes three for which a gene abnormality is known (LGMD1A, LGMD1B, and LGMD1C) and three with linkage only. As experience accumulates in LGMD1A, LGMD1B, and LGMD1C, it is clear that with all three an LGMD phenotype is only one of the possible presentations with mutations in the causative genes. A careful family history is important in all cases, with particular attention paid to the possible additional or alternative phenotypes that may be observed in individual family members.

LGMD1A was recognized first in two large American families in whom the disease (a proximal muscular dystrophy with Achilles tendon contractures and dysarthria) was linked to chromosome 5. Subsequent work confirmed that the causative gene was *myotilin* [98,99], which is now known to be part of a family of genes responsible for a group of diseases known as the myofibrillar myopathies (MFM) [100]. The phenotypes in these patients are quite variable, and as well as a possible proximal myopathy, may include distal muscle weakness, respiratory impairment, cardiomyopathy or arrhythmia, and dysarthria [101,102]. The diagnosis may be further helped by examination of the muscle biopsy, which may show the presence of vacuoles and accumulation of desmin and myotilin. Electron microscopy may be useful in demonstrating the presence of Z-line streaming [103]. Creatine kinase levels in these patients are variable. In the presence of suggestive clinical or muscle biopsy findings, the diagnosis needs to be confirmed by the systematic screening of the genes known to be involved in MFM (to date, *desmin*, *alpha b crystallin*, *myotilin*, *ZASP*, *filamin C*, and *Bag3*). Even with this screening, in approximately 45% of likely patients, the underlying mutation cannot be identified, indicating the likely existence of other genes responsible for an MFM phenotype. Management in all of these patients should include a high level of suspicion and surveillance for cardiac and respiratory complications.

LGMD1B is one of a broad range of phenotypes associated with mutations in lamin A/C [54,104]. Approximately 60% of lamin A/C mutations are associated with a predominantly skeletal or cardiac muscle phenotype, 25% involve adipose tissue (for example lipodystrophy), 6% with premature aging, and 3% with an axonal neuropathy (www.umd.be:2000). LGMD1B describes a group of patients with a predominantly proximal muscular dystrophy associated with the development of cardiomyopathy and arrhythmia. Other skeletal muscle presentations of lamin A/C mutations include autosomal dominant Emery–Dreifuss muscular dystrophy, EDMD (see previous discussion), and the much more rare and clinically more severe autosomal recessive EDMD. Increasingly, lamin A/C mutations are being described in other muscle diseases, such as with a congenital presentation or with a Duchenne-like presentation in early childhood. Some patients may have overlap phenotypes with features of several of the lamin A/C related conditions or family members may manifest different skeletal or cardiac muscle phenotypes, including lipodystrophy, neuropathy, and mandibuloacral dysplasia [54,104]. Further complicating diagnosis and counseling in this group of diseases is the high rate of new dominant mutations and germline mosaicism. The wide phenotypic variability alongside the very clear implications for management and genetic advice means that there should be a low threshold for considering a diagnosis of laminopathy. Confirmation of the diagnosis relies on the demonstration of mutations in the lamin A/C gene (*LMNA*) as ancillary investigations are nonspecific. Serum CK levels are usually less than 10 times the upper limit of normal, although rarely they can be higher; analysis of the muscle biopsy is nonspecific, and lamin A/C protein immunoanalysis is abnormal only in the rare autosomal recessive cases. As with Bethlem myopathy, there may be a secondary abnormality in labeling for laminin beta 1, but this finding is very nonspecific. Most mutations in lamin

A/C are missense changes, and many are novel. Proof of pathogenicity of a given mutation may prove to be a challenge.

However, the management implications of these diseases are so important that this is a crucial differential diagnosis to consider with a low index of suspicion. These disorders share a very high risk of cardiac complications, which may present initially as arrhythmias and progress to cardiomyopathy. The arrhythmias are typically more serious with laminopathy than with the X-linked form of EDMD, with a high risk of sudden death even following pacemaker insertion, so that recommendations for management in this condition include the early consideration of use of an implantable defibrillator [105,106]. Respiratory failure may also be a major complication requiring the initiation of nocturnal ventilatory support to reduce symptoms and prolong life.

LGMD1C is a result of mutations in the gene for caveolin 3 [107]. As with LGMD1A and LGMD1B, LGMD is only one of a variety of presentations with mutations in this gene, which include hyperCKaemia, muscle hypertrophy, distal myopathy, myalgia, and rippling muscle disease [108–111]. Patients presenting with hyperCKaemia, rippling muscle disease, or myalgia may be very strong indeed. Two families with caveolin 3 mutations and cardiomyopathy have been reported [112,113], but cardiac involvement otherwise appears rare in these conditions, which are typically relatively mild.

There undoubtedly exist a number of families with an autosomal dominant muscle disease in whom a diagnosis cannot be reached. One such phenotype that has recently been associated with an underlying gene defect is the rare combination of MD, dementia, and Paget's disease, now known to be caused by mutations in the valosin-containing protein gene [114–116].

Conclusions

This chapter has concentrated on the types of MD for which a clear genetic basis has been established and where diagnosis may be possible. Once all of these types of MD have been taken into consideration, there remains approximately 25% of patients for whom no clear diagnosis can be established [72]. They may have forms of MD for which only linkage analysis is available but family size may preclude this, or a type of MD for which no genetic cause has yet been established. It should be pointed out that it is always worth revisiting potential differential diagnoses, such as inflammatory causes of muscle disease, spinal muscular atrophy, and metabolic muscle diseases, if diagnosis of a specific MD cannot be confirmed. Alternative genetic causes of myopathy may also need to be revisited; for example, the distal myopathies and congenital myopathies which, confusingly, may present later in life in some cases. Confirmation of a specific diagnosis is already bringing benefits to affected patients and their families with respect to genetic counseling and management, and as the era of specific molecular therapies becomes a reality, these benefits are very likely to increase.

References

1. Bushby K, Straub V. Nonmolecular treatment for muscular dystrophies. *Curr Opin Neurol* 2005; **18**: 511–518.

2. Bushby KM, Hill A, Steele JG. Failure of early diagnosis in symptomatic Duchenne muscular dystrophy. *Lancet* 1999; **353**: 557–558.

3. Parsons EP, Clarke AJ, Bradley DM. Developmental progress in Duchenne muscular dystrophy: lessons for earlier detection. *Eur J Paediatr Neurol* 2004; **8**: 145–153.

4. Eagle M, Baudouin SV, Chandler C, *et al.* Survival in Duchenne muscular dystrophy: improvements in life expectancy since 1967 and the impact of home nocturnal ventilation. *Neuromuscul Disord* 2002; **12**: 926–929.

5. Bushby K, Bourke J, Bullock R, *et al.* The multidisciplinary management of Duchenne muscular dystrophy. *Current Paediatrics* 2005; **15**: 292–300.

6. Bushby K, Muntoni F, Bourke JP. 107th ENMC International Workshop. The management of cardiac involvement in muscular dystrophy and myotonic dystrophy. Naarden, the Netherlands, 2002. *Neuromuscul Disord* 2003; **13**: 166–172.

7. Campbell C, Jacob P. Deflazacort for the treatment of Duchenne dystrophy: a systematic review. *BMC Neurol* 2003; **3**: 7.

8. Bushby K, Muntoni F, Urtizberea A, Hughes R, Griggs R. Report on the 124th ENMC International Workshop. Treatment of Duchenne muscular dystrophy; defining the gold standards of management in the use of

corticosteroids. Naarden, the Netherlands, 2004. *Neuromuscul Disord* 2004; **14**: 526–534.

9. Manzur AY, Kuntzer T, Pike M, Swan A. Glucocorticoid corticosteroids for Duchenne muscular dystrophy. *Cochrane Database Syst Rev* 2004; **2**: CD003725.

10. Moxley RT 3rd, Ashwal S, Pandya S, *et al.* Practice parameter: corticosteroid treatment of Duchenne dystrophy: report of the Quality Standards Subcommittee of the American Academy of Neurology and the Practice Committee of the Child Neurology Society. *Neurology* 2005; **64**: 13–20.

11. Bushby K, Finkel R, Birnkrant DJ, *et al.* Diagnosis and management of Duchenne muscular dystrophy. Part 1: Diagnosis, and pharmacological and psychosocial management. *Lancet Neurol* 2010; **9**: 77–93.

12. Duboc D, Meune C, Lerebours G, *et al.* Effect of perindopril on the onset and progression of left ventricular dysfunction in Duchenne muscular dystrophy. *J Am Coll Cardiol* 2005; **45**: 855–857.

13. Hirano M. Does ACE inhibitor therapy delay onset and progression of cardiac dysfunction in Duchenne muscular dystrophy? *Curr Neurol Neurosci Rep* 2006; **6**: 35–36.

14. Eagle M, Bourke J, Bullock R, *et al.* Managing Duchenne muscular dystrophy – the additive effect of spinal surgery and home nocturnal ventilation in improving survival. *Neuromuscul Disord* 2007; **17**: 470–475.

15. Bushby KM, Thambyayah M, Gardner-Medwin D. Prevalence and incidence of Becker muscular dystrophy. *Lancet* 1991; **337**: 1022–1024.

16. Bushby KM, Gardner-Medwin D. The clinical, genetic and dystrophin characteristics of Becker muscular dystrophy. I. Natural history. *J Neurol* 1993; **240**: 98–104.

17. Bushby KM, Gardner-Medwin D, Nicholson LV, *et al.* The clinical, genetic and dystrophin characteristics of Becker muscular dystrophy. II. Correlation of phenotype with genetic and protein abnormalities. *J Neurol* 1993; **240**: 105–112.

18. Nicholson LV, Johnson MA, Bushby KM, Gardner-Medwin D. Functional significance of dystrophin positive fibres in Duchenne muscular dystrophy. *Arch Dis Child* 1993; **68**: 632–636.

19. Comi LI, Nigro G, Politano L, Petretta VR. The cardiomyopathy of Duchenne/Becker consultands. *Int J Cardiol* 1992; **34**: 297–305.

20. Hoffman EP, Arahata K, Minetti C, Bonilla E, Rowland LP. Dystrophinopathy in isolated cases of myopathy in females. *Neurology* 1992; **42**: 967–975.

21. Muntoni F, Mateddu A, Marosu MG, *et al.* Variable dystrophin expression in different muscles of a Duchenne muscular dystrophy carrier. *Clin Genet* 1992; **42**: 35–38.

22. Bushby KM, Goodship JA, Nicholson LV, *et al.* Variability in clinical, genetic and protein abnormalities in manifesting carriers of Duchenne and Becker muscular dystrophy. *Neuromuscul Disord* 1993; **3**: 57–64.

23. Sewry CA, Matsumura K, Campbell KP, Dubowitz V. Expression of dystrophin-associated glycoproteins and utrophin in carriers of Duchenne muscular dystrophy. *Neuromuscul Disord* 1994; **4**: 401–409.

24. Doriguzzi C, Palmucci L, Mongini T, *et al.* Systematic use of dystrophin testing in muscle biopsies: results in 201 cases. *Eur J Clin Invest* 1997; **27**: 352–358.

25. Sumita DR, Vainzof M, Campiotto S, *et al.* Absence of correlation between skewed X inactivation in blood and serum creatine-kinase levels in Duchenne/Becker female carriers. *Am J Med Genet* 1998; **80**: 356–361.

26. Yoshioka M, Yorifuji T, Mituyoshi I. Skewed X inactivation in manifesting carriers of Duchenne muscular dystrophy. *Clin Genet* 1998; **53**: 102–107.

27. Finsterer J, Stollberger C. The heart in human dystrophinopathies. *Cardiology* 2003; **99**: 1–19.

28. Muntoni F, Torelli S, Ferlini A. Dystrophin and mutations: one gene, several proteins, multiple phenotypes. *Lancet Neurol* 2003; **2**: 731–740.

29. Cohen N, Muntoni F. Multiple pathogenetic mechanisms in X-linked dilated cardiomyopathy. *Heart* 2004; **90**: 835–841.

30. Cohen N, Rimessi P, Gualandi F, Ferlini A, Muntoni F. In vivo study of an aberrant dystrophin exon inclusion in X-linked dilated cardiomyopathy. *Biochem Biophys Res Commun* 2004; **317**: 1215–1220.

31. Wu JY, Kuban KC, Allred E, Shapiro F, Darras BT. Association of Duchenne muscular dystrophy with autism spectrum disorder. *J Child Neurol* 2005; **20**: 790–795.

32. Hendriksen JG, Vles JS. Neuropsychiatric disorders in males with Duchenne muscular dystrophy: frequency rate of attention-deficit hyperactivity disorder (ADHD), autism spectrum

disorder, and obsessive-compulsive disorder. *J Child Neurol* 2008; **23**: 477–481.

33. Nicholson LV, Bushby KM, Johnson MA, Gardner-Medwin D, Ginjaar IB. Dystrophin expression in Duchenne patients with "in-frame" gene deletions. *Neuropediatrics* 1993; **24**: 93–97.

34. Nicholson LV, Johnson MA, Bushby KM, *et al.* Integrated study of 100 patients with Xp21 linked muscular dystrophy using clinical, genetic, immunochemical, and histopathological data. Part 1. Trends across the clinical groups. *J Med Genet* 1993; **30**: 728–736.

35. Nicholson LV, Johnson MA, Bushby KM, *et al.* Integrated study of 100 patients with Xp21 linked muscular dystrophy using clinical, genetic, immunochemical, and histopathological data. Part 2. Correlations within individual patients. *J Med Genet* 1993; **30**: 737–744.

36. Nicholson LV, Johnson MA, Bushby KM, *et al.* Integrated study of 100 patients with Xp21 linked muscular dystrophy using clinical, genetic, immunochemical, and histopathological data. Part 3. Differential diagnosis and prognosis. *J Med Genet* 1993; **30**: 745–751.

37. Schwartz M, Duno M. Improved molecular diagnosis of dystrophin gene mutations using the multiplex ligation-dependent probe amplification method. *Genet Test* 2004; **8**: 361–367.

38. Gatta V, Scarciolla O, Gaspari AR, *et al.* Identification of deletions and duplications of the DMD gene in affected males and carrier females by multiple ligation probe amplification (MLPA). *Hum Genet* 2005; **117**: 92–98.

39. Janssen B, Hartmann C, Scholz V, Jauch A, Zschocke J. MLPA analysis for the detection of deletions, duplications and complex rearrangements in the dystrophin gene: potential and pitfalls. *Neurogenetics* 2005; **6**: 29–35.

40. Flanigan KM, von Niederhausern A, Dunn DM, *et al.* Rapid direct sequence analysis of the dystrophin gene. *Am J Hum Genet* 2003; **72**: 931–939.

41. Dent KM, Dunn DM, von Niederhausern A, *et al.* Improved molecular diagnosis of dystrophinopathies in an unselected clinical cohort. *Am J Med Genet A* 2005; **134**: 295–298.

42. Prior TW, Papp AC, Snyder PJ, Mendell JR. Case of the month: germline mosaicism in carriers of Duchenne muscular dystrophy. *Muscle Nerve* 1992; **15**: 960–963.

43. Mukherjee M, Chaturvedi LS, Srivastava S, Mittal RD, Mittal B. *De novo* mutations in sporadic deletional Duchenne muscular dystrophy (DMD) cases. *Exp Mol Med* 2003; **35**: 113–117.

44. Ferreiro V, Szijan I, Giliberto F. Detection of germline mosaicism in two Duchenne muscular dystrophy families using polymorphic dinucleotide (CA)n repeat loci within the dystrophin gene. *Mol Diagn* 2004; **8**: 115–121.

45. Fischer C, Kruger J, Gross W. RISCALW: a Windows program for risk calculation in families with Duchenne muscular dystrophy. *Ann Hum Genet* 2006; **70**: 249–253.

46. Passos-Bueno MR, Bakker E, Kneppers AL, *et al.* Different mosaicism frequencies for proximal and distal Duchenne muscular dystrophy (DMD) mutations indicate difference in etiology and recurrence risk. *Am J Hum Genet* 1992; **51**: 1150–1155.

47. Helderman-van den Enden AT, de Jong R, den Dunnen JT, *et al.* Recurrence risk due to germ line mosaicism: Duchenne and Becker muscular dystrophy. *Clin Genet* 2009; **75**: 465–472.

48. American Academy of Pediatrics Section on Cardiology and Cardiac Surgery. Cardiovascular health supervision for individuals affected by Duchenne or Becker muscular dystrophy. *Pediatrics* 2005; **116**: 1569–1573.

49. Bione S, Maestrini E, Rivella S, *et al.* Identification of a novel X-linked gene responsible for Emery–Dreifuss muscular dystrophy. *Nat Genet* 1994; **8**: 323–327.

50. Manilal S, Nguyen TM, Sewry CA, Morris GE. The Emery–Dreifuss muscular dystrophy protein, emerin, is a nuclear membrane protein. *Hum Mol Genet* 1996; **5**: 801–808.

51. Manilal S, Sewry CA, Pereboev A, *et al.* Distribution of emerin and lamins in the heart and implications for Emery–Dreifuss muscular dystrophy. *Hum Mol Genet* 1999; **8**: 353–359.

52. Hayashi YK. X-linked form of Emery–Dreifuss muscular dystrophy. *Acta Myol* 2005; **24**: 98–103.

53. Wilson KL, Holaska JM, Montes de Oca R, *et al.* Nuclear membrane protein emerin: roles in gene regulation, actin dynamics and human disease. *Novartis Found Symp* 2005; **264**: 51–58; discussion 58–62, 227–230.

54. Worman HJ. Components of the nuclear envelope and their role in human disease. *Novartis Found Symp* 2005; **264**: 35–42; discussion 42–50, 227–230.

55. Roux KJ, Burke B. Nuclear envelope defects in muscular dystrophy. *Biochim Biophys Acta* 2007; **1772**: 118–127.

56. Muntoni F, Valero de Bernabe B, Bittner R, *et al.* 114th ENMC International Workshop on Congenital Muscular Dystrophy (CMD), Naarden, the Netherlands (8th Workshop of

the International Consortium on CMD; 3rd Workshop of the MYO-CLUSTER project GENRE). *Neuromuscul Disord* 2003; **13**: 579–588.

57. Di Blasi C, Piga D, Brioschi P, *et al.* LAMA2 gene analysis in congenital muscular dystrophy: new mutations, prenatal diagnosis, and founder effect. *Arch Neurol* 2005; **62**: 1582–1586.

58. Mercuri E, Longman C. Congenital muscular dystrophy. *Pediatr Ann* 2005; **34**: 560–562, 564–568.

59. Flanigan KM, Kerr L, Bromberg MB, *et al.* Congenital muscular dystrophy with rigid spine syndrome: a clinical, pathological, radiological, and genetic study. *Ann Neurol* 2000; **47**: 152–161.

60. Grewal PK, Hewitt JE. Glycosylation defects: a new mechanism for muscular dystrophy? *Hum Mol Genet* 2003; **12**: R259–R264.

61. Topaloglu H, Brockington M, Yuva Y, *et al.* FKRP gene mutations cause congenital muscular dystrophy, mental retardation, and cerebellar cysts. *Neurology* 2003; **60**: 988–992.

62. Jimenez-Mallebrera C, Brown SC, Sewry CA, Muntoni F. Congenital muscular dystrophy: molecular and cellular aspects. *Cell Mol Life Sci* 2005; **62**: 809–823.

63. Lampe AK, Bushby KM. Collagen VI related muscle disorders. *J Med Genet* 2005; **42**: 673–685.

64. Lampe AK, Dunn DM, Von Niederhausern AC, *et al.* Automated genomic sequence analysis of the three collagen VI genes: applications to Ullrich congenital muscular dystrophy and Bethlem myopathy. *J Med Genet* 2005; **42**: 108–120.

65. Senderek J, Krieger M, Stendel C, *et al.* Mutations in SIL1 cause

Marinesco-Sjogren syndrome, a cerebellar ataxia with cataract and myopathy. *Nat Genet* 2005; **37**: 1312–1314.

66. Moghadaszadeh B, Petit N, Jaillard C, *et al.* Mutations in SEPN1 cause congenital muscular dystrophy with spinal rigidity and restrictive respiratory syndrome. *Nat Genet* 2001; **29**: 17–18.

67. Ferreiro A, Ceuterick-de Groote C, Marks JJ, *et al.* Desmin-related myopathy with Mallory body-like inclusions is caused by mutations of the selenoprotein N gene. *Ann Neurol* 2004; **55**: 676–686.

68. Nucci A, Queiroz LS, Zambelli HJ, Martins Filho J. Multi-minicore disease revisited. *Arq Neuropsiquiatr* 2004; **62**: 935–939.

69. Jungbluth H, Zhou H, Hartley L, *et al.* Minicore myopathy with ophthalmoplegia caused by mutations in the ryanodine receptor type 1 gene. *Neurology* 2005; **65**: 1930–1935.

70. Philpot J, Bagnall A, King C, Dubowitz V, Muntoni F. Feeding problems in merosin deficient congenital muscular dystrophy. *Arch Dis Child* 1999; **80**: 542–547.

71. Mellies U, Dohna-Schwake C, Voit T. Respiratory function assessment and intervention in neuromuscular disorders. *Curr Opin Neurol* 2005; **18**: 543–547.

72. Bushby K, Norwood F, Straub V. The limb-girdle muscular dsytrophies – diagnostic strategies. *Biochim Biophys Acta* 2007; **1772**: 238–242.

73. Laval SH, Bushby KM. Limb-girdle muscular dystrophies – from genetics to molecular pathology. *Neuropathol Appl Neurobiol* 2004; **30**: 91–105.

74. Brouwer OF, Padberg GW, Ruys CJ, *et al.* Hearing loss in facioscapulohumeral muscular

dystrophy. *Neurology* 1991; **41**: 1878–1881.

75. Brouwer OF, Padberg GW, Wijmenga C, Frants RR. Facioscapulohumeral muscular dystrophy in early childhood. *Arch Neurol* 1994; **51**: 387–394.

76. Brouwer OF, Padberg GW, Bakker E, Wijmenga C, Frants RR. Early onset facioscapulohumeral muscular dystrophy. *Muscle Nerve* 1995; **2**: S67–S72.

77. Bindoff LAM, Sommerfelt N, Krossnes K, *et al.* Severe facioscapulohumeral muscular dystrophy presenting with Coats' disease and mental retardation. *Neuromuscul Disord* 2006; **16**: 559–563.

78. Klinge LE, Eagle M, Haggerty ID, *et al.* Severe phenotype in infantile facioscapulohumeral muscular dystrophy. *Neuromuscul Disord* 2006; **16**: 553–558.

79. van der Maarel SM, Frants RR. The D4Z4 repeat-mediated pathogenesis of facioscapulohumeral muscular dystrophy. *Am J Hum Genet* 2005; **76**: 375–386.

80. Lemmers RJ, van der Wielen MJ, Bakker E, Frants RR, van der Maarel SM. Rapid and accurate diagnosis of facioscapulohumeral muscular dystrophy. *Neuromuscul Disord* 2006; **16**: 615–617.

81. van der Maarel SM, Frants RR, Padberg GW. Facioscapulohumeral muscular dystrophy. *Biochim Biophys Acta* 2007; **1772**: 186–194.

82. Buzhov BT, Lemmers RJ, Tournev I, *et al.* Recurrent somatic mosaicism for D4Z4 contractions in a family with facioscapulohumeral muscular dystrophy. *Neuromuscul Disord* 2005; **15**: 471–475.

83. Bushby KM, Pollitt C, Johnxon MJ, Rogers MT, Chinnery PF. Muscle

pain as a prominent feature of facioscapulohumeral muscular dystrophy (FSHD): four illustrative case reports. *Neuromuscul Disord* 1998; **8**: 574–579.

84. Jensen MP, Hoffman AJ, Stoelb BL, *et al*. Chronic pain in persons with myotonic dystrophy and facioscapulohumeral dystrophy. *Arch Phys Med Rehabil* 2008; **89**: 320–328.

85. Jobsis GJ, Boers JM, Barth PG, de Visser M. Bethlem myopathy: a slowly progressive congenital muscular dystrophy with contractures. *Brain* 1999; **122**: 649–655.

86. Pepe G, Bertini E, Bonaldo P, *et al*. Bethlem myopathy (BETHLEM) and Ullrich scleroatonic muscular dystrophy: 100th ENMC International Workshop, Naarden, the Netherlands, 2001. *Neuromuscul Disord* 2002; **12**: 984–993.

87. Jobsis GJ, Bolhuis PA, Boers JM, *et al*. Genetic localization of Bethlem myopathy. *Neurology* 1996; **46**: 779–782.

88. Jobsis GJ, Keizers H, Vreijling JP, *et al*. Type VI collagen mutations in Bethlem myopathy, an autosomal dominant myopathy with contractures. *Nat Genet* 1996; **14**: 113–115.

89. Speer MC, Tandan R, Rao PN, *et al*. Evidence for locus heterogeneity in the Bethlem myopathy and linkage to 2q37. *Hum Mol Genet* 1996; **5**: 1043–1046.

90. Lamande SR, Bateman JF, Hutchison W, *et al*. Reduced collagen VI causes Bethlem myopathy: a heterozygous COL6A1 nonsense mutation results in mRNA decay and functional haploinsufficiency. *Hum Mol Genet* 1998; **7**: 981–989.

91. Pan TC, Zhang RZ, Pericak-Vance MA, *et al*. Missense mutation in a von Willebrand factor type A domain of the alpha 3(VI) collagen gene (COL6A3) in a family with Bethlem myopathy. *Hum Mol Genet* 1998; **7**: 807–812.

92. Pepe G, Bertini E, Giusti B, *et al*. A novel de novo mutation in the triple helix of the COL6A3 gene in a two-generation Italian family affected by Bethlem myopathy. A diagnostic approach in the mutations' screening of type VI collagen. *Neuromuscul Disord* 1999; **9**: 264–271.

93. Pepe G, Giusti B, Bertini E, *et al*. A heterozygous splice site mutation in COL6A1 leading to an in-frame deletion of the alpha1(VI) collagen chain in an Italian family affected by Bethlem myopathy. *Biochem Biophys Res Commun* 1999; **258**: 802–807.

94. Haq RU, Speer MC, Chu ML, Tandan R. Respiratory muscle involvement in Bethlem myopathy. *Neurology* 1999; **52**: 174–176.

95. Mercuri E, Lampe A, Allsop J, *et al*. Muscle MRI in Ullrich congenital muscular dystrophy and Bethlem myopathy. *Neuromuscul Disord* 2005; **15**: 303–310.

96. Hicks D, Lampe AK, Barresi R, *et al*. A refined diagnostic algorithm for Bethlem myopathy. *Neurology* 2008; **70**: 1192–1199.

97. Merlini L, Villanova M, Sabatelli P, Malandrini A, Maraldi NM. Decreased expression of laminin beta 1 in chromosome 21-linked Bethlem myopathy. *Neuromuscul Disord* 1999; **9**: 326–329.

98. Hauser MA, Horrigan SK, Salmikangas P, *et al*. Myotilin is mutated in limb girdle muscular dystrophy 1A. *Hum Mol Genet* 2000; **9**: 2141–2147.

99. Hauser MA, Conde CB, Kowaljow V, *et al*. Myotilin mutation found in second pedigree with LGMD1A. *Am J Hum Genet* 2002; **71**: 1428–1432.

100. Selcen D, Engel AG. Mutations in myotilin cause myofibrillar myopathy. *Neurology* 2004; **62**: 1363–1371.

101. Selcen D, Ohno K, Engel AG. Myofibrillar myopathy: clinical, morphological and genetic studies in 63 patients. *Brain* 2004; **127**: 439–451.

102. Olive M, Goldfarb LG, Shatunov A, Fischer D, Ferrer I. Myotilinopathy: refining the clinical and myopathological phenotype. *Brain* 2005; **128**: 2315–2326.

103. Fernandez C, Figarella-Branger D, Meyronet D, *et al*. Electron microscopy in neuromuscular disorders. *Ultrastruct Pathol* 2005; **29**: 437–450.

104. Ben Yaou R, Muchir A, Arimura T, *et al*. Genetics of laminopathies. *Novartis Found Symp* 2005; **264**: 81–90; discussion 90–97, 227–230.

105. van Berlo JH, de Voogt WG, van der Kooi AJ, *et al*. Meta-analysis of clinical characteristics of 299 carriers of LMNA gene mutations: do lamin A/C mutations portend a high risk of sudden death? *J Mol Med* 2005; **83**: 79–83.

106. Meune C, Van Berlo JH, Anselme F, *et al*. Primary prevention of sudden death in patients with lamin A/C gene mutations. *N Engl J Med* 2006; **354**: 209–210.

107. Minetti C, Sotgia F, Bruno C, *et al*. Mutations in the caveolin-3 gene cause autosomal dominant limb-girdle muscular dystrophy. *Nat Genet* 1998; **18**: 365–368.

108. Galbiati F, Razani B, Lisanti MP. Caveolae and caveolin-3 in muscular dystrophy. *Trends Mol Med* 2001; 7: 435–441.

109. Fischer D, Schroers A, Blümcke I, *et al*. Consequences of a novel caveolin-3 mutation in a large German family. *Ann Neurol* 2003; **53**: 233–241.

110. Woodman SE, Sotgia F, Galbiati F, Minetti C, Lisanti MP. Caveolinopathies: mutations in caveolin-3 cause four distinct autosomal dominant muscle diseases. *Neurology* 2004; **62**: 538–543.

111. Dabby R, Sadeh M, Herman O, *et al.* Asymptomatic or minimally symptomatic hyperCKemia: histopathologic correlates. *Isr Med Assoc J* 2006; **8**: 110–113.

112. Hayashi T, Arimura T, Ueda K, *et al.* Identification and functional analysis of a caveolin-3 mutation associated with familial hypertrophic cardiomyopathy.

Biochem Biophys Res Commun 2004; **313**: 178–184.

113. Catteruccia M, Sanna T, Santorelli FM, *et al.* Rippling muscle disease and cardiomyopathy associated with a mutation in the CAV3 gene. *Neuromuscul Disord* 2009; **19**: 779–783.

114. Guyant-Marechal L, Laquerriere A, Duyckaerts C, *et al.* Valosin-containing protein gene mutations: clinical and neuropathologic features. *Neurology* 2006; **67**: 644–651.

115. Mehta SG, Watts GD, McGillivray B, *et al.* Manifestations in a family

with autosomal dominant bone fragility and limb-girdle myopathy. *Am J Med Genet A* 2006; **140**: 322–330.

116. Kumar KR, Needham M, Mina K, *et al.* Two Australian families with inclusion-body myopathy, Paget's disease of bone and frontotemporal dementia: novel clinical and genetic findings. *Neuromuscul Disord* 2010; **20**: 330–334.

117. Norwood FL, Harling C, Chinnery PF, *et al.* Prevalence of genetic muscle disease in Northern England: in-depth analysis of a muscle clinic population. *Brain* 2009; **132**: 3175–3186.

Charcot–Marie–Tooth diseases

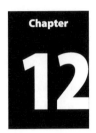

Odile Dubourg, Alexis Brice, and Eric LeGuern

Introduction

Charcot–Marie–Tooth (CMT) diseases constitute a clinically and genetically heterogeneous group of motor and sensory neuropathies. They represent the most common inherited peripheral neuropathies and have a prevalence of about 1 per 2500. They are clinically characterized by atrophy and weakness of the distal limbs. Tendon reflexes are diminished or abolished. Sensory deficit is present in the distal limbs, involving the different sensory modalities. Skeletal deformities such as pes cavus and scoliosis

are frequently observed (Figure 12.1). Disease onset is generally in childhood or adolescence but may occur later in life. In the vast majority of cases, the disease course is slowly progressive and does not affect life-span. However, functional disability is highly variable from one individual to another, even within the same family. The current classification is based on the mode of inheritance and electrophysiological criteria, and whenever possible, on the responsible gene. Long before the advent of molecular genetics, genetic heterogeneity was suspected by observing the segregation

(a)

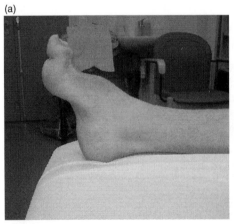

(b)

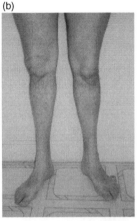

(c)

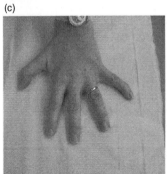

(d)

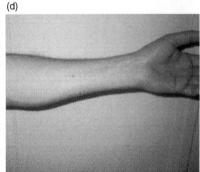

Figure 12.1. (a)–(d), clinical characteristics of Charcot–Marie–Tooth disease.

of the disease in pedigrees [1]. Indeed, the mode of inheritance may be autosomal dominant, autosomal recessive, or X-linked. Dominant forms are more frequent in Western countries, whereas autosomal recessive inheritance is observed mainly in North Africa and the Middle East, where it is a result of the high percentage of consanguineous marriages. Today, after more than 15 years of extensive studies in molecular genetics, nearly 30 responsible genes have been identified and others remain to be determined, making CMT a model of genetic heterogeneity. Moreover, at a very early stage, authors defined at least two different pathological processes, demyelinating and axonal, on the basis of histological examination of nerve biopsies. Electroneuromyographic examination also enables the demyelinating forms to be distinguished from the axonal forms. Because axonal loss is often very severe in the distal lower limbs, the motor nerve conduction velocity (MNCV) of the median nerve (in normal subjects, equal to or above 48 m/s) is generally taken as the reference value. Depending on the authors, the cutoff value for median MNCV that distinguishes between demyelinating and axonal CMT is reported to be either 30 or 38 m/s [2,3]. Most authors now recognize the existence of intermediate forms of CMT. Currently, there is no consensus on the MNCV range for intermediate CMT, but values between 30 and 40 m/s are generally accepted. In our center, we discriminate three ranges of MNCVs: (1) demyelinating CMT with median MNCVs below 30 m/s; (2) intermediate CMT with median MNCVs between 30 and 40 m/s; (3) axonal CMT with median MNCVs above 40 m/s. Owing to the increasing complexity of the classification, rational diagnostic approaches must be established in order to perform accurate molecular testing. These approaches are quite different according to the mode of transmission. The purpose of this chapter is to give an overview of the different forms of CMT and some practical guidelines on the diagnostic approach.

The nomenclature for the different forms of CMT is complex, because of the great genetic heterogeneity of these diseases and because it developed as the loci and genes were discovered. Globally, the autosomal dominant forms of demyelinating CMT are termed CMT1 and the autosomal dominant forms of axonal CMT are known as CMT2, with a letter corresponding to the locus (A, B, C, D, etc.). Autosomal recessive forms of demyelinating CMT are designated CMT4. The nomenclature for the axonal forms has not yet been codified. Both AR (autosomal recessive)-CMT2 and CMT2 are used, although the latter can be confused with autosomal dominant axonal CMT. CMT3, which corresponds to Dejerine–Sottas syndrome, was originally described in two siblings with a very severe phenotype with two non-affected parents, suggesting an autosomal recessive mode of inheritance. For this reason, many sporadic cases with severe phenotypes were also classified as CMT3, but electrophysiological studies have demonstrated that a large proportion of these patients had autosomal dominant CMT and that the asymptomatic parent had low conduction velocities and was found to carry the mutation. Therefore, CMT3 no longer exists in the classification.

Dominant forms of Charcot–Marie–Tooth disease

The dominant forms of CMT are the most frequent in Western populations. In a study of 270 CMT families examined at the Salpêtrière Hospital between 1991 and 1997, we found that 53% had dominant transmission, either autosomal dominant or X-linked dominant, compared to only 4% with demonstrated autosomal recessive mode of inheritance (at least two affected siblings with clinically and electrophysiologically unaffected parents, or a patient with related and clinically and electrophysiologically healthy parents). In addition, we observed a high frequency (35%) of isolated cases, without any obvious familial history, whatever the range of median MNCVs [4]. Purely motor forms, the so-called spinal CMT, were encountered in 7% of the families and CMT with involvement of the central nervous system were found in 1.5% of the families. Because these rare phenotypes are also very heterogeneous, they will not be dealt with in this chapter. In a study by Skre (1974) [5] in a western Norway population, autosomal recessive forms were far less frequent (1.4 per 100 000) than autosomal dominant forms (36 per 100 000). Autosomal dominant forms are either demyelinating (CMT1), intermediate, or axonal (CMT2). In the classification, a letter is added to indicate the different loci (CMT1A, CMT1B, etc.), according to the order in which they were identified. The two most frequent dominant forms are CMT1A, associated with a duplication of the chromosomal 17p11.2 region, and CMTX, owing to GJB1 mutations, the latter corresponding chiefly to an intermediate form of CMT.

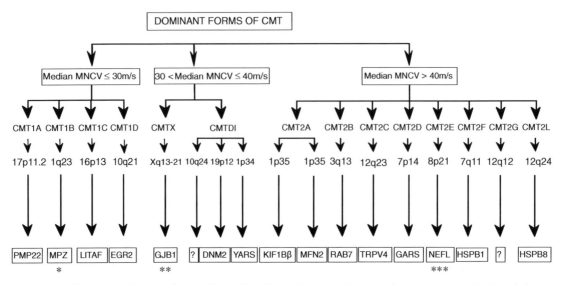

Figure 12.2. Classification of dominant forms of Charcot–Marie–Tooth disease according to median motor nerve conduction velocity. *MPZ; **GJB1; ***NEFL. Gene mutations are also encountered in CMT2, CMT1 and CMT2, and CMT1, respectively. CMT, Charcot–Marie–Tooth disease; MNCV, motor nerve conduction velocity.

Figure 12.2 summarizes the different loci and genes responsible for dominant forms of CMT.

Autosomal dominant forms of demyelinating Charcot–Marie–Tooth disease (CMT1)

CMT1 owing to the duplication of the 17p11.2 region (CMT1A)

CMT1A is the most frequent form of the disease and accounts for approximately 30% of all CMT and 70% of CMT1 cases. The gene responsible for CMT1A was mapped in 1990 to chromosome 17p11.2 [6]. Several studies have demonstrated that CMT1A is almost always associated with a 1.5 Mb duplication of this region [7,8], owing to unequal recombination between two homologous flanking sequences named CMT1A-REP [9,10] (Figure 12.3). This genomic region contains the *PMP22* gene, which encodes peripheral myelin protein 22 (PMP22), a transmembrane glycoprotein accounting for 5% of the proteins of the peripheral nervous system [11,12]. It is composed of 160 amino acids with four membrane domains. Its role is not yet fully understood. Point mutations in the same gene also cause a CMT1A phenotype, but they are very rare. A distinct neuropathy, the hereditary neuropathy with liability to

pressure palsies, is a result of a deletion of the 1.5 Mb region that is duplicated in CMT1A [13]. The phenotype in CMT1A patients results from a gene dosage effect owing to the presence of three copies of the *PMP22* gene instead of two [14]. In a study of 119 CMT1A patients, Birouk *et al.* (1997) [15] defined the clinical and electrophysiological phenotype associated with this rearrangement. Age at onset is highly variable, ranging from infancy to the eighth decade of life. However, 70% of patients develop the first symptoms before the age of 20 years. The predominant clinical signs are muscle weakness and wasting in the distal lower limbs. Pes cavus and lower limb areflexia are nearly always observed. Functional disability is variable from one individual to another, but loss of the ability to walk is rare in CMT1A. In the study by Birouk *et al.* (1997) [15], 96% of the patients were able to walk at the time of examination and 25% of duplication carriers were asymptomatic. The factors responsible for this phenotypical variability are not yet known, but a role of modulating genes and environmental factors is suspected. Electroneuromyographic testing shows a motor and sensory demyelinating neuropathy, characterized by a diffuse and homogeneous slowing of nerve conduction. Classically, conduction blocks or temporal dispersion are not observed in CMT1A,

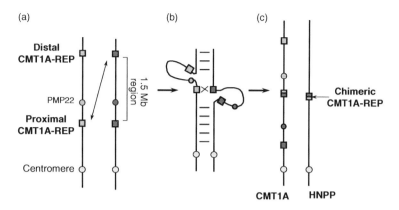

Figure 12.3. Unequal recombinations between chromosome 17 homologs leading to 17p11.2 rearrangements. CMT1A, in most cases, is a result of a tandem duplication of a 1.5 Mb region in 17p11.2 containing the peripheral myelin protein 22 gene (*PMP22*) [7,8]. The phenotype seems to result from dosage of the *PMP22* gene. This hypothesis was supported by the existence of another sensory and motor inherited neuropathy, the hereditary neuropathy with liability to pressure palsies (HNPP), which is caused by a deletion of the same 1.5 Mb region [13,161]. HNPP is also an autosomal dominant peripheral neuropathy characterized by variously located recurrent peripheral nerve palsies or sensory loss, often precipitated by minor trauma or compression. It was hypothesized that unequal crossing-over would generate both duplications and deletions of the 1.5 Mb region in 17p11.2. The identification of two highly homologous sequences of 24 kb flanking the 1.5 Mb CMT1A/HNPP monomer unit, the CMT1A-REPs, supported this hypothesis. At the prophase of the first division of meiosis, there is a misalignment (a) between the proximal CMT1A-REP of one homolog 17 with the distal CMT1A-REP of the other homolog 17, leading to the tetrad structure presented in (b). If a physiological recombination occurred between these two REPs (indicated by a cross in [b]), it would result in the formation of both a chromosome 17 with a duplication and another 17 with the deletion of the same 1.5 Mb region (c). If fertilization takes place with the gamete with either the duplicated or the deleted chromosome 17, the fetus will be affected by CMT1A or HNPP, respectively. Reiter *et al.* (1998) [9] and Lopes *et al.* (1998) [10] reported that about 70 cross-over breakpoints occurred in a 1.7 kb region of the CMT1A-REPs in both CMT1A and HNPP patients.

in contrast to chronic inflammatory demyelinating polyneuropathy (CIDP), an acquired dysimmune demyelinating polyneuropathy [16]. Sensory nerve action potential amplitudes are profoundly reduced or even abolished. These findings are identical in asymptomatic carriers, making median MNCV a reliable tool for screening at-risk individuals. Motor nerve CVs are diminished early, from the age of two years, and remain unchanged throughout the patient's life [17,18]. Motor nerve CVs vary among affected individuals in the same family [15]. Although MNCVs are inferior or equal to 30 m/s in most patients, intermediate MNCVs are observed in rare cases [15,19]. Secondary axonal loss is always observed and is correlated with neurological dysfunction and disease progression [20]. Nerve biopsy, which is no longer used for the diagnosis of CMT1A as the 17p11.2 duplication is routinely detected in molecular diagnosis laboratories using various molecular tools (Figure 12.3), shows a characteristic demyelinating neuropathy with the presence of onion bulb formations, associated with a secondary loss of myelinated fibers and especially of large diameter fibers [21].

Other subtypes of CMT1

CMT1 owing to mutations in *PMP22* (CMT1A)

Some rare missense mutations in one of the four coding exons of the *PMP22* gene have been associated with CMT1A and seem to cause a more severe phenotype than the 17p11.2 duplication, called Dejerine–Sottas disease (DSD) or congenital hypomyelinating neuropathy (CHN) [22]. Dejerine–Sottas disease corresponds to a severe hypertrophic neuropathy of early onset (before three years of age) with delayed motor milestones, very slowed MNCVs, and evidence of severe hypomyelination on nerve biopsy. Congenital hypomyelinating neuropathy is characterized by hypotonia and muscle weakness at birth, a severe course, very slowed or unobtainable MNCVs, and an absence or marked reduction of myelin on nerve biopsy. The missense mutation frequency of *PMP22* varies from 2% in a Russian CMT population to 5% in a Japanese CMT population [23,24].

CMT1 owing to mutations in *MPZ* (CMT1B)

Mutations in the *MPZ* (myelin protein zero) gene, encoding a major protein of the compact myelin, have been identified in demyelinating CMT with variable severity. MPZ protein is the most abundant protein (50%) in the myelin of peripheral nerve with an extracellular fold similar to immunoglobulin variable chain, and a transmembrane and cytoplasmic domain. The extracellular domains interact with each other in apposing myelin sheaths in order to maintain myelin compaction. The *MPZ* gene, which is localized to chromosome 1q22–q23, contains six coding exons. More than 60 mutations have been described, which are most commonly located in exons 2 and 3, encoding the immunoglobulin-like extracellular domain. The frequency of *MPZ* gene mutations is about 3%–4% in some reported series [23,25], but reached 9% of CMT in a Japanese population [24]. The clinical phenotype ranges from CHN to CMT1B [26,27]. Nerve pathology differs according to the site of the mutation, and may show features of uncompacted myelin or focal folding and thickening of myelin [28,29].

CMT1 owing to mutations in *LITAF/SIMPLE* (CMT1C)

Street *et al.* (2003) [30] identified the gene responsible for CMT1C, called *LITAF* (lipopolysaccharide-induced tumor necrosis factor-α)/*SIMPLE* (small integral membrane protein of lysosome/late endosome). The LITAF protein is a stimulator of monocytes and macrophages, causing secretion of tumor necrosis factor-α, and may play a role in protein degradation pathways. In a study of 12 non-duplicated CMTI patients from Chinese ancestry, no mutation was found in the *LITAF* gene, whereas a study in a French population found six families with missense mutations in the *LITAF* gene among a cohort of 968 unrelated dominant demyelinating CMT cases (0.6%) [31,32]. These data suggest that CMT1C is a rare cause of CMT1. The phenotype is similar to that of CMT1A. Electrophysiological studies show a diffuse demyelinating neuropathy with, in some patients, temporal dispersion and irregularity of nerve conduction slowing [30,33].

CMT1 owing to mutations in *EGR2* (CMT1D)

Mutations in the *EGR2* gene (early growth response 2 gene), a key factor for myelination, are responsible for CMT1D [34]. Very few mutations have been reported to date, and CMT1D appears to represent less than 1% of CMT cases in large cohorts [24,25]. EGR2 is a transcription factor with zinc fingers, which binds DNA regulatory domains of target genes. It is expressed at a high level early in the myelination of the peripheral nervous system and is mainly implicated in the regulation of the expression of the myelin genes, such as *MPZ*, *PMP22*, and *GJB1*. *EGR2* gene mutations are associated with a large spectrum of CMT phenotypes, ranging from CHN to late-onset CMT1 [35,36]. They may be transmitted in an autosomal dominant or autosomal recessive fashion [34].

CMT1 owing to mutations in *NEFL* (CMT1F)

A missense mutation in the neurofilament light chain (*NEFL*) gene at chromosome 8p21 was reported initially in a large Russian family diagnosed with CMT2, and the corresponding locus was called CMT2E [37]. This gene encodes a 62 kDa protein of the axonal cytoskeleton. In two subsequent papers, however, *NEFL* gene mutations were reported in families that could be classified as CMT1 on the basis of the electrophysiological examination [38,39]. Jordanova *et al.* (2003) [39] screened a cohort of 323 CMT patients and found six missense mutations, representing a frequency of 2%. They studied the clinical and electrophysiological phenotype in nine patients. They showed that the age at onset was before 13 years in all patients, and in early infancy (before five years) in four of them, and was sometimes associated with delayed motor milestones. The phenotype was that of a severe CMT, as in the Belgian family reported by De Jonghe *et al.* (2001) [38].

X-linked Charcot–Marie–Tooth disease (CMTX) owing to mutations in the *GJB1* gene

X-linked CMT is the second most common form of CMT and accounts for approximately 10% of all CMT cases [40]. It is caused by mutations in the second exon of the *GJB1* gene, encoding a gap junction protein localized in non-compact myelin, such as paranodal loops and Schmidt–Lantermann incisures [41]. GJB1 forms reflexive intracellular channels in Schwann cells and provides a radial pathway traversing the myelin sheath and connecting the perinuclear to the adaxonal cytoplasmic region [42]. More than 200 mutations of the *GJB1* gene have been described. The mutational type is variable, and includes missense, nonsense, and frameshift mutations and even deletion of the entire coding sequence [43]. X-linked CMT is characterized genetically by the absence of father-to-son transmission in pedigrees and clinically by a more severe disease course in men than in women. The mean age at onset in both genders is between 10 and 20 years. The clinical phenotype is similar to that of CMT1A. Interestingly, involvement of intrinsic hand muscles is often severe and sometimes inaugural [44]. In a few patients, additional features are observed, such as deafness or white matter abnormalities in the central nervous system [45–49]. Electroneuromyographic examination shows that MNCVs are more reduced in men than in women [40]. Indeed, in a series of 93 CMTX patients, we found that MNCVs were between 20 m/s and 40 m/s in 90% of men, whereas they were 40 m/s and above in 80% of women. Moreover, 75% of men had intermediate MNCVs (intermediate CMT) [43]. Mutations in GJB1 are identified in more than 40% of families where the index case presents intermediate MNCVs. Birouk et al. (1998) [50] found that the neuropathy in CMTX was mostly owing to an axonal process. In contrast, later observations showed that some patients may have merely a demyelinating neuropathy, similar to that observed in CIDP. Thus, a heterogeneity of MNCVs among nerve trunks, occasional conduction blocks, and temporal dispersion have been described [51,52]. Moreover, we showed that motor nerve conduction was heterogeneous between nerves in females and postulated that this finding reflected the process of chromosome X lyonization [43]. These observations brought controversy to the dogma of the uniformity of the demyelinating process in hereditary neuropathy, which remains true for CMT1A [53]. Hahn et al. (2001) [54], in a series of 13 nerve biopsies from CMTX patients, demonstrated a loss of myelinated fibers and the presence of clusters of regeneration, reflecting an axonal process, subtle abnormalities of myelin sheaths consisting of a widening of Schmidt–Lantermann incisures and nodes of Ranvier, and abnormalities reflecting the axon–Schwann cell interaction failure with widening of the adaxonal space and axonal cytoskeleton modifications. Identical aspects are observed in GJB1 knockout mice [55]. Nerve biopsy, however, is no longer useful for the diagnosis of CMTX.

Autosomal dominant forms of axonal Charcot–Marie–Tooth disease (CMT2)

CMT2 families represent 15% of our CMT families with median MNCV superior or equal to 40 m/s [4]. To date, eight responsible genes and one additional locus have been identified [37,55–65]. Table 12.1 summarizes the main phenotypical features of the different CMT2 subtypes, in terms of age at onset, disease course, topography of weakness, and associated signs.

CMT2A

CMT2A was initially mapped to chromosome 1p35–p36 and was subsequently associated with a missense mutation in the KIF1Bβ (kinesin family member 1Bβ) gene in a single Japanese family [56]. KIF1Bβ protein is a member of the kinesin superfamily and is implicated in the anterograde transport of synaptic vesicle precursors. Bissar-Tadmouri et al. (2004) [66] reported the absence of the KIF1Bβ mutation in a large Turkish family with linkage to CMT2A, which suggested the involvement of another gene at this locus. Concurrently, Zuchner et al. (2004) [57] reported that mutations in the MFN2 (mitochondrial GTPase mitofusin 2) gene, encoding a mitochondrial transmembrane GTPase that regulates the mitochondrial network architecture by fusion of mitochondria, were responsible for the phenotype in seven CMT2 families with diverse ethnic backgrounds. The authors emphasized that MFN2 gene mutations could represent a frequent cause of CMT2. This was confirmed by other studies. Kijima et al. (2004) [67] reported that they found seven MFN2 gene mutations in seven (8.6%) unrelated patients out of a subset of 81 patients with axonal or unclassified CMT. Verhoeven et al. (2006) [68] performed a large study in 323 families and isolated patients with distinct CMT phenotypes, including 249 CMT2 patients. They found mutations in the MFN2 gene in 29 patients, 28 with a CMT2 (11%) and one with an intermediate CMT. The frequency of MFN2 gene mutations increased to 33% when a familial history of CMT2 was present. Age at onset in this large cohort was between 1 and 45 years (mean: 8 years). The phenotype was rather severe, as 33% of patients with early onset (before five years of age) became wheelchair bound. The classical CMT phenotype was observed in these patients, but optic atrophy with subacute onset was present in some of them. This particular feature has also been reported in six additional families with MFN2 gene mutations [69]. Central nervous system involvement has been reported in some families, either clinically with the presence of pyramidal signs, or radiologically with the presence of periventricular and subcortical hyperintense lesions on brain MRI [70,71]. To date,

Table 12.1. Main characteristics of autosomal dominant Charcot–Marie–Tooth disease or CMT2

Locus Gene	Reference	Origin	Age at onset	Clinical characteristics	Course	Associated signs
CMT2A *KIF1B-β*	Zhao et al. (2001) [56]	Japan	1–50 years	Distal limbs LL>UL Anterior and posterior tibial muscles	Variable, may be severe	
CMT2A *MFN2*	Zuchner et al. (2004) [57]	Ubiquitous	1–62 years	Distal limbs LL>UL	Severe: onset <10 years, benign to moderate, onset >10 years	Optic atrophy, pyramidal signs, hearing loss
CMT2B *RAB7*	Verhoeven et al. (2003) [58]	Austria, Scotland, Belgium, United States	2nd and 3rd decade	Distal limbs LL>UL No dysautonomia	Variable, may be severe	Ulcers, infections, limb amputations
CMT2C *TRPV4* (allelic to congenital dSMA and scapuloperoneal SMA)	Auer-Grumbach et al. (2010) [59] Deng et al. (2010) [60] Landouré et al. (2010) [61]	Holland, New England, United States	2–57 years	Distal limbs LL>UL	May be severe	Vocal cords paresis Diaphragm and intercostal muscle weakness
CMT2D (allelic to dHMN type V) *GARS*	Antonellis et al. (2003) [62]	United States, Bulgaria, Mongolia, Algeria	16–30 years	Inaugural and predominant in UL	Slow	
CMT2E *NEFL*	Mersiyanova et al. (2000) [37]	Russia, Slovenia, Italy, Austria	1st to 5th decade	Distal limbs LL>UL	Slow	Hearing loss
CMT2F *HSPB1*	Evgarov et al. (2004) [63]	England, India, Pakistan, Russia, Belgium	6–54 years	Distal limbs LL>UL	Slow, may be severe	
CMT2G	Nelis et al. (2004) [64]	Spain	9–76 years	Distal limbs LL>UL	Slow	
CMT2L *HSPB8* (allelic to dHMN type II)	Tang et al. (2004b) [65]	China	15–33 years	Distal limbs LL>UL	Slow	

dSMA, distal spinal muscular atrophy; dHMN, distal hereditary motor neuropathy; LL, lower limbs; UL, upper limbs.

no other family has been reported with a mutation in the *KIF1Bβ* gene.

CMT2B

CMT2B was assigned to chromosome 3q13–q22 before the responsible gene, *RAB7*, encoding a small GTP-ase late endosomal protein, was identified by Verhoeven *et al.* (2003) [58]. CMT2B is clinically characterized by marked distal weakness and wasting, and a high frequency of foot ulcers, infections, and toe amputations because of recurrent infections [72,73]. Sensory loss of all modalities is observed. This particular phenotype may place CMT2B in the group of ulcero-mutilating neuropathies, with hereditary sensitive and dysautonomic neuropathy type 1 (HSAN type 1) [74], owing to mutations within the *SPTLC1* gene [75,76]. Verhoeven *et al.* (2003) [58] identified two missense mutations in six families from diverse geographical origins. Three of these CMT2B families were selected among a set of 24 unrelated families with a phenotype of ulcero-mutilating neuropathy, showing that *RAB7* gene mutations account for a significant fraction of CMT2 families with this phenotype, but that this group is genetically heterogeneous.

CMT2C

CMT2C was mapped to 12q23–24 in a large American family of English and Scottish ethnicity by Klein *et al.* (2003) [77]. CMT2C is a rare phenotype characterized by distal motor weakness and sensory loss, vocal cord paresis and, sometimes, diaphragmatic and intercostal muscle involvement. Age at onset and disease severity are variable among affected individuals within the same family [78]. Four missense mutations in the *TRPV4* gene have been identified in families with different phenotypes, including CMT2C, congenital distal spinal muscular atrophy (SMA), and scapuloperoneal SMA [59–61]. The gene encodes the transient receptor potential cation channel, subfamily V, member 4 protein. Mutations lie within the intracellular N-terminal ankyrin domain and alter calcium homeostasis in transfected cell lines.

CMT2D

CMT2D was first mapped to chromosome 7p in a large North American family [79], and is allelic to distal hereditary neuropathy type V (d-HMN type V). These disorders share a phenotype characterized by an inaugural and predominantly distal upper limb involvement that affects the thenar and interosseous muscles. The difference between them lies in the absence of clinical and electrophysiological sensory loss in d-HMN type V. Antonellis *et al.* (2003) [62] identified four missense mutations in the glycyl tRNA synthetase (*GARS*) gene in five families with either CMT2D or d-HMN type V.

CMT2E

As stated previously, CMT2E is a result of a mutation in the *NEFL* gene [37]. These authors did not find other *NEFL* gene mutations in 20 unrelated CMT2 patients or in 26 others with an undetermined form of CMT, which suggests that the *NEFL* gene mutation is a rare cause of CMT. In a study of four individuals from a three-generational family, Zuchner *et al.* (2004) [80] found a variable age at onset ranging from early infancy to the fifth decade of life. The phenotype was moderate, with selective weakness and atrophy in the distal lower limbs and a slowly progressive course. Median MNCVs were normal in all individuals. Two sural nerve biopsies showed a reduction of large myelinated axons and several clusters of regenerated myelinated fibers, reflecting an axonal process. In addition, onion bulb formations were observed indicating previous demyelination and remyelination. These findings led the authors to postulate that the primary axonal lesions were followed by a secondary process of demyelination.

CMT2F, 2G, and 2L

CMT2F was mapped to 7q11–q21 in a Russian family [81]. Subsequently, a missense mutation in the gene encoding the 27 kDa small heat-shock protein B1 (*HSPB1*) was reported in the same family by Evgarov *et al.* (2004) [63]. The authors identified four additional mutations in four families with distal HMN and in one individual with CMT2 in a panel of 416 families (1.2%). CMT2G was mapped to chromosome 12q12–q13.3 by Nelis *et al.* (2004) [64], but the disease-causing gene has not yet been identified. CMT2L was mapped to chromosome 12q24–qter in a Chinese family and the responsible mutation was then identified in the *HSPB8* (heat-shock 22 kDa protein 8) gene [65,82]. The same gene is mutated in distal hereditary motor neuropathy type II (dHMN type 2) [83].

CMT2 caused by *MPZ* gene mutations (CMT2I and CMT2J)

There have been numerous reports of predominantly axonal neuropathy associated with *MPZ* gene mutations [84–92]. These publications stressed the distinct clinical features associated with these MPZ mutations: late onset neuropathy, slow progression and, in some patients, deafness. Patients with the Thr124Met mutation have a late onset neuropathy starting in the fourth or fifth decade of life, marked sensory abnormalities and, in some cases, hearing loss and pupillary abnormalities [85]. MNCVs showed variable slowing and could be assigned to the intermediate or axonal range. Senderek *et al.* (2000) [89] reported a frequency of *MPZ* gene mutations of 6% in a cohort of 49 CMT2 patients. Shy *et al.* (2004) [93] reviewed the data of 64 patients with *MPZ* gene mutations reported in the literature, to which they added the data of 13 of their own patients. They showed that most individuals with an *MPZ* gene mutation develop one of the two phenotypes: an early onset neuropathy (infancy) with very slowed MNCVs and predominant dysmyelination on nerve biopsy, or a late-onset neuropathy (adult) with minimally or moderately slowed MNCVs and a predominant axonal neuropathy on nerve biopsy.

CMT2K

Autosomal dominant axonal CMT associated with a heterozygous mutation in the *GDAP1* gene has been reported in few families [94,95]. The onset is in the second or third decade of life, the phenotype is much milder than that observed in patients with recessive *GDAP1* gene mutations, and the progression is slow.

Autosomal dominant forms of intermediate Charcot–Marie–Tooth disease

Three loci on chromosome 10q24.1–q25.1 (CMTDIA) [96], 19p12–p13.2 (CMTDIB) [97], and 1p34–p35 (CMTDIC) [98] were identified in families with autosomal dominant intermediate CMT. Mutations in the *DNM2* gene encoding dynamin-2 were found in several families with CMTDIB [99]. Dynamin-2 is a GTPase implicated in endocytosis and cell motility, composed of three domains: a pleckstrin homology (PH), a middle, and a proline-rich domain. CMT-related mutations in dynamin-2 are located mostly in the PH domain, but two mutations have also been described in the middle and proline-rich domains [100]. Patients present with a classical CMT phenotype, which is mild to moderately severe. In two pedigrees with two different mutations affecting the lys558 residue, the disease cosegregated with neutropenia. In addition, early onset cataract was observed in one of the six families described by Claeys *et al.* (2009) [100]. MNCVs may range from intermediate to normal values, indicating that patients with axonal CMT without mutations in more common genes should have investigations for DNM2 mutations [101]. Two heterozygous missense mutations (G41R and E196K) and one *de novo* deletion (153–156delVKQV) in the tyrosyl-tRNA synthetase (*YARS*) gene were identified in three families with CMTDIC. Mutated proteins have a partial loss of aminoacylation activity in yeast. The specific distribution of YARS in axonal termini is significantly reduced in differentiating primary motor neuron and neuroblastoma cultures [102].

Autosomal recessive forms of Charcot–Marie–Tooth disease

Pedigrees with a proven autosomal recessive form of CMT account for only 4% of the families in our CMT population. In contrast, in communities with a high percentage of consanguineous marriages, autosomal recessive CMT (AR-CMT) is likely to account for 30%–50% of all CMT cases [103]. It should be noted that patients in western countries who are affected by autosomal recessive disease often appear as isolated cases because of the small number of siblings. Autosomal recessive CMT forms are demyelinating or axonal, or even intermediate, as in dominant forms, but are generally distinguished by an earlier onset and a more severe disease course. Numerous genes have been identified, mostly in inbred families originating from North Africa or the Middle East. Figure 12.4 summarizes the different loci and genes identified in AR-CMT. All mutations cause a loss of function, many of them leading to a truncated protein (nonsense, frameshift, deletions, etc.). In many patients, owing to the severity of the secondary axonal loss, electroneuromyographic examination is often incomplete or does not allow MNCVs to be measured. In such cases, a nerve biopsy may be needed to determine the nature of the neuropathy – axonal or demyelinating – and, if demyelinating, the pattern of myelin abnormalities may help to guide the molecular

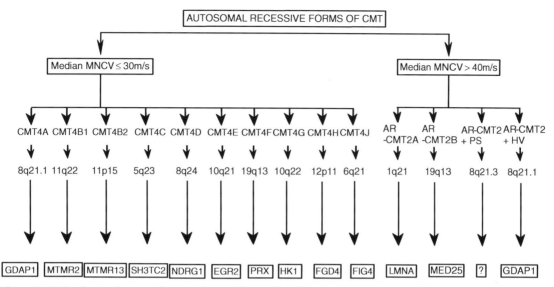

Figure 12.4. Classification of autosomal recessive forms of Charcot–Marie–Tooth disease according to median motor nerve conduction velocity. CMT, Charcot–Marie–Tooth disease; MNCV, motor nerve conduction velocity; AR, autosomal recessive; PS, pyramidal signs; HV, hoarse voice.

diagnosis. For this reason, nerve biopsy features will be mentioned for each of the CMT4 subtypes.

Autosomal recessive demyelinating forms of Charcot–Marie–Tooth disease (CMT4)

Most CMT4 subtypes are clinically characterized by an onset in early infancy, sometimes congenital, or with delayed motor milestones. The atrophy and weakness initially involve the distal limbs but may progress to the proximal limbs, especially in the lower limbs, resulting in the loss of ambulation. The involvement of peripheral nerves may be more widespread in CMT4. Thus, vocal cord paresis; bulbar, facial, and diaphragmatic weakness; and sensorineural deafness may sometimes be observed. Some of these associated signs are closely related to a given CMT4 subtype and, therefore, must be carefully investigated in order to guide the molecular diagnosis. Table 12.2 indicates the different CMT4 subtypes in terms of age at onset, disease course, associated signs, MNCV values, and histopathological features.

CMT4A

CMT4A was originally mapped to chromosome 8q21.3 in four Tunisian families displaying a severe phenotype [104], and was subsequently shown to be

a result of mutations in the *GDAP1* gene encoding ganglioside-induced, differentiation-associated protein 1 [105]. GDAP1 is expressed in Schwann cells and the central nervous system and has sequence similarities to glutathione-S-transferase. It is localized on the outer mitochondrial membrane where it may play a role in mitochondrial network dynamics by promoting mitochondrial fission [106,107]. CMT4A is characterized by a severe neuropathy beginning in early childhood (before the age of three years), and rapidly progressive distal (and further proximal) weakness and atrophy of the limbs, leading to an inability to walk in adolescence or early adulthood. Motor nerve CVs range from 25 m/s to 35 m/s. Histopathological features include loss of myelinated fibers, especially those of large diameter axons, hypomyelination, segmental demyelination, and onion bulb formations. The same gene is responsible for autosomal recessive axonal [108–110] as well as intermediate CMT [111]. The locus is also close to that responsible for autosomal recessive CMT with pyramidal signs [112].

CMT4B1

CMT4B1 is associated with mutations in the gene encoding the MTMR2 protein (myotubularin-related protein 2) [113]. This protein is expressed at high

Table 12.2. Main characteristics of autosomal recessive demyelinating Charcot–Marie–Tooth disease or CMT4

Locus Gene	Reference	Origin	Age at onset	Clinical characteristics	Median MNCV	Histopathological features
CMT4A GDAP1	Baxter et al. (2002) [105]	Ubiquitous	<3 years	Distal + proximal limbs, diaphragm	27–35 m/s	Hypomyelination, onion bulbs, loss of myelinated fibers
CMT4B1 MTMR2	Bolino et al. (2000) [113]	Italy, Saudi Arabia, England, India	<4 years	Distal + proximal limbs, facial, bulbar, and diaphragmatic weakness	9–20 m/s	Myelin outfolding, loss of myelinated fibers
CMT4B2 SBF2 MTMR13	Senderek et al. (2003) [120] Azzedine et al. (2003) [121]	Tunisia, Morocco, Turkey, Japan	1st decade	Distal ± proximal, congenital glaucoma	15–30 m/s	Myelin outfolding, loss of myelinated fibers
CMT4C SH3TC2	Senderek et al. (2003c) [124]	Ubiquitous	1st or 2nd decade	Distal ± proximal limbs, severe and early scoliosis, hearing loss, tongue atrophy, facial weakness	4–37 m/s	Basal membrane, onion bulbs, cytoplasmic expansions of Schwann cells, loss of myelinated fibers
CMT4D NDRG1	Kalaydjieva et al. (2000) [129]	Gypsies from Bulgaria, Slovenia, Spain, Italy	<10 years	Distal + proximal limbs, sensorineural deafness, tongue atrophy,	10–20 m/s	Hypomyelination, onion bulbs, myelin decompaction, axonal inclusions, loss of myelinated fibers
CMT4E EGR2	Warner et al. (1998) [34]	United States	Birth	Congenital hypotonia	5–20 m/s	Congenital hypomyelination
CMT4F PRX	Guilbot et al. (2001) [133] Boerkoel et al. (2001) [134]	Libya, United States, northern Europe	<7 years	Distal + proximal limbs	< 5 m/s	Onion bulbs, myelin outfolding, loss of myelinated fibers
CMT4G HK1	Hantke et al. (2009) [141]	Bulgaria, Romania, gypsies from Spain	5–16 years	Distal + proximal limbs	30–35 m/s	Hypomyelination, regenerating clusters
CMT4H FGD4	De Sandre-Giovannoli et al. (2005) [142]	Lebanon, Algeria	<2 years	Distal limbs	<15 m/s	Hypomyelination, onion bulbs, myelin outfolding, loss of myelinated fibers
CMT4J FIG4	Chow et al. (2007) [146]	Caucasus	Childhood or adulthood	Rapidly progressive, asymmetric motor neuron degeneration	2–50 m/s	Loss of myelinated fibers, thinly myelinated axons, onion bulbs

levels in Schwann cells as well as in neurons and is a member of the dual specificity phosphatase superfamily, characterized by a protein/tyrosine phosphatase domain and an SID (SET-interacting domain). The latter interacts with proteins containing a SET (Suvar 3–9, Enhancer-of-zeste, Trithorax) domain that associates with chromatin. MTMR1, another member of the myotubularin family, is responsible for X-linked myotubular myopathy [114]. Disease onset is in early infancy (before the age of four years). Early developmental milestones are normal. The atrophy and weakness initially involve the distal parts of the four limbs and progress toward proximal muscles, resulting in the patient requiring a wheelchair from late childhood or adolescence. Facial, bulbar, and diaphragmatic involvement has been reported in some families [115–117]. Lifespan was shortened in the large Italian family reported by Quattrone et al. (1996) [115], with death occurring in the fourth or fifth decade of life. Motor nerve CVs range from 9 m/s to 20 m/s and are often undetectable in adult patients. Histopathological examination shows irregular folding and redundant loops of myelin, the so-called myelin outfolding, and a secondary axonal loss [118].

CMT4B2

Genetic heterogeneity of CMT4B (i.e. CMT4 with focally folded myelin sheaths) was demonstrated by the absence of linkage to the 11q22.1 locus in Tunisian families, and was subsequently mapped to chromosome 11p15 [119]. This locus has been named CMT4B2. The responsible gene was identified concurrently by two teams in consanguineous families with varying phenotypical features. In the German and Turkish families reported by Senderek et al. (2003) [120], the phenotype was less severe than in CMT4B1 patients. Disease onset was around five years of age and the patients had a severe distal motor and sensory neuropathy, but the proximal muscles were spared and, for two patients, walking was still possible with an aid in the third decade of life. The responsible gene was called SBF2 (SET binding factor 2). In the two families from Tunisia and Morocco reported by Azzedine et al. (2003) [121], the demyelinating motor and sensory neuropathy segregated with a congenital glaucoma. They called the responsible gene MTMR13 (myotubularin-related protein-13) as it clearly belonged to the MTM1-related protein family. The same association has been reported in a Japanese family with an SBF2/MTMR13 gene mutation [122].

Azzedine et al. (2003) [121] postulated that MTMR13 could be involved in both the differentiation of Schwann cells of peripheral nerves during myelination and in the formation and development of the trabeculum meshwork, which permits the outflow of the aqueous humor, both types of cells being derived from the neural crest.

CMT4C

CMT4C was mapped to chromosome 5q23–q33 [123] and was found to be associated with mutations in the KIAA1985 gene [124]. This gene encodes a protein of unknown function containing SH3 and TPR motifs and is expressed in neural tissues, including peripheral nerve. It could represent a relatively common cause of CMT4. This gene was then named SH3TC2. Mutations in the SH3TC2 gene have been found in families of diverse geographic origin: Algeria, France, Germany, Greece, Iran, Italy, the Netherlands, and Turkey [123–126]. The age at walking may be delayed. Disease onset is variable, from the first decade of life to adulthood. The progression of the neuropathy is generally slow, but some patients become wheelchair dependent because of involvement of the proximal lower limbs. The hallmark of CMT2C is the presence of early and severe scoliosis, which is reported to be the presenting sign in the majority of patients [125,127], and may require surgery. Median MNCVs range from 4 m/s to 37 m/s, with a mean of 22 m/s. Nerve biopsies show a loss of myelinated fibers, relatively few and small classical onion bulbs as observed in CMT1A, but also basal membrane onion bulbs, made of concentric Schwann cell lamellae intermingled with single and duplicated basal membranes or concentric basal membranes alone, and multiple cytoplasmic processes of Schwann cells of unmyelinated axons [125,127]. Gabreëls-Festen et al. (1999) [125] considered this combination of morphological features to be unique among demyelinating CMT.

HMSNL or CMT4D

CMT4D was originally designated HMSNL (hereditary motor and sensory neuropathy – Lom) because it was first diagnosed in Bulgarian gypsies from Lom, a small town on the river Danube. It was mapped to chromosome 8q24 [128]. The responsible gene is NDRG1 (N-myc downstream regulated gene 1), which encodes a protein highly expressed in Schwann cells [129]. Disease onset is in the first decade, with delayed walking in some patients. Difficulty in using

177

the hands is noted between 5 and 15 years of age. Distal lower limb involvement is usually severe and may compromise the ability to walk. Tongue atrophy is a frequent finding. Sensorineural deafness generally develops during the second or third decade of life. Brainstem auditory evoked potentials (BAEPs) show an increase in I–V interpeak latency. Nerve conduction studies show a profound and diffuse demyelinating neuropathy with median MNCVs of about 14 m/s [130]. Nerve biopsies show a severe depletion of myelinated fibers, with a complete loss of large diameter fibers, hypomyelination, and multiple poorly developed onion bulbs, which tend to disappear in older individuals [130]. Myelin decompaction and axonal inclusions with curvilinear structures have also been described [131,132].

CMT4E

CMT4E is a result of *EGR2* gene mutations and is discussed in a previous section.

CMT4F

CMT4F is because of mutations within the periaxin gene (*PRX*) [133,134]. It encodes two proteins with PDZ domains, L- and S-periaxin. They are expressed in myelinating Schwann cells. During myelination, L-periaxin is predominantly located at the adaxonal membrane but, once myelination is achieved, it is localized at the abaxonal membrane, Schmidt–Lantermann incisures, and paranodal membranes [135]. Periaxins interact via PDZ domains with the dystroglycan–dystrophin-related protein-2 complex linking the Schwann cell cytoskeleton to the extracellular matrix [136]. Periaxins are thought to be essential for the maintenance of peripheral nerve myelin. The phenotype has been reported as Dejerine–Sottas disease, because the onset is in early infancy and delayed motor milestones are frequently noted [134,137]. However, the disease course can be quite variable, severe in some patients with distal and proximal involvement of the limbs in the first decade or slow in others with predominantly distal sensory signs [137,138]. In a cohort of 66 Japanese demyelinating CMT patients who were negative for the gene mutation causing dominant or X-linked demyelinating CMT, Kijima *et al.* (2004) [138] found three (4.5%) *PRX* gene mutations. Motor nerve CVs are unrecordable or very slowed (<5 m/s) with a marked temporal dispersion of compound muscle action potentials (CMAPs). Nerve biopsies show a severe

loss of axons of all diameters, tomacula, and onion bulbs. Paranodal abnormalities, including a reduced number of myelin loops and absence of septate-like junctions between the paranodal myelin and axon, have been reported in a single patient [137].

HMSN–Russe (HMSNR) or CMT4G

HMSNR has been reported in Bulgarian, Romanian, and Spanish gypsy families [139,140] and mapped to chromosome 10q23, close to the *EGR2* gene. Distal lower limb weakness begins between the ages of 8 and 16 years and distal upper limb involvement between 10 and 43 years. This progresses toward a severe distal weakness of the four limbs. Motor nerve CVs are moderately reduced in the upper limbs (32 m/s). Nerve biopsies show a loss of large myelinated fibers, abnormally thinly myelinated fibers, and profuse regenerating activity [140]. Hantke *et al.* (2009) [141] identified a G>C substitution in a highly conserved alternative untranslated exon of hexokinase 1 (HK1), which catalyzes the first step of glucose metabolism.

CMT4H

CMT4H was mapped to chromosome 12p11.21–q13.11 in two consanguineous Lebanese and Algerian families with a severe form of CMT [142]. Mutations in the gene *FGD4*, encoding FGD4 or Frabin (FGD1-related F-actin binding protein), were found in both families [143]. Frabin is a GDP/GTP nucleotide exchange factor (GEF), specific to Cdc42, a member of the Rho family of small guanosine triphosphate (GTP)-binding proteins (Rho GTPases). These proteins play a key role in regulating signal-transduction pathways in eukaryotes. Other families with *FGD4* gene mutations had a milder phenotype and slow disease progression [144,145].

CMT4J

CMT4J was reported in four unrelated patients with AR-CMT and mutations in the *FIG4* gene [146]. The authors screened for the *FIG4* gene in 95 patients with CMT lacking mutations in known genes, because of phenotypical similarities between CMT and pale tremor (plt) mice. These mice have a spontaneous mutation that eliminates the expression of FIG4. Homozygous plt mice have a neuronopathy with extensive neuronal degeneration in the central and peripheral nervous systems, including loss of dorsal root ganglion (DRG) neurons and large myelinated axons in the sciatic nerve. The phenotype of CMT4J patients differs from the classical CMT phenotype. Effectively, Zhang *et al.* (2008) [147] gave a detailed description of two patients carrying the truncation mutation R183X and the missense mutation I41T in the *FIG4* gene. They develop rapidly progressive, asymmetric motor neuron degeneration, without clinical sensory loss or upper motor neuron signs. Onset of the disease was in the fourth decade of life. Electrophysiological studies demonstrated progressive and asymmetric reduction of motor and sensory responses accompanied by features of a demyelinating neuropathy. A sural nerve biopsy demonstrated axonal loss and features of demyelination and remyelination. The postulated mechanism for neurodegeneration is impaired cellular vesicle trafficking as shown in human cultured fibroblasts and in mice.

Autosomal recessive axonal forms of Charcot–Marie–Tooth disease (AR-CMT2)

AR-CMT2A

AR-CMT2A was mapped to chromosome 1q21.1 in a large Moroccan family [148], before the responsible gene was found in 2002 by De Sandre-Giovannoli *et al.* [149] in Algerian families. Mutations of this gene, *LMNA*, encoding lamin A/C, a nuclear envelope protein, had already been implicated in autosomal dominant diseases: Emery–Dreifuss muscular dystrophy type 2, dilated cardiomyopathy with atrioventricular block, familial partial lipodystrophy (Köbberling–Dunnigan syndrome), limb-girdle muscular dystrophy 1B, mandibuloacral dysplasia, and progeria [150]. In AR-CMT2A, a unique homozygous mutation, R298C, causes the phenotype. The age at onset ranges from 6 to 27 years. Weakness initially involves the distal limbs and then progresses to the proximal limbs after 10 to 15 years in 60% of the patients [151,152]. However, as in the other forms of CMT, phenotypical variability is the rule and the functional disability may remain mild after a disease course of ten years [152]. The mutation is found in individuals originating from a restricted region of north-western Africa (northwest of Algeria and east of Morocco), which results from a founder effect [152]. Motor nerve CVs and nerve biopsy findings are those of an axonal neuropathy.

AR-CMT2B

AR-CMT2B has been mapped to chromosome 19q13.3 in a large Costa Rican family with a mild phenotype [153]. A homozygous missense mutation has been identified in the *MED25* gene [154]. The onset is in the third, fourth, or fifth decade of life and the course is slowly progressive, most patients remaining ambulatory.

AR-CMT with pyramidal signs

AR-CMT2C has been mapped to chromosome 8q21.3, close to the CMT4A or axonal AR-CMT with the hoarseness locus, in a Tunisian family with a motor and sensory neuropathy associated with pyramidal signs [112].

AR-CMT with hoarseness

This form of AR-CMT2 is a result of *GDAP1* gene mutations and has been reported by Cuesta *et al.* (2002) [108] in Spanish families. The phenotype is similar to that reported for CMT4A, except that most patients develop vocal cord paresis in the second decade of life. It is not yet clear if the presence of vocal cord paresis results from the association of the recurrent S194X mutation with other mutations [110]. Diaphragmatic involvement has also been described in some patients [110,155]. Motor nerve CVs are in the axonal range but are often unrecordable. Nerve biopsies show a severe loss of myelinated fibers, with disappearance of fibers with a diameter of more than 7 μm, and the presence of pseudo-onion bulb formations, made of concentrically arranged Schwann cell processes around clusters of thinly myelinated fibers or enclosing numerous unmyelinated fibers around a single myelinated fiber, and occasional onion bulbs [109,110,156].

Conclusion

The molecular diagnosis of CMT is very complex and time consuming owing to its very great genetic heterogeneity. As the systematic screening of all responsible genes is not technically feasible today, molecular strategies based on the phenotype, after a detailed clinical and electrophysiological examination, and the mode of transmission have been developed. Indeed, many molecular geneticists take into account the type of CMT, demyelinating or axonal based on the MNCV of the median nerve, and the putative mode of inheritance, namely dominant or autosomal recessive.

In demyelinating CMT, systematic screening, first for the 17p11.2 duplication and second for the *GJB1* gene mutation, enables a molecular diagnosis to be made in about 70% of patients [4]. Taken together, MPZ and PMP22 mutations have been shown to account in Caucasian populations for 9% to 14% of CMT1 patients without 17p11.2 duplication [23,157]. EGR2 mutations are very rare and account for less than 1% of CMT1 cases [24,25]. When all these genes have been excluded in families with dominant demyelinating CMT, the other genes, such as NEFL and LITAF, can be explored. Sequencing of the GJB1 gene in families without father-to-son transmission has identified a mutation in 44% and 17% of the patients with MNCVs between 30 and 40 m/s (intermediate CMT) and over 40 m/s (axonal CMT), respectively [4]. MFN2 gene mutations account for 11 to 24% of the CMT2 families [68,71]. Moreover, in axonal CMT with dominant inheritance, mutations in the MPZ gene have been identified in 6% of patients [89]. Thus, after having excluded MFN2, GJB1, and MPZ gene mutations in CMT2 families, a molecular diagnosis still has to be made in the remaining 55%–65% of families. As we have shown, a precise phenotypical study may help to orientate the molecular testing; for example, an ulcero-mutilating neuropathy will lead to the search for a mutation within the RAB7 gene, and the presence of a predominant or inaugural involvement of the hands points to a possible mutation of the GARS gene. However, it must be stressed that these phenotypes are very rare and that a case-by-case approach is technically difficult, even in centers with a large recruitment of CMT families.

Genetic counseling remains highly problematic in isolated patients with CMT for whom various hypotheses can be made regarding the mode of inheritance: (1) a de novo mutation (as described for the 17p11.2 duplication and for PMP22, MPZ, GJB1, EGR2, and NEFL gene mutations); (2) a dominant CMT with incomplete penetrance, which is difficult to validate when the parents are not available for clinical and electrophysiological studies; or (3) an autosomal recessive CMT. Patients with isolated demyelinating CMT should be systematically tested for the presence of the 17p11.2 duplication, as this accounts for 40% of cases. Mutations in the MPZ, GJB1, and PMP22 genes account for an additional 10%. In other cases of demyelinating CMT without a familial history, molecular diagnosis may be oriented by particular clinical features and/or by nerve biopsy results. The presence of vocal cord paresis, facial and bulbar paralysis, early glaucoma, severe scoliosis, associated with either an early onset and/or a severe course, reinforces the hypothesis of an autosomal recessive CMT (in the absence of a clear familial history), and will lead to an exploration of the GDAP1, MTMR2, MTMR13, and SH3TC2 genes, respectively. Moreover, when an autosomal recessive demyelinating CMT is suspected, the nerve biopsy can be extremely helpful – the presence of myelin outfoldings points to mutations in the MTMR2, MTMR13, or PRX genes, the presence of basal membrane onion bulbs points to a mutation in the SH3TC2 gene, and the observation of pseudo-onion bulbs will lead to an exploration of the GDAP1 gene. The situation is much more complex for cases with axonal CMT without a familial history, particularly when onset is in adulthood. Molecular studies rarely help to elucidate the molecular basis of these cases and it should be kept in mind that the diagnosis of axonal CMT is made only after exclusion of acquired forms of chronic neuropathy.

The large spectrum of proteins responsible for CMT and the great variety of their functions in Schwann cells (structural or regulator proteins of myelin, such as PMP22 and MPZ; zinc transcription factor, such as EGR2; the protein forming channels, such as GJB1; etc.) or in axons (proteins of the axonal cytoskeleton, such as NEFL; proteins involved in the vesicular traffic, such as RAB7 and KIF1Bβ; etc.) make it difficult to develop specific therapeutic approaches aimed at correcting each dysfunction. Nevertheless, such approaches are already being developed for the most frequent form of CMT, namely CMT1A. For example, Sereda et al. (2003) [158] reported that, in a rat model, treatment with onapristone, a progesterone antagonist, was able to down-regulate PMP22 expression and decrease the motor deficit. Ascorbic acid treatment has demonstrated similar effects in a CMT1A mouse model [159]. However, a 12-month, randomized, double-blind, placebo-controlled French study in patients with CMT1A did not show any significant difference between the effects of placebo, 1 g ascorbic acid per day, and 3 g ascorbic acid per day on the CMT neuropathy score [160]. A more global approach may be to prevent or decrease the axonal loss, which is common to all forms of CMT and responsible for the functional disability, through the use of neuroprotective or neurotrophic factors.

References

1. Dyck PJ, Lambert EH. Lower motor and primary sensory neuron diseases with peroneal muscular atrophy. I. Neurologic, genetic, and electrophysiologic findings in hereditary polyneuropathies. *Arch Neurol* 1968; **18**: 603–618.

2. Harding AE, Thomas PK. The clinical features of hereditary motor and sensory neuropathy types I and II. *Brain* 1980; **103**: 259–280.

3. Bouche P, Gherardi R, Cathala HP, Lhermitte F, Castaigne P. Peroneal muscular atrophy. Part 1. Clinical and electrophysiological study. *J Neurol Sci* 1983; **61**: 389–399.

4. Dubourg O, Tardieu S, Birouk N, *et al.* The frequency of 17p11.2 duplication and connexin 32 mutations in 282 Charcot–Marie–Tooth families in relation to the mode of inheritance and motor nerve conduction velocity. *Neuromuscul Disord* 2001; **11**: 458–463.

5. Skre H. Genetic and clinical aspects of Charcot-Marie-Tooth disease. *Clin Genet* 1974; **6**: 98–118.

6. Chance PF, Bird TD, O'Connell P, *et al.* Genetic linkage and heterogeneity in type I Charcot–Marie–Tooth disease (hereditary motor and sensory neuropathy type I). *Am J Hum Genet* 1990; **47**: 915–925.

7. Lupski JR, de Oca-Luna RM, Slaugenhaupt S, *et al.* DNA duplication associated with Charcot–Marie–Tooth disease type 1A. *Cell* 1991; **66**: 219–232.

8. Raeymaekers P, Timmerman V, Nelis E, *et al.* Duplication in chromosome 17p11.2 in Charcot–Marie–Tooth neuropathy type 1a (CMT 1a). The HMSN Collaborative Research Group. *Neuromuscul Disord* 1991; **1**: 93–97.

9. Reiter LT, Hastings PJ, Nelis E, *et al.* Human meiotic recombination products revealed by sequencing a hotspot for homologous strand exchange in multiple HNPP deletion patients. *Am J Hum Genet* 1998; **62**: 1023–1033.

10. Lopes J, Ravise N, Vandenberghe A, *et al.* Fine mapping of de novo CMT1A and HNPP rearrangements within CMT1A-REPs evidences two distinct sex-dependent mechanisms and candidate sequences involved in recombination. *Hum Mol Genet* 1998; 7: 141–148.

11. Timmerman V, Nelis E, Van Hul W, *et al.* The peripheral myelin gene PMP-22 is contained within the Charcot–Marie–Tooth disease type 1A duplication. *Nat Genet* 1992; **1**: 171–175.

12. Valentijn LJ, Bolhuis PA, Zorn I, *et al.* The peripheral myelin gene PMP-22/GAS-3 is duplicated in Charcot–Marie–Tooth type 1A. *Nat Genet* 1992; **1**: 166–170.

13. Chance PF, Alderson MK, Leppig KA, *et al.* DNA deletion associated with hereditary neuropathy with liability to pressure palsies. *Cell* 1993; **72**: 143–151.

14. Lupski JR, Wise CA, Kuwano A, *et al.* Gene dosage is a mechanism for Charcot–Marie–Tooth disease type 1A. *Nat Genet* 1992; **1**: 29–33.

15. Birouk N, Gouider R, LeGuern E, *et al.* Charcot–Marie–Tooth disease type 1A with 17p11.2 duplication. Clinical and electrophysiological phenotype study and factors influencing disease severity in 119 cases. *Brain* 1997; **120**: 813–823.

16. Lewis RA, Sumner AJ. The electrodiagnostic distinctions between chronic familial and acquired demyelinative neuropathies. *Neurology* 1982; **32**: 592–596.

17. Garcia A, Combarros O, Calleja J, Berciano J. Charcot–Marie–Tooth disease type 1A with 17p duplication in infancy and early childhood: a longitudinal clinical and electrophysiologic study. *Neurology* 1998; **50**: 1061–1067.

18. Killian JM, Tiwari PS, Jacobson S, Jackson RD, Lupski JR. Longitudinal studies of the duplication form of Charcot–Marie–Tooth polyneuropathy. *Muscle Nerve* 1996; **19**: 74–78.

19. Hattori N, Yamamoto M, Yoshihara T, *et al.* Study Group for Hereditary Neuropathy in Japan. Demyelinating and axonal features of Charcot-Marie-Tooth disease with mutations of myelin-related proteins (PMP22, MPZ and Cx32): a clinicopathological study of 205 Japanese patients. *Brain* 2003; **126**: 134–151.

20. Krajewski KM, Lewis RA, Fuerst DR, *et al.* Neurological dysfunction and axonal degeneration in Charcot–Marie–Tooth disease type 1A. *Brain* 2000; **123**: 1516–1527.

21. Gabreëls-Festen AAWM, Joosten EMG, Gabreëls FJM, Jennekens FGI, Janssen van Kempen TW. Early morphological features in dominantly inherited demyelinating motor and sensory neuropathy (HMSN type I). *J Neurol Sci* 1992; **107**: 145–154.

22. Roa BB, Warner LE, Garcia CA, *et al.* Dejerine–Sottas syndrome associated with point mutation in the peripheral myelin protein 22 (PMP22) gene. *Nat Genet* 1993; **5**: 269–273.

23. Mersiyanova IV, Ismailov SM, Polyakov AV, *et al.* Screening for mutations in the peripheral myelin genes PMP22, MPZ and Cx32 (GJB1) in Russian Charcot–Marie–Tooth neuropathy patients. *Hum Mutat* 2000a; **15**: 340–347.

181

24. Numakura C, Shirahahta E, Yamashita S, *et al.* Screening of the early growth response 2 gene in Japanese patients with Charcot–Marie–Tooth disease type 1. *J Neurol Sci* 2003; **15**: 61–64.

25. Boerkoel CF, Takashima H, Garcia CA, *et al.* Charcot–Marie–Tooth disease and related neuropathies: mutation distribution and genotype-phenotype correlation. *Ann Neurol* 2002; **51**: 190–201.

26. Warner LE, Hilz MJ, Appel SH, *et al.* Clinical phenotypes of different MPZ (P0) mutations may include Charcot–Marie–Tooth type 1B, Dejerine–Sottas, and congenital hypomyelination. *Neuron* 1996; **17**: 451–460.

27. Roa BB, Warner LE, Garcia CA, *et al.* Myelin protein zero (MPZ) gene mutations in nonduplication type 1 Charcot–Marie–Tooth disease. *Hum Mutat* 1996; **7**: 36–45.

28. Gabreëls-Festen AA, Hoogendijk JE, Meijerink PH, *et al.* Two divergent types of nerve pathology in patients with different P0 mutations in Charcot–Marie–Tooth disease. *Neurology* 1996; **47**: 761–765.

29. Lagueny A, Latour P, Vital A, *et al.* Peripheral myelin modification in CMT1B correlates with MPZ gene mutations. *Neuromuscul Disord* 1999; **9**: 361–367.

30. Street VA, Bennett CL, Goldy JD, *et al.* Mutation of a putative protein degradation gene LITAF/SIMPLE in Charcot–Marie–Tooth disease 1C. *Neurology* 2003; **60**: 22–26.

31. Song S, Zhang Y, Chen B, *et al.* Mutation frequency for Charcot–Marie–Tooth disease type 1 in the Chinese population is similar to that in the global ethnic patients. *Genet Med* 2006; **8**: 532–535.

32. Latour P, Gonnaud PM, Ollagnon E, *et al.* SIMPLE mutation analysis in dominant demyelinating Charcot–Marie–Tooth disease: three novel mutations. *J Peripher Nerv Syst* 2006; **11**: 148–155.

33. Bennett CL, Shirk AJ, Huynh HM, *et al.* SIMPLE mutation in demyelinating neuropathy and distribution in sciatic nerve. *Ann Neurol* 2004; **55**: 713–720.

34. Warner LE, Mancias P, Butler IJ, *et al.* Mutations in the early growth response 2 (EGR2) gene are associated with hereditary myelinopathies. *Nat Genet* 1998; **18**: 382–384.

35. Boerkoel CF, Takashima H, Bacino CA, Daentl D, Lupski JR. EGR2 mutation R359W causes a spectrum of Dejerine–Sottas neuropathy. *Neurogenetics* 2001a; **3**: 153–157.

36. Yoshihara T, Kanda F, Yamamoto M, *et al.* A novel missense mutation in the early growth response 2 gene associated with late-onset Charcot–Marie–Tooth disease type 1. *J Neurol Sci* 2001; **184**: 149–153.

37. Mersiyanova IV, Perepelov AV, Polyakov AV, *et al.* A new variant of Charcot–Marie–Tooth disease type 2 is probably the result of a mutation in the neurofilament-light gene. *Am J Hum Genet* 2000; **67**: 37–46.

38. De Jonghe P, Mersivanova I, Nelis E, *et al.* Further evidence that neurofilament light chain gene mutations can cause Charcot–Marie–Tooth disease type 2E. *Ann Neurol* 2001; **49**: 245–249.

39. Jordanova A, De Jonghe P, Boerkoel CF, *et al.* Mutations in the neurofilament light chain gene (NEFL) cause early onset severe Charcot–Marie–Tooth disease. *Brain* 2003; **126**: 590–597.

40. Nicholson G, Nash J. Intermediate nerve conduction velocities define X-linked Charcot–Marie–Tooth neuropathy families. *Neurology* 1993; **43**: 2558–2564.

41. Bergoffen J, Scherer SS, Wang S, *et al.* Connexin mutations in X-linked Charcot–Marie–Tooth disease. *Science* 1993; **262**: 2039–2042.

42. Scherer SS, Deschenes SM, Xu YT, *et al.* Connexin32 is a myelin-related protein in the PNS and CNS. *J Neurosci* 1995; **15**: 8281–8294.

43. Dubourg O, Tardieu S, Birouk N, *et al.* Clinical, electrophysiological and molecular genetic characteristics of 93 patients with X-linked Charcot–Marie–Tooth disease. *Brain* 2001; **124**: 1958–1967.

44. Hahn AF, Brown WF, Koopman WJ, Feasby TE. X-linked dominant hereditary motor and sensory neuropathy. *Brain* 1990; **113**: 1511–1525.

45. Stojkovic T, Latour P, Vandenberghe A, Hurtevent JF, Vermersch P. Sensorineural deafness in X-linked Charcot–Marie–Tooth disease with connexin 32 mutation (R142Q). *Neurology* 1999; **52**: 1010–1014.

46. Bahr M, Andres F, Timmerman V, *et al.* Central visual, acoustic, and motor pathway involvement in a Charcot–Marie–Tooth family with an Asn205Ser mutation in the connexin 32 gene. *J Neurol Neurosurg Psychiatry* 1999; **66**: 202–206.

47. Paulson HL, Garbern JY, Hoban TF, *et al.* Transient central nervous system white matter abnormality in X-linked Charcot–Marie–Tooth disease. *Ann Neurol* 2002; **52**: 429–434.

48. Hanemann CO, Bergmann C, Senderek J, Zerres K, Sperfeld AD. Transient, recurrent, white matter lesions in X-linked Charcot–Marie–Tooth disease

with novel connexin 32 mutation. *Arch Neurol* 2003; **60**: 605–609.

49. Takashima H, Nakagawa M, Umehara F, *et al.* Gap junction protein beta 1 (GJB1) mutations and central nervous system symptoms in X-linked Charcot–Marie–Tooth disease. *Acta Neurol Scand* 2003; **107**: 31–37.

50. Birouk N, LeGuern E, Maisonobe T, *et al.* X-linked Charcot–Marie–Tooth disease with connexin-32 mutations: clinical and electrophysiologic study. *Neurology* 1998; **50**: 1074–1082.

51. Tabaraud F, Lagrange E, Sindou P, *et al.* Demyelinating X-linked Charcot–Marie–Tooth disease: unusual electrophysiological findings. *Muscle Nerve* 1999; **22**: 1442–1447.

52. Gutierrez A, England JD, Sumner AJ, *et al.* Unusual electrophysiological findings in X-linked dominant Charcot–Marie–Tooth disease. *Muscle Nerve* 2000; **23**: 182–188.

53. Lewis RA, Sumner AJ, Shy ME. Electrophysiological features of inherited demyelinating neuropathies: a reappraisal in the era of molecular diagnosis. *Muscle Nerve* 2000; **23**: 1472–1487.

54. Hahn AF, Ainsworth PJ, Bolton CF, Bilbao JM, Vallat JM. Pathological findings in the X-linked form of Charcot–Marie–Tooth disease: a morphometric and ultrastructural analysis. *Acta Neuropathol* 2001; **101**: 129–139.

55. Scherer SS, Xu YT, Nelles E, *et al.* Connexin32-null mice develop demyelinating peripheral neuropathy. *Glia* 1998; **24**: 8–20.

56. Zhao C, Takita J, Tanaka Y, *et al.* Charcot–Marie–Tooth disease type 2A caused by mutation in a microtubule motor KIF1B-beta. *Cell* 2001; **105**: 587–597.

57. Zuchner S, Mersiyanova IV, Muglia M, *et al.* Mutations in the mitochondrial GTPase mitofusin 2 cause Charcot–Marie–Tooth neuropathy type 2A. *Nature Genet* 2004; **36**: 449–441.

58. Verhoeven K, De Jonghe P, Coen K, *et al.* Mutations in the small GTP-ase late endosomal protein RAB7 cause Charcot–Marie–Tooth type 2B neuropathy. *Am J Hum Genet* 2003; **72**: 722–727.

59. Auer-Grumbach M, Olschewski A, Papić L, *et al.* Alterations in the ankyrin domain of TRPV4 cause congenital distal SMA, scapuloperoneal SMA and HMSN2C. *Nat Genet* 2010; **42**: 160–164.

60. Deng HX, Klein CJ, Yan J, *et al.* Scapuloperoneal spinal muscular atrophy and CMT2C are allelic disorders caused by alterations in TRPV4. *Nat Genet* 2010; **42**: 165–169.

61. Landouré G, Zdebik AA, Martinez TL, *et al.* Mutations in TRPV4 cause Charcot–Marie–Tooth disease type 2C. *Nat Genet* 2010; **42**: 170–174.

62. Antonellis A, Ellsworth RE, Sambuughin N, *et al.* Glycyl tRNA synthetase mutations in Charcot–Marie–Tooth disease type 2D and distal spinal muscular atrophy type V. *Am J Hum Genet* 2003; **72**: 1293–1299.

63. Evgarov OV, Mersiyanova I, Irobi J, *et al.* Mutant small heat shock protein 27 causes axonal Charcot–Marie–Tooth disease and distal hereditary motor neuropathy. *Nat Genet* 2004; **36**: 602–606.

64. Nelis E, Berciano J, Verpoorten N, *et al.* Autosomal dominant axonal Charcot–Marie–Tooth disease type 2 (CMT2G) maps to chromosome 12q12-q13.3. *J Med Genet* 2004; **41**: 193–197.

65. Tang BS, Luo W, Xia K, *et al.* A new locus for autosomal dominant Charcot–Marie–Tooth disease type 2 (CMT2L) maps to chromosome 12q24. *Hum Genet* 2004; **114**: 527–533.

66. Bissar-Tadmouri N, Nelis E, Zuchner S, *et al.* Absence of KIF1B mutation in a large Turkish CMT2A family suggests involvement of a second gene. *Neurology* 2004; **62**: 522–1525.

67. Kijima K, Numakura C, Izumino H, *et al.* Mitochondrial GTPase mitofusin 2 mutation in Charcot–Marie–Tooth neuropathy type 2A. *Hum Genet* 2004; **116**: 23–27.

68. Verhoeven K, Claeys KG, Zuchner S, *et al.* MFN2 mutation distribution and genotype/phenotype correlation in Charcot–Marie–Tooth type 2. *Brain* 2006; **129**: 2093–2102.

69. Zuchner S, De Jonghe P, Jordanova A, *et al.* Axonal neuropathy with optic atrophy is caused by mutations in mitofusin 2. *Ann Neurol* 2006; **59**: 276–281.

70. Zhu D, Kennerson ML, Walizada G, *et al.* Charcot–Marie–Tooth with pyramidal signs is genetically heterogeneous: families with and without MFN2 mutations. *Neurology* 2005; **65**: 496–497.

71. Chung KW, Kim SB, Park KD, *et al.* Early onset severe and late-onset mild Charcot–Marie–Tooth disease with mitofusin 2 (MFN2) mutations. *Brain* 2006; **129**: 2103–2118.

72. Kwon JM, Elliott JL, Yee WC, *et al.* Assignment of a second Charcot–Marie–Tooth type II locus to chromosome 3q. *Am J Hum Genet* 1995; **57**: 853–858.

73. De Jonghe P, Timmerman V, FitzPatrick D, *et al.* Mutilating neuropathic ulcerations in a chromosome 3q13-q22 linked Charcot–Marie–Tooth disease type 2B family. *J Neurol Neurosurg Psychiatry* 1997; **62**: 570–573.

74. Auer-Grumbach M. Hereditary sensory neuropathies. *Drugs Today* 2004; **40**: 385–394.

75. Bejaoui K, Wu C, Scheffler MD, *et al.* SPTLC1 is mutated in hereditary sensory neuropathy, type 1. *Nat Genet* 2001; **27**: 261–262.

76. Dawkins JL, Hulme DJ, Brahmbhatt SB, Auer-Grumbach M, Nicholson GA. Mutations in SPTLC1, encoding serine palmitoyltransferase, long chain base subunit-1, cause hereditary sensory neuropathy type I. *Nat Genet* 2001; **27**: 309–312.

77. Klein CJ, Cunningham JM, Atkinson EJ, *et al.* The gene for HMSN2C maps to 12q23–24: a region for neuromuscular disorders. *Neurology* 2003; **60**: 1151–1156.

78. Santoro L, Manganelli F, Di Maio L, *et al.* Charcot–Marie–Tooth disease type 2C: a distinct genetic entity. Clinical and molecular characterization of the first European family. *Neuromuscul Disord* 2002; **12**: 399–404.

79. Ionasescu V, Searby C, Sheffield VC, *et al.* Autosomal dominant Charcot–Marie–Tooth axonal neuropathy mapped on chromosome 7p (CMT2D). *Hum Mol Genet* 1996; **5**: 1373–1375.

80. Zuchner S, Vorgerd M, Sindern E, Schroder JM. The novel neurofilament light (NEFL) mutation Glu397Lys is associated with a clinically and morpho-logically heterogeneous type of Charcot–Marie–Tooth neuropathy. *Neuromuscul Disord* 2004; **14**: 147–157.

81. Ismailov SM, Fedotov VP, Dadali EL, *et al.* A new locus for autosomal dominant Charcot–Marie–Tooth disease type 2 (CMT2F) maps to chromosome 7q11-q21. *Europ J Hum Genet* 2001; **9**: 646–650.

82. Tang BS, Zhao GH, Luo W, *et al.* Small heat-shock protein 22 mutated in autosomal dominant Charcot–Marie–Tooth disease type 2L. *Hum Genet* 2005; **116**: 222–224.

83. Irobi J, Van Impe K, Seeman P, *et al.* Hot-spot residue in small heat-shock protein 22 causes distal motor neuropathy. *Nat Genet* 2004; **36**: 597–601.

84. Marrosu MG, Vaccargiu S, Marrosu G, *et al.* Charcot–Marie–Tooth disease type 2 associated with mutation of the myelin protein zero gene. *Neurology* 1998; **50**: 1397–1401.

85. De Jonghe P, Timmerman V, Ceuterick C, *et al.* The Thr124Met mutation in the peripheral myelin protein zero (MPZ) gene is associated with a clinically distinct Charcot–Marie–Tooth phenotype. *Brain* 1999; **122**: 281–290.

86. Chapon F, Latour P, Diraison P, Schaeffer S, Vandenberghe A. Axonal phenotype of Charcot–Marie–Tooth disease associated with a mutation in the myelin protein zero gene. *J Neurol Neurosurg Psychiatry* 1999; **66**: 779–782.

87. Mastaglia FL, Nowak KJ, Stell R, *et al.* Novel mutation in the myelin protein zero gene in a family with intermediate hereditary motor and sensory neuropathy. *J Neurol Neurosurg Psychiatry* 1999; **67**: 174–179.

88. Misu K, Yoshihara T, Shikama Y, *et al.* An axonal form of Charcot–Marie–Tooth disease showing distinctive features in association with mutations in the peripheral myelin protein zero gene (Thr124Met or Asp75Val). *J Neurol Neurosurg Psychiatry* 2000; **69**: 806–811.

89. Senderek J, Hermanns B, Lehmann U, *et al.* Charcot–Marie–Tooth neuropathy type 2 and P0 point mutations: two novel amino acid substitutions (Asp61Gly; Tyr119Cys) and a possible "hotspot" on Thr124Met. *Brain Pathol* 2000; **10**: 235–248.

90. Young P, Grote K, Kuhlenbaumer G, *et al.* Mutation analysis in Chariot–Marie–Tooth disease type 1: point mutations in the MPZ gene and the GJB1 gene cause comparable phenotypic heterogeneity. *J Neurol* 2001; **248**: 410–415.

91. Auer-Grumbach M, Strasser-Fuchs S, Robl T, Windpassinger C, Wagner K. Late onset Charcot–Marie–Tooth 2 syndrome caused by two novel mutations in the MPZ gene. *Neurology* 2003; **61**: 1435–1437.

92. Santoro L, Manganelli F, Di Maria E, *et al.* A novel mutation of myelin protein zero associated with an axonal form of Charcot–Marie–Tooth disease. *J Neurol Neurosurg Psychiatry* 2004; **75**: 262–265.

93. Shy ME, Jani A, Krajewski K, *et al.* Phenotypic clustering in MPZ mutations. *Brain* 2004; **127**: 371–384.

94. Claramunt R, Pedrola L, Sevilla T, *et al.* Genetics of Charcot–Marie–Tooth disease type 4A: mutations, inheritance, phenotypic variability, and founder effect. *J Med Genet* 2005; **42**: 358–365.

95. Chung KW, Kim SM, Sunwoo IN, *et al.* A novel GDAP1 Q218E mutation in autosomal dominant Charcot–Marie–Tooth disease. *J Hum Genet* 2008; **53**: 360–364.

96. Verhoeven K, Villanova M, Rossi A, *et al.* Localization of the gene for the intermediate form of Charcot–Marie–Tooth to chromosome 10q24.1-q25.1. *Am J Hum Genet* 2001; **69**: 889–894.

97. Kennerson ML, Zhu D, Gardner RJ, *et al.* Dominant intermediate Charcot–Marie–Tooth neuropathy maps to chromosome 19p12-p13.2. *Am J Hum Genet* 2001; **69**: 883–888.

98. Jordanova A, Thomas FP, Guergueltcheva V, *et al.* Dominant intermediate Charcot–Marie–Tooth type C maps to chromosome 1p34-p35. *Am J Hum Genet* 2003b; **73**: 1423–1430.

99. Zuchner S, Noureddine M, Kennerson M, *et al.* Mutations in the pleckstrin homology domain of dynamin 2 cause dominant intermediate Charcot–Marie–Tooth disease. *Nat Genet* 2005; **37**: 289–294.

100. Claeys KG, Züchner S, Kennerson M, *et al.* Phenotypic spectrum of dynamin 2 mutations in Charcot–Marie–Tooth neuropathy. *Brain* 2009; **132**: 1741–1752.

101. Fabrizi GM, Ferrarini M, Cavallaro T, *et al.* Two novel mutations in dynamin-2 cause axonal Charcot–Marie–Tooth disease. *Neurology* 2007; **69**: 291–295.

102. Jordanova A, Irobi J, Thomas FP, *et al.* Disrupted function and axonal distribution of mutant tyrosyl-tRNA synthetase in dominant intermediate Charcot–Marie–Tooth neuropathy. *Nat Genet* 2006; **38**: 197–202.

103. Martin JJ, Brice A, Van Broeckhoven C. 4th Workshop of the European CMT-Consortium – 62nd ENMC International Workshop. Rare forms of Charcot–Marie–Tooth disease and related disorders. Soestduinen, the Netherlands, 1998. *Neuromuscul Disord* 1999; **9**: 279–287.

104. Ben Othmane K, Hentati F, Lennon F, *et al.* Linkage of a locus (CMT4A) for autosomal recessive Charcot–Marie–Tooth disease to chromosome 8q. *Hum Mol Genet* 1993; **2**: 1625–1628.

105. Baxter RV, Ben Othmane K, Rochelle JM, *et al.* Ganglioside-induced differentiation-associated protein-1 is mutant in Charcot–Marie–Tooth disease

type 4A/8q21. *Nat Genet* 2002; **30**: 21–22.

106. Niemann A, Ruegg M, La Padula V, Schenone A, Suter U. Ganglioside-induced differentiation associated protein 1 is a regulator of the mitochondrial network: new implications for Charcot–Marie–Tooth disease. *J Cell Biol* 2005; **170**; 1067–1078.

107. Pedrola L, Espert A, Wu X, *et al.* GDAP1, the protein causing Charcot–Marie–Tooth disease type 4A, is expressed in neurons and is associated with mitochondria. *Hum Mol Genet* 2005; **14**: 1087–1094.

108. Cuesta A, Pedrola L, Sevilla T, *et al.* The gene encoding ganglioside-induced differentiation-associated protein 1 is mutated in axonal Charcot–Marie–Tooth type 4A disease. *Nat Genet* 2002; **30**: 22–25.

109. Birouk N, Azzedine H, Dubourg O, *et al.* Phenotypical features of a Moroccan family with autosomal recessive Charcot–Marie–Tooth disease associated with the S194X mutation in the GDAP1 gene. *Arch Neurol* 2003; **60**: 598–604.

110. Azzedine H, Ruberg M, Ente D, *et al.* Variability of disease progression in a family with autosomal recessive CMT associated with a S194X and new R310Q mutation in the GDAP1 gene. *Neuromuscul Disord* 2003a; **13**: 341–346.

111. Senderek J, Bergmann C, Ramaekers VT, *et al.* Mutations in the ganglioside-induced differentiation-associated protein-1 (GDAP1) gene in intermediate type autosomal recessive Charcot–Marie–Tooth neuropathy. *Brain* 2003a; **126**: 642–649.

112. Barhoumi C, Amouri R, Ben Hamida C, *et al.* Linkage of a new locus for autosomal recessive axonal form of

Charcot–Marie–Tooth disease to chromosome 8q21.3. *Neuromuscul Disord* 2001; **11**: 27–34.

113. Bolino A, Muglia M, Conforti FL, *et al.* Charcot–Marie–Tooth type 4B is caused by mutations in the gene encoding myotubularin-related protein-2. *Nat Genet* 2000; **25**: 17–19.

114. Laporte J, Hu LJ, Kretz C, *et al.* A gene mutated in X-linked myotubular myopathy defines a new putative tyrosine phosphatase family conserved in yeast. *Nat Genet* 1996; **13**: 175–182.

115. Quattrone A, Gambardella A, Bono F, *et al.* Autosomal recessive hereditary motor and sensory neuropathy with focally folded myelin sheaths: clinical, electrophysiologic, and genetic aspects of a large family. *Neurology* 1996; **46**: 1318–1324.

116. Houlden H, King RH, Wood NW, Thomas PK, Reilly MM. Mutations in the 5′ region of the myotubularin-related protein 2 (MTMR2) gene in autosomal recessive hereditary neuropathy with focally folded myelin. *Brain* 2001; **124**: 907–915.

117. Verny C, Ravise N, Leutenegger AL, *et al.* Coincidence of two genetic forms of Charcot–Marie–Tooth disease in a single family. *Neurology* 2004; **63**: 1527–1529.

118. Tyson J, Ellis D, Fairbrother U, *et al.* Hereditary demyelinating neuropathy of infancy. A genetically complex syndrome. *Brain* 1997; **120**: 47–63.

119. Othmane KB, Johnson E, Menold M, *et al.* Identification of a new locus for autosomal recessive Charcot–Marie–Tooth disease with focally folded myelin on chromosome 11p15. *Genomics* 1999; **62**: 344–349.

120. Senderek J, Bergmann C, Weber S, *et al.* Mutation of the SBF2 gene, encoding a novel member of the myotubularin

family, in Charcot–Marie–Tooth neuropathy type 4B2/11p15. *Hum Mol Genet* 2003; **12**: 349–356.

121. Azzedine H, Bolino A, Taieb T, *et al.* Mutations in MTMR13, a new pseudophosphatase homolog of MTMR2 and Sbf1, in two families with an autosomal recessive demyelinating form of Charcot–Marie–Tooth disease associated with early onset glaucoma. *Am J Hum Genet* 2003; **72**: 1141–1153.

122. Hirano R, Takashima H, Umehara F, *et al.* SET binding factor 2 (SBF2) mutation causes CMT4B with juvenile onset glaucoma. *Neurology* 2004; **63**: 577–580.

123. LeGuern E, Guilbot A, Kessali M, *et al.* Homozygosity mapping of an autosomal recessive form of demyelinating Charcot–Marie–Tooth disease to chromosome 5q23-q33. *Hum Mol Genet* 1996; **5**: 1685–1688.

124. Senderek J, Bergmann C, Stendel C, *et al.* Mutations in a gene encoding a novel SH3/TPR domain protein cause autosomal recessive Charcot–Marie–Tooth type 4C neuropathy. *Am J Hum Genet* 2003c; **73**: 1106–1119.

125. Gabreels-Festen A, van Beersum S, Eshuis L, *et al.* Study on the gene and phenotypic characterisation of autosomal recessive demyelinating motor and sensory neuropathy (Charcot–Marie–Tooth disease) with a gene locus on chromosome 5q23-q33. *J Neurol Neurosurg Psychiatry* 1999; **66**: 569–574.

126. Guilbot A, Kessali M, Ravise N, *et al.* The autosomal recessive form of CMT disease linked to 5q31-q33. *Ann NY Acad Sci* 1999; **883**: 453–456.

127. Kessali M, Zemmouri R, Guilbot A, *et al.* A clinical, electrophysiologic, neuropathologic, and genetic study of two large Algerian

families with an autosomal recessive demyelinating form of Charcot–Marie–Tooth disease. *Neurology* 1997; **48**: 867–873.

128. Kalaydjieva L, Hallmayer J, Chandler D, *et al.* Gene mapping in gypsies identifies a novel demyelinating neuropathy on chromosome 8q24. *Nat Genet* 1996; **14**: 214–217.

129. Kalaydjieva L, Gresham D, Gooding R, *et al.* N-myc downstream-regulated gene 1 is mutated in hereditary motor and sensory neuropathy-Lom. *Am J Hum Genet* 2000; **67**: 47–58.

130. Kalaydjieva L, Nikolova A, Turnev I, *et al.* Hereditary motor and sensory neuropathy-Lom, a novel demyelinating neuropathy associated with deafness in gypsies. Clinical, electrophysiological and nerve biopsy findings. *Brain* 1998; **121**: 399–408.

131. Baethmann M, Gohlich-Ratmann G, Schroder JM, Kalaydjieva L, Voit T. HMSNL in a 13-year-old Bulgarian girl. *Neuromuscul Disord* 1998; **8**: 90–94.

132. King RH, Tournev I, Colomer J, *et al.* Ultrastructural changes in peripheral nerve in hereditary motor and sensory neuropathy-Lom. *Neuropathol Appl Neurobiol* 1999; **25**: 306–312.

133. Guilbot A, Williams A, Ravise N, *et al.* A mutation in periaxin is responsible for CMT4F, an autosomal recessive form of Charcot–Marie–Tooth disease. *Hum Mol Genet* 2001; **10**: 415–421.

134. Boerkoel CF, Takashima H, Stankiewicz P, *et al.* Periaxin mutations cause recessive Dejerine–Sottas neuropathy. *Am J Hum Genet* 2001; **68**: 325–333.

135. Gillespie CS, Sherman DL, Blair GE, Brophy PJ. Periaxin, a novel protein of myelinating Schwann cells with a possible role in

axonal ensheathment. *Neuron* 1994; **12**: 497–508.

136. Sherman DL, Fabrizi C, Gillespie CS, Brophy PJ. Specific disruption of a Schwann cell dystrophin-related protein complex in a demyelinating neuropathy. *Neuron* 2001; **30**: 677–687.

137. Takashima H, Boerkoel CF, De Jonghe P, *et al.* Periaxin mutations cause a broad spectrum of demyelinating neuropathies. *Ann Neurol* 2002; **51**: 709–715.

138. Kijima K, Numakura C, Shirahata E, *et al.* Periaxin mutations causes early onset but slow-progressive Charcot–Marie–Tooth disease. *J Hum Genet* 2004; **49**: 376–379.

139. Rogers T, Chandler D, Angelicheva D, *et al.* A novel locus for autosomal recessive peripheral neuropathy in the EGR2 region on 10q23. *Am J Hum Genet* 2000; **67**: 664–667.

140. Thomas PK, Kalaydjieva L, Youl B, *et al.* Hereditary motor and sensory neuropathy-Russe: new autosomal recessive neuropathy in Balkan gypsies. *Ann Neurol* 2001; **50**: 452–457.

141. Hantke J, Chandler D, King R, *et al.* A mutation in an alternative untranslated exon of hexokinase 1 associated with hereditary motor and sensory neuropathy – Russe (HMSNR). *Eur J Hum Genet* 2009; **17**: 1606–1614.

142. De Sandre-Giovannoli A, Delague V, Hamadouche T, *et al.* Homozygosity mapping of autosomal recessive demyelinating Charcot–Marie–Tooth neuropathy (CMT4H) to a novel locus on chromosome 12p11.21-q13.11. *J Med Genet* 2005; **42**: 260–265.

143. Delague V, Jacquier A, Hamadouche T, *et al.* Mutations in FGD4 encoding the Rho GDP/GTP exchange factor FRABIN

cause autosomal recessive Charcot–Marie–Tooth type 4H. *Am J Hum Genet* 2007; **81**: 1–16.

144. Houlden H, Hammans S, Katifi H, Reilly MM. A novel frabin (FGD4) nonsense mutation p.R275X associated with phenotypic variability in CMT4H. *Neurology* 2009; **72**: 617–620.

145. Fabrizi GM, Taioli F, Cavallaro T, *et al.* Further evidence that mutations in FGD4/frabin cause Charcot–Marie–Tooth disease type 4H. *Neurology* 2009; **72**: 1160–1164.

146. Chow CY, Zhang Y, Dowling JJ, *et al.* Mutation of FIG4 causes neurodegeneration in the pale tremor mouse and patients with CMT4J. *Nature* 2007; **448**: 68–72.

147. Zhang X, Chow CY, Sahenk Z, *et al.* Mutation of FIG4 causes a rapidly progressive, asymmetric neuronal degeneration. *Brain* 2008; **131**: 1990–2001.

148. Bouhouche A, Benomar A, Birouk N, *et al.* A locus for an axonal form of autosomal recessive Charcot–Marie–Tooth disease maps to chromosome 1q21.2-q21.3. *Am J Hum Genet* 1999; **65**: 722–727.

149. De Sandre-Giovannoli A, Chaouch M, Kozlov S, *et al.* Homozygous defects in LMNA, encoding lamin A/C nuclear-envelope proteins, cause autosomal recessive axonal neuropathy in human (Charcot–Marie–Tooth disorder type 2) and mouse. *Am J Hum Genet* 2002; **70**: 726–736.

150. Worman HJ, Courvalin JC. How do mutations in lamins A and C cause disease? *J Clin Invest* 2004; **113**: 349–351.

151. Chaouch M, Allal Y, De Sandre-Giovannoli A, *et al.* The phenotypic manifestation of autosomal recessive axonal Charcot–Marie–Tooth due to a mutation in lamin A/C gene. *Neuromusc Disord* 2003; **13**: 60–67.

152. Tazir M, Azzedine H, Assami S, *et al.* Phenotypic variability in autosomal recessive axonal Charcot–Marie–Tooth disease due to the R298C mutation in lamin A/C. *Brain* 2004; **127**: 154–163.

153. Leal A, Morera B, Del Valle G, *et al.* A second locus for an axonal form of autosomal recessive Charcot–Marie–Tooth disease maps to chromosome 19q13.3. *Am J Hum Genet* 2001; **68**: 269–274.

154. Leal A, Huehne K, Bauer F, *et al.* Identification of the variant Ala335Val of MED25 as responsible for CMT2B2: molecular data, functional studies of the SH3 recognition motif and correlation between wild-type MED25 and PMP22 RNA levels in CMT1A animal models. *Neurogenetics* 2009; **10**: 275–287.

155. Stojkovic T, Latour P, Viet G, *et al.* Vocal cord and diaphragm paralysis, as clinical features of a French family with autosomal recessive Charcot–Marie–Tooth disease, associated with a new mutation in the GDAP1 gene. *Neuromuscul Disord* 2004; **14**: 261–264.

156. Sevilla T, Cuesta A, Chumillas MJ, *et al.* Clinical, electrophysiological and morphological findings of Charcot–Marie–Tooth neuropathy with vocal cord palsy and mutations in the GDAP1 gene. *Brain* 2003; **126**: 2023–2033.

157. Mostacciuolo ML, Righetti E, Zortea M, *et al.* Charcot–Marie–Tooth disease type I and related demyelinating neuropathies: mutation analysis in a large cohort of Italian families. *Hum Mutat* 2001; **18**: 32–41.

158. Sereda MW, Meyer zu Hörste G, Suter U, Uzma N, Nave KA. Therapeutic administration of progesterone antagonist in a model of Charcot–Marie–Tooth disease (CMT-1A). *Nat Med* 2003; **9**: 1533–1537.

159. Passage E, Norreel JC, Noack-Fraissignes P, *et al.* Ascorbic acid treatment corrects the phenotype of a mouse model of Charcot–Marie–Tooth disease. *Nat Med* 2004; **10**: 396–401.

160. Micallef J, Attarian S, Dubourg O, *et al.* Effect of ascorbic acid in patients with Charcot–Marie–Tooth disease type 1A: a multicentre, randomised, double-blind, placebo-controlled trial. *Lancet Neurol* 2009; **12**: 1103–1110.

161. LeGuern E, Sturtz F, Gugenheim M, *et al.* Detection of deletion within 17p11.2 in 7 French families with hereditary neuropathy with liability to pressure palsies (HNPP). *Cytogenet Cell Genet* 1994; **65**: 261–264.

Mitochondrial disorders

Robert McFarland, Robert Taylor, Andrew Schaefer, and Doug Turnbull

Introduction

Mitochondrial diseases that primarily affect oxidative metabolism are increasingly recognized as one of the most common genetic disorders seen in neurology. These disorders may be a result of the involvement of either the nuclear or the mitochondrial genome. Mitochondrial DNA genetics is particularly complicated because of the presence of multiple copies of mitochondrial DNA in the cell, the presence of both heteroplasmic and homoplasmic mutations, and the maternal pattern of transmission. The clinical features of mitochondrial disease are also extremely variable and make both clinical and laboratory diagnosis a challenge. In this chapter, we review the basics of mitochondrial genetics and the clinical features and investigation of mitochondrial disease and, finally, we discuss the management of these patients.

Genetics of mitochondrial disorders

Mitochondria are intracellular organelles the major (but not only) function of which is the generation of ATP from the metabolic fuels. This process is called oxidative phosphorylation and results in the formation of adenosine triphosphate (ATP), a readily utilizable energy source. It is dependent on five multi-subunit polypeptide complexes (I–V) located within the inner mitochondrial membrane. Only one complex, complex II, is entirely encoded by the nuclear genome, the others comprising subunits encoded by both the nuclear and mitochondrial genomes. The mitochondrial genome (mtDNA) is small (16.6 kb) and encodes only 13 proteins of the respiratory chain and 24 RNAs required for intramitochondrial protein synthesis [1] (Figure 13.1). It is present in multiple copies within cells, and thus any defect may involve all copies of the mitochondrial genome (homoplasmy) or only a proportion of it (heteroplasmy) [2] (Figure 13.2). In the presence of heteroplasmy, the severity of the biochemical defect is linked to the level of mutated mtDNA. The rest of the proteins involved in the respiratory chain and the proteins responsible for maintenance of the mitochondrial genome are nuclear encoded and transported into the mitochondrial matrix. Thus, the genetic defect in patients with mitochondrial disease may occur in either the mitochondrial or the nuclear genome [3].

MtDNA is thought to be strictly maternally inherited and, certainly from a clinical perspective, this guidance is still valid. A patient with a myopathy and a microdeletion in the *MTND2* gene had inherited most of his muscle mtDNA (but not the deletion) from his father [4]. This has subsequently been shown to be a very uncommon (if not unique) finding that should not change our advice to patients [5–7].

Defects of the mitochondrial genome take the form of either rearrangements (deletions and duplications) or point mutations. MtDNA deletions usually occur in the major arc of the mitochondrial genome [8]. A 4977 bp deletion is the most commonly detected and is described as the common deletion [9]. There are also several different pathogenic mtDNA point mutations involving either the protein coding or tRNA genes. Point mutations may be either heteroplasmic or homoplasmic, as described earlier. Over the last few years, an increasing number of nuclear genetic defects have been identified. The genetic defect may involve one of the subunit proteins, proteins involved in complex assembly, proteins involved in mtDNA maintenance, and the synthesis of non-protein respiratory chain components.

Epidemiology of mitochondrial disorders

The clinical variability of the mitochondrial disorders has made epidemiological studies very difficult. Genetic and phenotypic heterogeneity hamper attempts to ensure accurate ascertainment, and reliance on specialized diagnostic techniques limits the feasibility

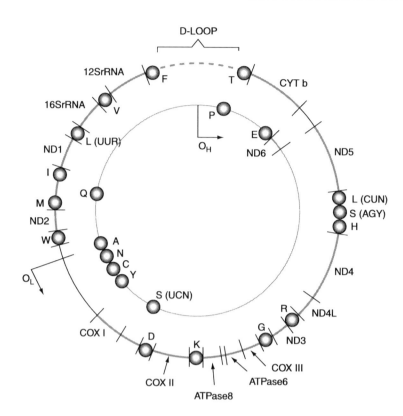

Figure 13.1. Schematic representation of the mitochondrial genome. The mitochondrial genome is a small (16 569 bases) DNA molecule made up of two DNA strands, the inner light or L-strand and the outer heavy or H-strand. The only non-coding region of the mitochondrial genome is called the displacement or D-loop and is shown at the top of the figure. The polypeptide-encoding genes are represented by the thicker purple lines that are distributed throughout the coding region of the mtDNA. The genes encoding subunits of complex I are: *ND1, ND2, ND3, ND4L, ND4, ND5,* and *ND6.* The *CYT b* gene encodes one subunit of complex III, and *COXI, COXII,* and *COXIII* encode subunits of complex IV. *ATPase6* and *ATPase8* encode complex V subunits. The tRNA genes are represented by the circles and are labeled according to the standard tRNA single letter abbreviation coding system. The two rRNA genes are labeled *12S rRNA* and *16S rRNA.*

of such studies in all but a few specialized centers. Furthermore, population genetic bottlenecks and founder effects can lead to the under- or over-representation of specific mtDNA [10] and recessive nuclear [11] disorders in any given study.

The first population-based study of a single pathogenic mtDNA mutation was carried out in northern Finland [12]. Majamaa and colleagues (1998) estimated the frequency of the m.3243A>G mutation in the general population to be 16.3 per 100 000 (95% C.I. = 11.3–21.4/100 000) or 1 in 6135 [12]. The frequency of the m.3243A>G mutation was particularly high in certain disease groups, including those with deafness and a family history of hearing loss (7.4%), occipital stroke (6.9%), ophthalmoplegia (13%), and hypertrophic cardiomyopathy (14%). The first population-based study of all mitochondrial disorders was carried out in the northeast of England [13]. This study has recently been updated with all adults with suspected mitochondrial disease in the northeast of England having been referred to a single neurology center for investigation from 1990 to 2004 [14]. Those with pathogenic mtDNA mutations were identified and

their families traced. For the mid-year period of 2001, the minimum point prevalence of clinically manifest mtDNA disease for adults of working age (>16 and <60–65 years) was 9.2 in 100 000 people. In addition, a further 16.5 in 100 000 children and adults younger than retirement age are at risk for development of mtDNA disease. The m.3243A>G mutation was the most common pathogenic mtDNA mutation identified (40%). A further 34% of adults with disease (predominantly Leber's hereditary optic neuropathy [LHON]) were affected by the m.11778G>A or m.3460G>A point mutations. Single large-scale deletions of mtDNA were rarely inherited, but despite this, represented 13% of disease cases. The m.8344A>G mutation caused disease (myoclonic epilepsy with ragged red fibers, MERRF) in a further 4%, whereas the remaining 9% of affected adults had 10 different point mutations.

The population frequency of different mtDNA point mutations has also been studied recently. The frequency of 10 mitochondrial point mutations in 3168 neonatal cord blood samples from sequential live births has been studied. MtDNA mutations were detected in 15 offspring, giving an incidence of

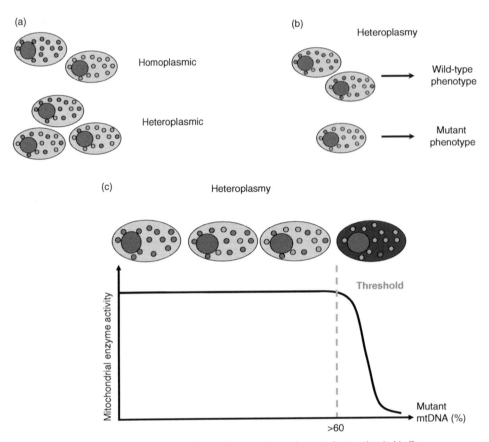

Figure 13.2a–c. Schematic representation of heteroplasmy and homoplasmy, indicating threshold effect.

approximately 1 in 200 healthy humans with a pathogenic mtDNA point mutation [15]. The most commonly detected mutation was m.3243A>G. In other studies, two groups have looked at the prevalence of the m.1555A>G mutation [16,17]. Carriers of this mutation develop permanent, profound hearing loss after receiving aminoglycoside antibiotics, even when drug levels are within the therapeutic range. The prevalence of this mutation both in children from the United Kingdom and adults from Australia was about 1 in 500 of the population.

Clinical features of patients with defects of mitochondrial oxidation

Neurological features

Neurological disease is one of the most consistently reported features of mitochondrial dysfunction,

and often one of the most disabling aspects. A number of syndromes have been characterized, many of them associated with but not exclusive to a specific type of mtDNA or nuclear defect. There are, however, a very large proportion of patients with mitochondrial disease who either do not conform to the clinical criteria for a particular syndrome or present with only some of the features. This group of patients presents a considerable clinical and diagnostic challenge and many patients remain without a diagnosis for years. Neurological presentations such as migraine, seizures, stroke-like episodes, myopathy, or neuropathy are not uncommon, but clinicians often only consider mitochondrial disease when these features occur in conjunction with other prompts such as deafness, diabetes, or a clear history of maternal transmission. Isolated nonspecific symptoms such as fatigue

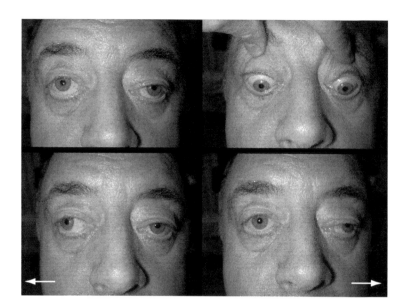

Figure 13.3. External ophthalmoplegia in a patient with a single deletion.

and myalgia probably result in many patients not being referred or investigated initially. In contrast, some patients with what seem like cardinal signs of respiratory chain dysfunction are extensively investigated without any firm conclusions being reached.

Mitochondrial myopathy

Myopathy is an important finding in patients with mitochondrial disease and a prominent clinical feature of the syndromes described later. A significant number of patients with mitochondrial disease present with nonspecific symptoms, but proximal weakness and exercise intolerance are the principle clinical features. Some of these patients progress to having involvement of other organ systems, and their symptoms become more obviously mitochondrial in origin; the symptoms of others remain confined to muscle with gradual deterioration in power and involvement of muscle groups outside the shoulder and hip girdles, including the diaphragm. The finding of a proximal myopathy, in conjunction with other clinical features such as diabetes, sensory organ impairment, or progressive multisystem disease, should prompt further investigation for mitochondrial disorders. Symptoms compatible with mtDNA disease in maternal relatives should also raise suspicion, even if the pedigree appears to exhibit variable penetrance.

Chronic progressive external ophthalmoplegia

One of the commonest presentations in adults, CPEO is defined by a slowly progressive ophthalmoparesis and ptosis [18,19] (Figure 13.3). Adults with a single mtDNA deletion, or multiple mtDNA deletions secondary to a nuclear defect, often present with ptosis and CPEO, although the ophthalmoplegia may be well advanced, having developed insidiously without intrusive diplopia. Despite this, diplopia is commonly reported during the course of the disease but tends to be mild. Ptosis and CPEO also occur in a number of the mtDNA point mutations but are seen less frequently and often constitute part of a broader phenotype. Many of our patients first notice ptosis in their third or fourth decade of life, but the age of onset is variable. Contrary to early textbook descriptions, marked asymmetry is not uncommon, but most patients go on to develop bilateral disease. As the disease progresses, there is often associated proximal muscle weakness and fatigue although rarely to a debilitating extent. Cardiac conduction defects and respiratory insufficiency are relatively uncommon but can occur in severe cases (see Kearns–Sayre syndrome).

Either recessive or dominant families with CPEO are well recognized and are associated with multiple species of deleted mtDNA [20,21]. A number of causative nuclear gene mutations, including *ANT1* [22], *PEO1* [23], and *POLG* [24], have now been described in these families. In these patients, the clinical features show more variability than those seen in patients with single mtDNA deletions, likely reflecting the variation in the causative nuclear defect. Many patients exhibit mild disease, with onset in the fifth or sixth decade of life. Optic atrophy, cataracts, deafness, cerebellar ataxia, cardiomyopathy, and depression may also occur where other systems are involved. In some pedigrees, patients develop a Parkinsonian syndrome [25,26] or a severe sensorimotor neuropathy [27].

Kearns–Sayre syndrome

The onset of ophthalmoparesis and pigmentary retinopathy before the age of 20 years is characteristic of the Kearns–Sayre syndrome (KSS). This predominantly sporadic condition is usually the result of either a large-scale single deletion or complex rearrangements of mtDNA. Other clinical features include cerebellar ataxia, proximal myopathy, complete heart block, cardiomyopathy, endocrinopathies, short stature, deafness, and an elevated cerebrospinal fluid (CSF) protein. As may be predicted from the early onset of this multisystem disorder, life expectancy is considerably reduced.

Pearson (bone marrow pancreas) syndrome

Pearson syndrome is a rare disorder resulting from large-scale rearrangements of mtDNA. In this instance, however, clinical features of sideroblastic anemia with pancytopenia and exocrine pancreatic dysfunction predominate in early life and frequently result in death during infancy. Survival through childhood leads to an improvement in anemia, but patients then develop the characteristic features of KSS.

For Pearson's syndrome, KSS, and CPEO, the clinical severity appears to correlate with the tissue localization of mutated mtDNA. In Pearson syndrome (and to a lesser extent, KSS), mutated mtDNA can be demonstrated in a wide variety of tissues whereas in CPEO, the defective mtDNA is confined to a limited number of tissues.

Mitochondrial neurogastrointestinal encephalopathy syndrome

This multisystem disorder (MNGIE) is characterized by the onset of chronic progressive external ophthalmoplegia, ptosis, gastrointestinal dysmotility (pseudo-obstruction), diffuse leukoencephalopathy, peripheral neuropathy, and myopathy. Histological and biochemical studies of patients with MNGIE have confirmed the involvement of mitochondria in this disorder. The inheritance is autosomal recessive and it is a result of mutations in the thymidine phosphorylase (TP) gene [28,29].

Mitochondrial DNA depletion syndrome

Mitochondrial DNA depletion, a decrease in the absolute amount of mtDNA within a tissue, is associated with several different genetic mutations and clinical phenotypes, predominantly affecting children [30]. Depletion syndromes often appear to be tissue specific, with both hepatocerebral and encephalomyopathic forms. Alpers–Huttenlocher syndrome is a form of hepatocerebral mtDNA depletion that occurs in infants and young children [31,32]. It is associated with the sudden onset of focal or generalized seizures, developmental delay or regression, and hepatic dysfunction. The latter is often a terminal event, but may pre-date the seizures and be precipitated by the use of sodium valproate therapy [33]. Neuroimaging reveals thalamic and parietooccipital cortical atrophy, reflecting the pathological correlate of spongiform degeneration of gray matter [34]. A large number of mutations in *POLG* have been identified in patients with Alpers–Huttenlocher syndrome, with almost invariable involvement of the linker region of this gene [35]. Three mutations (p.A467T, p.W748S, and p.G848S) occur with sufficient frequency, and some diagnostic centers screen for these mutations before sequencing the entire gene (Figure 13.4). Although seizures are a less prominent feature of other forms of hepatocerebral depletion, these should be considered in patients where *POLG* is normal and mutations should be sought in the *DGUOK*, *RRM2B*, *MPV17*, and *PEO1* genes [36–38].

In the muscular form, mutations should be sought in *TK2* [39] and the p53-controlled ribonucleotide reductase gene, *RRM2B* [37]. The latter is also associated with a phenotype that includes hypotonia, lactic acidosis, and renal tubulopathy. Other forms of depletion syndrome have a more prominent encephalopathy with additional clinical features such as hypotonia, dystonia, seizures, and neurodevelopmental regression. The presence of a mild methylmalonic aciduria should alert the clinician to the possibility of a mutation in *SUCLA2*, a gene encoding a subunit of the

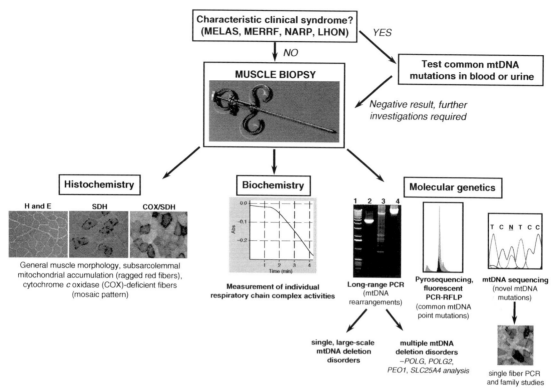

Figure 13.4. Algorithm for investigation in adults. Skeletal muscle biopsy has a pivotal role in the diagnosis of mitochondrial disease in adults. In the context of classic features of adult-onset mitochondrial disease, the histochemical analysis of skeletal muscle is particularly important in directing genetic investigation, and biochemistry is often unnecessary in establishing the diagnosis.

Krebs cycle enzyme succinyl CoA synthase [40]. Mutations in a related gene, *SUCLG1*, which encodes the α-subunit of the same Krebs cycle enzyme, also cause depletion and a fatal congenital lactic acidosis [41].

Mitochondrial encephalopathy lactic acidosis and stroke-like episodes

This clinical syndrome (MELAS) is characterized by parietooccipital stroke-like episodes, often associated (as the name implies) with concurrent encephalopathy and elevated plasma and CSF lactate. These events may herald the onset of clinical disease in an otherwise apparently healthy young adult, or represent a new facet to an already lengthy past medical history. Termed stroke-like episodes, these events are not a result of thromboembolic disease but of respiratory chain dysfunction within cerebral tissues. Consequently, the focal deficit is rarely of sudden onset, and often develops over hours or even days. Radiological lesions frequently fail to conform to a single recognized vascular territory and may exhibit rapid resolution associated with clinical improvement. Such events are commonly associated with a variable prodrome of headache, nausea, and encephalopathic features, further distinguishing them from most thromboembolic causes of stroke. Seizures commonly accompany the acute episodes, sometimes preceding any focal deficit, and should be actively sought. The presence of deafness, diabetes, myopathy, or a pigmentary retinopathy may contribute to the diagnostic process. It is not uncommon for patients to have been investigated for failure to thrive during childhood, and in adulthood to have short stature and long-standing gastrointestinal complaints (reflecting bowel dysmotility).

The m.3243A>G mutation in the mitochondrial tRNA$^{Leu(UUR)}$ gene was the first and most frequently described mtDNA mutation associated with this clinical phenotype [42]. However, other mutations including MTND subunit genes [43] have been described in association with this presentation. The m.3243A>G mutation also causes other distinct clinical phenotypes such as maternally inherited diabetes and deafness (MIDD) [44] or CPEO [45]. Variations in phenotype can occur between individuals in the same family harboring identical mutations [46]. A maternal mode of transmission, therefore, is not always apparent, and indeed, the mother of the patient may remain asymptomatic as a result of low levels of heteroplasmy in her tissues.

Myoclonic epilepsy with ragged red fibers

This disorder (MERRF) was initially reported in association with an A>G mutation in the gene encoding mitochondrial tRNA^{Lys} at position m.8344, and although other mutations in the same tRNA have been reported, this remains by far the most common cause of this disease [47,48]. In patients with MERRF, there is progressive myoclonus, focal and generalized epilepsy, cerebellar ataxia, cognitive impairment, and myopathy. Proximal muscle weakness can be pronounced, with gross wasting developing in a limb-girdle distribution. Sensory ataxia frequently occurs owing to a loss of proprioception as part of a progressive sensorimotor neuropathy. Occasionally, proprioception is lost without evidence of a neuropathy when the pathology is thought to be more proximal and owing to degeneration of the dorsal root ganglia or posterior columns. Pyramidal signs such as hyperreflexia, clonus, and upgoing plantar responses can also occur. In the later stages of the disease, severe cognitive impairment is common and often exhibits prominent frontal features. The m.8344A>G mutation has been identified as the cause of the original hereditary syndrome described by Ekbom, of cerebellar ataxia, photomyoclonus, skeletal deformities, and lipomata [49,50]. The reported aversion to flickering lights is almost uniform in these patients, while generalized seizures are surprisingly infrequent. Lipomas are common in patients with m.8344A>G, distributed in the neck region particularly.

Loss of mobility usually occurs owing to a combination of myopathy and cerebellar and sensory ataxia. The timescale for this is variable but rarely occurs earlier than two decades from the disease onset. Hypertrophic cardiomyopathy can occur but re-entrant atrioventricular tachycardias, such as Wolff–Parkinson–White syndrome, are reported more commonly. Life expectancy is usually reduced significantly, and pedigrees frequently contain individuals who have suffered sudden and unexplained deaths before their sixth decade of life.

Leigh syndrome

Leigh syndrome is a progressive neurodegenerative condition of infancy and childhood. The characteristic symmetric necrotic lesions distributed along the brainstem, diencephalon, and basal ganglia were first described in postmortem tissue [51] but are readily visible on magnetic resonance imaging (MRI) or computer tomography (CT) scans. The clinical presentation and course vary considerably but common features include signs of brainstem or basal ganglia dysfunction such as respiratory abnormalities, nystagmus, ataxia, dystonia, hypotonia, and optic atrophy. Developmental delay and, more particularly, regression are prominent clinical features of this disorder, and the latter may be evident only after a period of slow developmental progress. The clinical course can follow a stepwise deterioration with moderate recovery of developmental skills between episodes of regression, or alternatively, a slowly progressive decline.

A severe failure of oxidative metabolism within the mitochondria of the developing brain owing to a variety of biochemical and molecular defects, including nuclear and mtDNA mutations, have been described in Leigh syndrome [52,53]. Therefore, inheritance can be X-linked recessive, autosomal recessive, or maternal, depending on the defect responsible.

Neuropathy, ataxia, and retinitis pigmentosa

First described as a variable combination of developmental delay, retinitis pigmentosa, dementia, seizures, ataxia, proximal neurogenic muscle weakness, and sensory neuropathy in four members of a single family [54], the phenotype of NARP has been expanded now to include cardiomyopathy and Leigh syndrome. The original family had a heteroplasmic T>G transversion at the nucleotide pair m.8993 in subunit 6 of mitochondrial ATPase (ATP6). A T>C mutation at m.8993 has subsequently been described with a generally milder clinical phenotype but higher frequency of ataxia. Mutations in the mitochondrial ATPase subunits do not affect cytochrome oxidase activity and, therefore, NARP patients will have no evidence of mitochondrial myopathy on routine histochemical analysis.

Leber hereditary optic neuropathy

The first mitochondrial disease to be ascribed to a point mutation in mtDNA, LHON is an acute or subacute, bilateral, painless, central visual loss, and a common cause of blindness in young men. The clinical condition was described as a familial neuroophthalmologic disease in 1871, but it was not until over a century later that Wallace and colleagues (1988) [55] demonstrated that the majority of LHON families harbor the same mtDNA mutation (m.11778G>A). A number of mtDNA mutations have subsequently been described in association with LHON, but three mutations (m.11778G>A, m.3460G>A, and m.14484T>C) are present in at least 95% of families [56]. These mutations in the complex I (NADH: ubiquinone-oxidoreductase) encoding genes *ND4*, *ND1*, and *ND6*, respectively, are considered on the basis of their frequency, penetrance, and clinical severity to be primary LHON mutations. In this disorder, there is an excess of affected males, but no X-linked visual-loss susceptibility locus has been found.

Clinical examination reveals peripapillary telangiectasia (which gradually disappears with disease progression), microangiopathy, disk pseudo-edema, and tortuous retinal vessels in over half of the patients harboring the m.11778G>A mutation, with some apparently unaffected relatives demonstrating the same pathology. The onset of the disease is most common in the third or fourth decade of life, with initial unilateral involvement being typical. Sequential involvement of the other eye commonly occurs within a two-month period, and subsequent decline in visual acuity of both eyes may be very sudden or slowly progressive over a period of several years. Both the disease penetrance and the clinical course appear to be determined by the mutation responsible, with measurements of final visual acuity ranging from 20/60 to no light perception at all. Similarly, the extent of visual recovery varies in relation to the mutation, with only 4% of m.11778G>A patients showing recovery an average of 36 months after onset, while 37% of m.14484T>C patients recover after 16 months [57,58].

Occasionally, extra-ocular clinical features such as cardiac conduction defects (Wolff–Parkinson–White and Lown–Ganong–Levine syndromes [direct atrio-nodal pathway associated with a short PR interval and no delta wave]) are evident and minor neurological problems are also not uncommon. In some patients, there is a clinical syndrome indistinguishable from multiple sclerosis [59].

Cardiac features of mitochondrial disease

As highlighted earlier, many patients who present with neurological features may have cardiac involvement. This may include cardiomyopathy and conduction defects, both of which can be life threatening. In some patients, however, cardiomyopathy may be the presenting or only feature of mitochondrial disease. Familial cardiomyopathies have been described in which the predominant cardiac features are of hypertrophic cardiomyopathy, often with biventricular involvement. Patients with this pattern of cardiac involvement should be investigated further for the possibility of mitochondrial disease.

Diabetes

Diabetes is commonly present in patients with mtDNA mutations, particularly those with the m.3243A>G mutation, and may be the presenting feature [44,60,61]. The diabetes has a characteristic pattern in some patients and is a result of impaired insulin secretion by the β-islet cells of the pancreas. These patients often present with relatively mild diabetes in their 20s–40s, which rapidly progresses to insulin dependence. In patients with mitochondrial diabetes, deafness is a frequently associated clinical feature [44,62]. Other endocrinopathies such as hypoparathyroidism are less common but are well recognized in patients with Kearns–Sayre syndrome [63] and some point mutations [64].

Childhood presentations of mitochondrial disease

In general, childhood presentations of mitochondrial disease tend to be more severe than those with their onset in adult life and frequently involve many different organ systems. Hepatic dysfunction and hemopoeitic stem cell failure (Pearson's syndrome) are uncommon features of mitochondrial disease but are seen more often in children than adults. Renal disease also appears to be a more prominent clinical feature of pediatric mitochondrial disorders, evident in both mitochondrial DNA depletion syndrome and complex III deficiencies (*BCS1L* gene mutations) [65]. In addition, it is reported in m.3243A<G pedigrees and may be the presenting feature in children [66]. Developmental delay is a prominent but nonspecific finding that is much more discriminating as a diagnostic feature when found in conjunction with lactic acidemia. However, stepwise developmental regression, the loss of acquired skills, is a much more specific indicator of a mitochondrial disorder (Leigh's syndrome). Symptoms such as deafness, migraines, or failure to thrive are seen so frequently in pediatric practice that, prior to the development of other features of mtDNA disease, a maternal family history may provide the only clue as to the underlying genetic etiology.

Investigation of suspected mitochondrial disease

The differential diagnosis for patients with mitochondrial disease is extensive owing to the varied clinical presentation. In addition, the investigation of presumed mitochondrial disease is made more difficult, not only because the same genetic or biochemical defect may present in a variety of different ways, but also because the same clinical syndrome may be a result of a variety of different biochemical or molecular defects. Therefore, the detailed history and examination of a patient with suspected mitochondrial disease is crucial.

In some patients, the initial presentation alone may be sufficient to suggest a diagnosis of mtDNA disease. For example, stroke-like episodes (as described earlier) are usually accompanied by a number of features which help distinguish them from thromboembolic events. Chronic progressive external ophthalmoplegia (often presenting as ptosis) is relatively specific to mtDNA disease and usually can be differentiated clinically from other forms of ophthalmoplegia [67]. In the majority of cases, however, presentations are sufficiently nonspecific as to require the connection of several aspects of the history and examination to prompt the diagnosis. Strokes, seizures, diabetes, deafness, migraine, and gastrointestinal complaints are, on their own, common complaints. Together, whether in an individual or a pedigree, they may represent mtDNA disease. The obstetric history is

important, with particular reference to a previous miscarriage or infant death. Family history is of great importance but may be misleading. Limited pedigrees may appear dominant if the absence of male transmission is not appreciated. Detailed pedigree analysis, therefore, is vital. Variable levels of mutation (heteroplasmy) throughout the family may mean that the mother and siblings of an adult with m.3243 A>G MELAS remain asymptomatic, yet there is a history of deafness and failure to thrive in a maternal cousin. Mitochondrial pedigrees, therefore, are rarely as transparent as those associated with nuclear defects. Reports of other neurological conditions within the family should also be viewed with suspicion, particularly if their clinical course appears atypical.

Few individual features on examination are specific to mtDNA disease. Frequently, it is the combination of a number of clinical signs that point toward the diagnosis. Specific clues may be gained from the ophthalmological examination, however. The pigmentary retinopathy seen in some patients with mtDNA disease is typically more diffuse than the dense, spiculated pigment seen as a result of retinitis pigmentosa (RP) associated with a number of other neurological diseases. The retinopathy witnessed in mtDNA disease rarely results in visual loss, in contrast to RP. Chronic progressive external ophthalmoplegia, as discussed previously, is also relatively specific for mtDNA disease, although similarities do exist with other disorders of muscle, neuromuscular junction, and supranuclear structures [67]. High-frequency, sensorineural hearing loss is typical of mtDNA disease but may occur in a number of other genetic disorders. Mitochondrial myopathies can be particularly difficult to identify, especially in their early stages. Often assessment of proximal power appears normal but "give way" in nature. The fatiguability seen in myasthenia gravis does not occur, yet the ability to maintain full resistance is poorly sustained. EMG studies may be normal [68], and it is not uncommon for these myopathies to remain undiagnosed until "hard" signs have developed or other systems have become involved. Ataxia, dementia, and neuropathy rarely develop in isolation, more often forming part of a degenerative multisystem involvement.

Simple blood tests play only a minor role in the diagnosis of the mtDNA disorders. Instead, their purpose is to provide some supporting evidence for the clinical diagnosis and to detect potential complications associated with the disease. Initial investigations, therefore, should include creatine kinase, resting blood lactate, electrolytes, full blood count, thyroid and liver function, bone chemistry, fasting blood glucose, and glycosylated hemoglobin (HbA1c). Serum lactate levels may be elevated significantly in some patients, but frequently are normal. Creatine kinase levels can vary greatly, but are typically normal or only modestly elevated (below 500 U/L). Levels exceeding 1000 U/L are rare but can occur, particularly in the presence of renal disease or seizures, or in the patients who present with rhabdomyolysis. It is vital that all patients have an electrocardiogram (EKG) and echocardiogram (ECHO) at baseline, as cardiac conduction defects or hypertrophy may remain asymptomatic even at an advanced stage. Lumbar puncture in children is a valuable investigation as raised CSF lactate and mild protein elevation are consistent with mitochondrial dysfunction [68]. However, an increased CSF lactate following seizure activity or stroke, two common features of mitochondrial disease, should always be interpreted with caution. Electromyography may be normal, even in the presence of clinical myopathy, and nerve conduction studies can demonstrate either an axonal or a mixed axonal-demyelinating peripheral sensorimotor neuropathy. A pattern of generalized slow waves, indicative of a subacute encephalopathy, or subclinical seizure activity may be evident on the electroencephalogram (EEG). Cognitive impairment, central neurological signs, movement disorder, or abnormal EEG all warrant some form of cerebral imaging. A variety of changes can be seen on CT scans and MRI, but abnormalities are frequently nonspecific (e.g. cerebral or cerebellar atrophy). Certain findings may be characteristic for specific mitochondrial disorders; for example, the symmetrical hypodensities of brainstem, thalamus, and basal ganglia seen in Leigh syndrome. More often, however, changes strongly suggestive of mitochondrial dysfunction (e.g. basal ganglia calcification) are not unique to any one phenotype.

Even where these studies fail to reveal any specific abnormalities, a strong clinical suspicion of mtDNA disease should prompt further investigation. Where a particular phenotype exists, molecular studies may be possible from blood or epithelial samples (see following discussion). Where such studies are negative, or the phenotype is less clear, muscle biopsy may be warranted.

Laboratory investigations

The laboratory diagnosis of mitochondrial disease is led by clinical phenotype. In view of the very different presentations in children and adults, we have devised two different protocols for the investigation (Figures 13.4 and 13.5). If the history and examination are suggestive of a specific mitochondrial syndrome (e.g. MERRF or LHON), investigation for the common point mutations should be undertaken in blood. For patients with symptoms suggesting MELAS, investigation of m.3243A>G in cells taken from a urine sample is much more reliable, as levels of this mutation may be undetectable in blood [69]. Results of screening for specific mutations should be interpreted with caution as negative results do not exclude other forms of mitochondrial disease in a patient where there is a high index of clinical suspicion.

Histochemical studies

Muscle biopsy is a valuable investigation as mitochondrial defects may be detected by histochemistry or biochemistry. Histochemical techniques are particularly valuable in adults, and one method of detecting mitochondrial accumulation is the Gomori trichrome stain, which shows the subsarcolemmal collection of mitochondria – the so-called ragged red fiber. While this term has persisted, it is far better to evaluate mitochondrial involvement by using specific histochemical enzyme reactions for the mitochondrial enzymes succinate dehydrogenase (SDH) and cytochrome c oxidase (COX). The SDH reaction clearly shows the subsarcolemmal accumulation of mitochondria. The COX reaction is particularly useful in evaluation of mitochondrial disease because COX contains subunits encoded for by both the mitochondrial and nuclear genome. A mosaic pattern of COX activity is highly suggestive of a heteroplasmic mtDNA disorder. In cases where fibers are only partially COX deficient, or only a very low percentage of COX-deficient fibers are present, sequential COX/SDH histochemistry [70] is especially valuable for identifying abnormal fibers that may otherwise go undetected against a background of normal COX activity.

Biochemical analysis of mitochondrial respiratory chain complexes

A biochemical diagnosis of mitochondrial respiratory chain deficiency is invaluable in determining the presence of disease and identifying further molecular genetic testing strategies, particularly in the pediatric

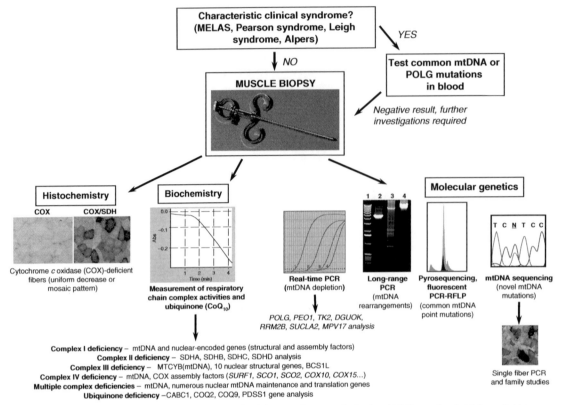

Figure 13.5. Algorithm for investigation in children. As with adult cases of suspected mitochondrial disease, the skeletal muscle biopsy is central to the investigative process. However, in contrast to adults, biochemical analysis of pediatric skeletal muscle is routine and extremely useful in prioritizing the genetic investigations.

population where isolated respiratory chain complex abnormalities are more common (see Figure 13.2). The spectrophotometric assays of enzyme activities in tissue homogenates are widely used and readily adaptable for the study of frozen tissues, allowing samples to be transported to specialist centers for analysis. Blue (or clear)-native polyacrylamide gel electrophoresis allows assessment of intact complexes "in-gel" and is particularly useful for investigating complex V activity (for which there is no spectrophotometric assay) and for assessing whether the assembly of specific respiratory chain complexes is perturbed.

Measurement of ubiquinone

Primary deficiency of ubiquinone (coenzyme Q_{10}) can result in a number of clinical phenotypes including encephalomyopathy, isolated myopathy, Leigh syndrome, and cerebellar ataxia [71]. Early replacement therapy, with a high dose of coenzyme Q_{10}

(20 mg/kg/day), may be of clinical benefit [72,73], and prompt diagnosis by measuring ubiquinone levels in skeletal muscle or blood leukocytes. The phenotype observed will influence the genetic investigations undertaken, but mutations have been observed in a variety of genes, including *COQ2*, *CABC1/ADCK3*, *COQ9*, *PDSS1*, *PDSS2*, *ETFDH*, and *APTX* [74].

Molecular genetic analyses

Pediatric cases are more likely to present with nuclear DNA defects than are adults [75], and nuclear genes encode the vast majority of information necessary for manufacturing the individual structural subunits of the mitochondrial respiratory chain complexes. Mutations have been documented in a number of structural genes for complexes I [76–82], II [83–85], III [86], and IV [87]. In addition, mutations in genes encoding assembly factors and chaperone proteins, essential for the formation of the complexes, have been identified for complexes I [88–92], II [93], III [94–96], IV [97–101], and V [102]. Recently, a mutation in the apoptosis related gene *FASTKD2* has been associated with complex IV deficiency [103]. While some of the resulting clinical problems such as cardiomyopathy, encephalopathy, and Leigh syndrome are indistinguishable from those caused by mtDNA mutations, other clinical phenotypes are unique to nuclear gene mutations: GRACILE (growth retardation, aminoaciduria, cholestasis, iron overload, lactic acidosis, and early death) syndrome caused by mutations in the *BCS1L* gene [95]; LBSL (leukoencephalopathy with brainstem and spinal cord involvement and high brain lactate) syndrome associated with mutations in the mitochondrial aspartyl-tRNA synthetase gene, *DARS2* [104]; or the deafness–dystonia (Mohr–Tranebjaerg) syndrome resulting from mutations in the *TIMM8A* gene [105] are three such examples.

Understanding of nuclear-mitochondrial interactions remains limited, but over the last decade it has become apparent that disruption or malfunction of this interaction has major pathological consequences. The compact mitochondrial genome has no capacity for independent replication and relies on a nuclear-encoded DNA polymerase gamma (pol-γ) helicase (Twinkle) and numerous other proteins, including ANT1 and thymidine phosphorylase (TP), involved in the transport and metabolism of substrates necessary for mtDNA synthesis. Defects in this replication and repair machinery result in either qualitative (multiple deletions of mtDNA), quantitative (mtDNA depletion), or both defects of mtDNA depending on the gene mutated. In some cases (*POLG* and *PEO1*), the site of the mutation within the gene determines the defect observed in mtDNA [106].

Searching for novel, pathogenic mtDNA mutations

The next stage in the investigation of patients who are negative for common mutations often involves the analysis of the entire mitochondrial genome, as this is more efficient and cost effective than screening for rarer mutations on an individual basis. By way of illustration, more than 80% of cases of MELAS are a result of the m.3243A>G tRNA$^{Leu(UUR)}$ gene mutation. However, four other mutations in the same gene (at positions 3252 [64], 3256 [107], 3271 [108], and

3291 [109]), together with others in tRNA^{Phe} ([110], tRNA^{Val} [111], *COIII* [111], and *ND5* [43,112]) have also been described as causes of MELAS. Many laboratories including our own now sequence the entire mitochondrial genome to search for novel mutations [113], or in some cases, to exclude mtDNA involvement before investigating candidate nuclear genes.

Assigning pathogenicity to an mtDNA mutation

The advent of rapid, high-throughput sequencing of mitochondrial genomes for diagnostic and other (e.g. evolutionary biology [114]) purposes has highlighted the extensive mtDNA sequence variation within human populations, with distinct clusters of sequence changes forming well-recognized haplogroups [115]. Because the majority of mtDNA sequence variants are neutral polymorphisms with no pathogenic significance, careful assessment of newly identified mutations must be made to establish a link with human disease. Consequently, DiMauro and Schon (2001) [116] put forward five canonical criteria, which they suggest should be met in order to support a pathogenic role for a novel mtDNA mutation. While these criteria provide valuable advice, the recent discovery of several homoplasmic mtDNA mutations has suggested that other scoring systems may also be valuable in assessing the pathogenic nature of individual mutations [117].

Novel point mutations in mtDNA continue to be described about 22 years after the first report. A disproportionately large number of these point mutations occur in mitochondrial tRNA (*MTT*) genes (MITOMAP: a human mitochondrial genome database: http://www.mitomap.org; 2010). Demonstrating the pathogenicity of novel mutations in these *MTT* genes can be extremely difficult [117], particularly if the mutations are associated with unusual characteristics such as dominance [118], skewed segregation within a tissue, and homoplasmy [119]. Other areas of the mitochondrial genome, such as the *MTND* genes encoding structural subunits of complex I, are also mutation hotspots [120,121]. Interestingly, while some of these mutations are readily transmitted through the germline (e.g. primary LHON mutations), many others are sporadic and recurrent [122,123]. Some of these sporadic mutations are present at high levels of tissue heteroplasmy, but cause severe (fatal), early onset disease, such as Leigh syndrome (subacute necrotizing encephalopathy), which limits their transmission.

Genetic counseling for mitochondrial disorders

For families with nuclear genetic defects, the implications are similar to those of the other genetic diseases described in this book and will not be discussed further. For patients with mtDNA defects, the advice is more difficult and will depend upon the specific mutation detected. Many single mtDNA deletions and some point mutations are sporadic and the risks to other family members or offspring are low, but transmission does occur and should be discussed [124]. Other mutations, especially homoplasmic mtDNA mutations, are transmitted to all maternal offspring and are often present in other maternal family members.

Advice for family members

For patients with point mutations known or likely to be maternally transmitted, the advice is difficult. This is mainly owing to heteroplasmy and the extreme clinical variability witnessed between individuals, even within the same family. The problem is compounded by the tendency for most mtDNA mutations to remain asymptomatic into adulthood, even where high levels of mutation are present and dramatic disease progression may occur thereafter. Despite the absence of a cure for mtDNA disease, a number of common complications are potentially treatable, yet may remain asymptomatic well into their course. Genetic testing is necessary to guide advice regarding prognosis and potential risks to offspring. These benefits must be considered in the context of a disease in which the majority of complications are incurable, and in which available prognostic information is imprecise. All concerned must balance the potential psychological effects of a positive diagnosis in an asymptomatic individual, versus the advantages of appropriate prognostic advice, screening, and the potential for presymptomatic treatment of serious complications. Our practice is to discuss openly the genetic implications with all family members, stressing the potential variability of these disorders and acknowledging the limitations of our current knowledge.

Genetic advice for mothers with mtDNA disease or mtDNA mutation

This falls into several different groups.

1. Genetic counseling: while the maternal transmission of the mtDNA defect is well established, the outcome for specific pregnancies remains unpredictable. For heteroplasmic disorders, this is largely owing to the genetic bottleneck [125,126] that occurs during development, which means that there is considerable variation in the mutated mtDNA load to different offspring [127]. As many of the clinical features are dependent upon the load of mutated to wild-type (or at least the absolute amount of wild-type) mtDNA, then the outcome for each pregnancy remains difficult to predict [128]. For homoplasmic mtDNA disorders, the situation is different because the mutation will be transmitted to all offspring, but even in these patients, the outcome is difficult to predict as there is variable expression [119,129] presumably owing to a combination of environmental and nuclear genetic factors. This leaves considerable uncertainty for families and definitive counseling is not possible; however, studies on patients with mtDNA deletions present data on the transmission of this genetic defect [124].

2. Oocyte donation: donation from an unrelated individual would certainly stop transmission of the mutation to the offspring, but the child would have the nuclear genotype of the donor female. Certainly this is a concern when we have discussed this with our potential mothers, particularly when there is always a chance of having their own normal offspring with low levels of mutated mtDNA. In addition, in most countries there is a considerable delay in obtaining donor oocytes and thus a long waiting period for the mother with an mtDNA mutation.

3. Chorionic villus sampling and amniocentesis: this type of investigation may be of value in mtDNA disorders. In some cases in which this technique has been used, the results have influenced the clinical management [130,131]. In many heteroplasmic mtDNA [18,132] disorders, there is often remarkable tissue-specific differences in the level of heteroplasmy, and thus a reasonable concern is whether a prenatal sample will reflect

the likely outcome for the fetus. The present evidence suggests this should not be a problem [133,134] but, of course, different mtDNA mutations may not all behave similarly. A major problem is that while we might be able to predict the outcome for either very high or very low levels of heteroplasmy, for intermediate levels prediction is extremely difficult and may even vary for the same mutation in different families.

4. Preimplantation genetic diagnosis: this allows analysis of mtDNA from one or two cells from each of several eight-cell embryos, followed by implantation of healthy embryos. The potential value of this technique is clear [135]. Again, there is a concern that individual cells may not be representative of total mutational load, although experiments in heteroplasmic mice have shown the levels of heteroplasmy were virtually identical between blastomeres of 2-, 4-, and 6–8-cell embryos [136]. There may be problems about which embryos should be re-implanted, and thus the number of oocyte stimulation cycles required [137].

5. Prevention of mtDNA transmission: many mtDNA diseases are severe and multisystem attempts to prevent transmission of mtDNA mutations are now being considered. Pro-nuclear transfer is a technique shown to be successful in animal models and allows transfer of both maternal and paternal chromosomes from an oocyte containing an mtDNA mutation to an enucleated normal donor oocyte; biparental nuclear genetic inheritance is preserved, but mtDNA is of donor origin [138]. A variation of this technique, using metaphase II spindle transfer, has been performed successfully in macaque monkeys, confirming its potential for safe use in humans [139].

Management of mitochondrial diseases

The management of patients with mitochondrial disease remains difficult and there is little evidence on which to base decisions. Most of the reports in the literature are anecdotal and there is very little information regarding the natural history of patients with mitochondrial disease. Many of the reported clinical improvements may simply reflect a fluctuating disease course, or a placebo effect, rather than a true result of treatment. Furthermore, mitochondrial disease commonly involves multiple systems and it is vital that management strategies reflect this. A Cochrane review confirmed the lack of suitably controlled clinical trials in this area [140].

Access to a specialist center – national commissioning model of referral and management

The National Commissioning Group (NCG) is a U.K. Government body that promotes equity of access to safe, sustainable, and highly specialized services across the U.K. High levels of clinical expertise are sustained through the development of national centers of excellence, where specialized investigations and assessments can be undertaken. Through the engagement of local care providers, expertise and clinical responsibility can be shared in a spoke-hub model. In England and Scotland, the NCG for Rare Mitochondrial Diseases of Adults and Children has improved equity of access by facilitating the referral of patients and samples to three national centers. The different expertise available at each center has avoided unnecessary duplication of services, encouraged the development of standardized laboratory and clinical practices, and stimulated a process of patient education and public engagement in mitochondrial disease.

Early detection of potentially treatable complications

An important aspect of the care of patients with mitochondrial disease is the prevention or early recognition of treatable clinical features. Diabetes mellitus and cardiac involvement are prime examples. Paradoxically, in some patients the chronicity of a complication may deter both patient and clinician from pursuing therapeutic intervention (e.g. ptosis surgery), despite a strong likelihood of a good outcome. Mitochondrial disease is a multisystem disorder and, as such, requires a relatively holistic approach to management. The major systems commonly involved are dealt with briefly as follows:

1. Ophthalmology – optic atrophy, pigmentary retinopathy, and cataracts can all lead to visual impairment and should be investigated. The apparent vulnerability of the occipital lobes in MELAS may leave some patients with field defects that may not be appreciated owing to coexistent cognitive decline. Ptosis is often tolerated for

surprisingly long periods despite major esthetic or functional consequences. Ptosis surgery can be very effective in the hands of an experienced surgeon but care must be taken to avoid corneal overexposure. This occurs more frequently in cases with poor eye closure owing to weakness of the orbicularis oculi muscle. Complaints of gritty eyes may suggest poor eye closure (irrespective of previous surgery), and this should be treated in the same way as for other causes of facial weakness. In some cases, surgery to elevate the lower lid may be indicated. Severe and intrusive diplopia is uncommon in CPEO but can occur and may require the prescription of prisms, or in severe cases, corrective surgery.

2. Hearing – this is another prominent and neglected feature of mitochondrial disease. In certain families, (ribosomal mtDNA) mutation deafness only occurs in the presence of aminoglycoside antibiotics, which clearly should be avoided [141]. In those patients with significant hearing loss, digital hearing aids help considerably, but in some patients, cochlear implants are needed.

3. Swallowing – weakness of the palate and bulbar musculature seems common in the later stages of CPEO. Mild dysphagia often progresses to nasal regurgitation and dysphonia. Cerebellar involvement and incoordination of the swallowing mechanism can be an additional problem in some phenotypes. Food may be aspirated and may compound preexisting respiratory impairment (see following discussion). Speech and swallowing assessments are important in this group. For those in whom aspiration is a recurrent problem, or nutritional status appears adversely affected, percutaneous endoscopic gastrostomy (PEG) may be indicated.

4. Respiratory – complications usually occur in the context of an advanced myopathy, in particular when axial weakness is pronounced. Associated bulbar weakness and swallowing difficulties can compound the situation. It should be remembered, however, that many patients with significantly reduced respiratory function may lack specific respiratory symptoms if motor activity is significantly reduced because of a proximal myopathy. The forced vital capacity (FVC) should, therefore, be measured annually in all patients with a significant myopathy, whether at the bedside or via formal pulmonary function tests. A supine FVC will help to identify diaphragmatic weakness. Respiratory muscle weakness will be relevant to any future anesthetic assessments and may warrant discussion regarding annual influenza immunization. Both nocturnal hypoventilation and obstructive sleep apnea can occur in these patients, and a compatible history (morning headaches, nausea, excessive daytime somnolescence) should be sought and overnight oximetry performed for confirmation. Formal respiratory referral may be warranted.

5. Cardiac – typically asymptomatic to an advanced stage of disease, cardiac involvement is a major indication for annual screening, even in asymptomatic mutation carriers. Complete heart block (and asystole) is most commonly reported in Kearns–Sayre syndrome but can occur in CPEO and other phenotypes. Re-entrant supraventicular tachycardias (e.g. Wolff–Parkinson–White syndrome) and concentric left ventricular hypertrophy (LVH) also occur, perhaps most frequently in MERRF and MELAS, respectively, and the latter may progress to a severe hypertrophic cardiomyopathy (HCM), left ventricular failure, and death. In the presence of LVH or HCM, β-blockade or ACE inhibitor therapy may be indicated, although no trials of their use in mitochondrial disease exist. We recommend an EKG and ECHO at baseline for all patients, with annual screening thereafter depending on changes and severity of the mitochondrial disease. Formal cardiology input is invaluable, particularly where such input incorporates prior experience of mitochondrial diseases.

6. Gastrointestinal – a variety of symptoms are common to and often overlooked in mitochondrial disease. These range from anorexia and failure to thrive in infancy, to chronic constipation in the elderly. In many patients, and in particular those with the m.3243A>G mutation, gastrointestinal symptoms can be severe, but often remain in the background, overshadowed by neurological features. Alternating bowel habits, and intermittent abdominal pain and bloating, often are given the label of irritable bowel syndrome. In other cases, investigations may have been extensive and invasive, on occasion to the extent of bowel

resection, without a diagnosis being reached. This is not surprising as reference to mitochondrial disease cannot be found in most gastroenterology textbooks, unless in acknowledgment of a well-defined syndrome such as MNGIE. Gastric stasis, pseudo-obstruction, and severe constipation should all be considered in patients with mtDNA disease, especially those with m.3243A>G mutations. Regular laxatives and enemas often are essential in this group.

7. Seizures – epilepsy is a prominent feature in some patients, sometimes associated with myoclonus. The only drug that should be avoided, if possible, is sodium valproate as this compound enters mitochondria and can inhibit mitochondrial oxidation reactions [142]. It is reasonable to be fairly aggressive in the treatment of epilepsy in this group of patients as seizures may induce brain damage in an already vulnerable brain. In patients with *POLG* gene mutations and an Alper's phenotype, valproate can induce liver failure.

8. Diabetes – impaired glucose tolerance is an integral part of some mitochondrial phenotypes (e.g. m.3243A>G and m.14709T>C mutations) but has been described in association with the majority of mutations. Diabetes onset may be atypical, fitting neither the classical type 1 nor type 2 pattern. Glucose intolerance may be diet or tablet controlled initially, and often occurs in individuals of normal or low body mass index. In some patients, the diabetes rapidly progresses to insulin dependence (often within 12 months of diagnosis). In others, diet or tablets may suffice, with the sulfonylureas appearing particularly effective. We advocate yearly screening for glucose intolerance, by way of fasting blood glucose. An oral glucose tolerance test and glycosylated hemoglobin measurement will detect additional individuals, if performed at baseline. In those pedigrees at particular risk of diabetes, presymptomatic dietary advice may help to delay the development of clinical glucose intolerance. Gestational diabetes is also likely to be more prevalent in this group.

9. Biochemical – a number of biochemical parameters may be deranged in mitochondrial disease. These are rarely severe but warrant acknowledgment. Hyponatremia may occur in patients with the m.3243A>G mutation. Renal disease has also been described in a number of mitochondrial diseases and may cause more widespread biochemical derangement. Calcium levels should be checked routinely, as hypoparathyroidism can occur and nonspecific symptoms may be attributed to the underlying mitochondrial dysfunction. Lactic acidosis is a feature of many phenotypes, but can be severe and life threatening, particularly in pediatric presentations and in the MELAS syndrome. Uncuffed serum lactate levels, in addition to an arterial blood gas sample, should be considered in cases exhibiting general malaise, vomiting, or encephalopathy (which may be subtle, initially presenting as apathy, blunted affect, or personality change). These tests should also be done routinely in cases of exercise intolerance or unexplained dyspnea.

10. Obstetric/surgical – it is important to stress to patients the need to declare their condition when contemplating future pregnancies or surgical procedures. This allows early discussion of genetic issues and the options available. Some patients with myopathy may have difficulty carrying a fetus to full term or pursuing a normal vaginal delivery. In some mutations, hypertension and glucose intolerance may be more common in pregnancy. Several features of mitochondrial DNA disease (e.g. LVH, respiratory insufficiency, bulbar symptoms) may complicate a surgical procedure and, more typically, the application of the anesthetic.

11. Supportive – the multisystem involvement of mitochondrial disease is sufficiently diffuse as to warrant a multidisciplinary approach to management, perhaps more so than in any other neurological disorder. The involvement of other medical and surgical specialties has been touched upon already, but an underestimated component of management is the provision of adequate support mechanisms for the disability that results from mitochondrial disease. Speech, occupational therapy, and physical therapy input is vital to many patients. Mobility issues can be complex, and require an understanding of the underlying pathology. Few other conditions combine the effects of myopathy, neuropathy, and cerebellar ataxia to limit upper and lower limb function to such an extent. Irrespective of the number of

systems involved, work and home circumstances as well as available benefits and local support services need to be addressed. The gradual onset of symptoms in many patients may disguise the desperate need for such input. The problem appears further compounded by a widespread paucity of information regarding mitochondrial disease, such that other health professionals and those involved in providing medical assessments may inadvertently base their judgments on inaccurate clinical and genetic information. The increasing profile of mitochondrial disorders and the development of specialist mitochondrial centers hopefully will provide much needed support for these patients.

Specific disease treatments and vitamin supplementation

Ubiquinone is specifically indicated for those rare patients in whom a primary deficiency of ubiquinone is suspected or proven [143–145]. For the other patients with mitochondrial disease, there are many anecdotal reports of improvement with ubiquinone (also known as coenzyme Q_{10}) and positive results from small open-label trials (doses vary from 90 to 240 mg/day). However, while there may be some improvements in surrogate markers such as lactate and pyruvate, there is little evidence for altering the clinical course of the disease. Ubiquinone has been used in the treatment of Friedreich's ataxia, a condition with mitochondrial involvement, with some evidence of clinical and biochemical improvement [146]. Idebenone, a short-chain quinone analogue, has also been used in patients with mitochondrial disease including Leber's hereditary optic neuropathy (5 mg/kg/day), and some clinicians prefer this preparation [147], although there is very little evidence to support the use of one quinone analogue over another.

Dichloroacetate (DCA) is an activator of pyruvate dehydrogenase and has been proposed in the treatment of many different conditions associated with lactic acidosis. There is good evidence that DCA lowers lactic acid in blood, but the evidence for prolonged clinical improvement is less clear [148] and, in clinical trials, it has been shown to be toxic [149].

Some clinicians try nicotinamide in children with lactic acidosis owing to respiratory chain disease (50–75 mg/kg/day) and report some improvement in biochemical parameters. There is a rationale for using riboflavin in patients with complex I and complex II deficiency as both complexes contain flavoproteins. Riboflavin responsive inborn errors of metabolism have been reported, but there is little evidence that this includes respiratory chain disease. Treatment is often tried in patients with complex I deficiency for up to six months. Vitamins E, C, and K have also been tried but, apart from anecdotal reports, there is no evidence of sustained clinical improvement.

In an attempt to replace thymidine phosphorylase, bone marrow transplantation has been used in patients with MNGIE, and has been shown to correct the biochemical abnormalities associated with the condition [150]. Prescription of arginine for both acute treatment of stroke-like episodes and as stroke prophylaxis is gaining favor following reports of success in the Japanese population [151]. However, the frequency of stroke-like episodes in these patients is widely variable and the results of these initial studies have yet to be replicated in placebo controlled double-blind trials.

Manipulating mtDNA mutation levels through exercise training

Insufficient evidence means that we are currently unable to argue for or against specific exercise regimens in mtDNA disease. In healthy individuals, it is known that lack of exercise (deconditioning) leads to an overall reduction in mitochondrial enzyme activity, whereas endurance training prompts an improvement in these parameters. Resistance training stimulates the incorporation of satellite cells (and their mtDNA) into existing muscle fibers. It is postulated that in sporadic mutations (such as single mtDNA deletions) this may lead to an overall reduction in the proportion of mutated mtDNA versus wild-type, as satellite cells contain low or negligible levels of mutated mtDNA. In all mutations, it is hypothesized that the overall amount of wild-type mtDNA is the crucial factor modulating respiratory chain function, rather than the relative proportion of wild-type versus mutated mtDNA. Endurance training may, therefore, improve function by increasing wild-type mtDNA levels. Concerns do exist, however, that the mutated mtDNA molecule may be amplified preferentially, and that this increase may become clinically relevant following deconditioning. Studies to date have been small [152,153], and a recent study has not shown any change in mutation load while there was a significant improvement in exercise tolerance in patients with single mtDNA deletions [154,155].

Conclusions

Mitochondrial disease is now widely accepted as a common genetic cause of disease. Much has changed over the last 22 years since the first genetic defect in the mitochondrial genome was identified, when such disorders were felt to be rare. Over the recent years, presentations of mtDNA disease have been reported by virtually every medical specialty, but most frequently in neurological practice. Conservative estimations of prevalence continue to increase, and are likely to continue doing so as our understanding and diagnostic techniques evolve.

The contribution of both nuclear and mitochondrial DNA mutations accounts for the unparalleled spectrum of disease seen in these multisystem disorders. Both the investigation and management of these disorders is complex, and best conducted in a specialist center with access to both laboratory and clinical expertise of mitochondrial disease. Although the genetic defect is currently incurable, this should not overshadow the many aspects of mitochondrial disease that are eminently treatable, or those the impact of which may be minimized through early detection and directed management strategies. The major challenge in mitochondrial disorders, as in so many neurogenetic diseases, is to prevent the transmission and to develop effective therapies for those patients affected clinically.

References

1. Anderson S, Bankier AT, Barrell BG, et al. Sequence and organization of the human mitochondrial genome. Nature 1981; 290: 457–465.

2. Lightowlers RN, Chinnery PF, Turnbull DM, Howell N. Mammalian mitochondrial genetics: heredity, heteroplasmy and disease. Trends Genet 1997; 13: 450–455.

3. DiMauro S, Schon EA. Mitochondrial respiratory-chain diseases. N Engl J Med 2003; 348: 2656–2668.

4. Schwartz M, Vissing J. Paternal inheritance of mitochondrial DNA. N Engl J Med 2002; 347: 576–580.

5. Taylor RW, McDonnell MT, Blakely EL, et al. Genotypes from patients indicate no paternal mitochondrial DNA contribution. Ann Neurol 2003; 54: 521–524.

6. Filosto M, Mancuso M, Vives-Bauza C, et al. Lack of paternal inheritance of muscle mitochondrial DNA in sporadic mitochondrial myopathies. Ann Neurol 2003; 54: 524–526.

7. Schwartz M, Vissing J. No evidence for paternal inheritance of mtDNA in patients with sporadic mtDNA mutations. J Neurol Sci 2004; 218: 99–101.

8. Samuels DC, Schon EA, Chinnery PF. Two direct repeats cause most human mtDNA deletions. Trends Genet 2004; 20: 393–398.

9. Schon EA, Rizzuto R, Moraes CT, et al. A direct repeat is a hotspot for large-scale deletion of human mitochondrial DNA. Science 1989; 244: 346–349.

10. Macmillan C, Kirkham T, Fu K, et al. Pedigree analysis of French Canadian families with T14484C Leber's hereditary optic neuropathy. Neurology 1998; 50: 417–422.

11. Skladal D, Bernier FP, Halliday JL, Thorburn DR. Birth prevalence of mitochondrial respiratory chain defects in children. J Inherit Metab Dis 2000; 23: 138.

12. Majamaa K, Moilanen JS, Uimonen S, et al. Epidemiology of A3243G, the mutation for mitochondrial encephalomyopathy, lactic acidosis, and strokelike episodes: prevalence of the mutation in an adult population. Am J Hum Genet 1998; 63: 447–454.

13. Chinnery PF, Johnson MA, Wardell TM, et al. Epidemiology of pathogenic mitochondrial DNA mutations. Ann Neurol 2000; 48: 188–193.

14. Schaefer AM, McFarland R, Blakely EL, et al. Prevalence of mitochondrial DNA disease in adults. Ann Neurol 2008; 63: 35–39.

15. Elliott HR, Samuels DC, Eden JA, et al. Pathogenic mitochondrial DNA mutations are common in the general population. Am J Hum Genet 2008; 83: 254–260.

16. Bitner-Glindzicz M, Pembrey M, Duncan A, et al. Prevalence of mitochondrial 1555A–>G mutation in European children. N Engl J Med 2009; 360: 640–642.

17. Vandebona H, Mitchell P, Manwaring N, et al. Prevalence of mitochondrial 1555A–>G mutation in adults of European descent. N Engl J Med 2009; 360: 642–644.

18. Moraes CT, DiMauro S, Zeviani M, et al. Mitochondrial DNA deletions in progressive external ophthalmoplegia and Kearns–Sayre syndrome. N Engl J Med 1989; 320: 1293–1299.

19. Laforet P, Lombes A, Eymard B, et al. Chronic progressive external ophthalmoplegia with ragged-red fibers: clinical, morphological and genetic investigations in 43 patients. Neuromuscul Disord 1995; 5: 399–413.

20. Zeviani M, Sevidei S, Gallera C, *et al.* An autosomal dominant disorder with multiple deletions of mitochondrial DNA starting in the D-loop region. *Nature* 1989; **339**: 309–311.

21. Bohlega S, Tanji K, Santorelli FM, *et al.* Multiple mitochondrial DNA deletions associated with autosomal recessive ophthalmoplegia and severe cardiomyopathy. *Neurology* 1996; **46**: 1329–1334.

22. Kaukonen J, Juselius JK, Tiranti V, *et al.* Role of adenine nucleotide translocator 1 in mtDNA maintenance. *Science* 2000; **289**: 782–785.

23. Spelbrink JN, Li FY, Tiranti V, *et al.* Human mitochondrial DNA deletions associated with mutations in the gene encoding Twinkle, a phage T7 gene 4-like protein localised in mitochondria. *Nat Genet* 2001; **28**: 223–231.

24. Van Goethem G, Dermaut B, Lofgren A, *et al.* Mutation of POLG is associated with progressive external ophthalmoplegia characterized by mtDNA deletions. *Nat Genet* 2001; **28**: 211–212.

25. Casali C, Bonifati V, Santorelli FM, *et al.* Mitochondrial myopathy, parkinsonism, and multiple mtDNA deletions in a Sephardic Jewish family. *Neurology* 2001; **56**: 802–805.

26. Siciliano G, Mancuso M, Ceravolo R, *et al.* Mitochondrial DNA rearrangements in young onset parkinsonism: two case reports. *J Neurol Neurosurg Psychiatry* 2001; **71**: 685–687.

27. Mancuso M, Filosto M, Bellan M, *et al.* POLG mutations causing ophthalmoplegia, sensorimotor polyneuropathy, ataxia, and deafness. *Neurology* 2004; **62**: 316–318.

28. Nishino I, Spinazzola A, Hirano M. Thymidine phosphorylase gene mutations in MNGIE, a human mitochondrial disorder. *Science* 1999; **283**: 689–692.

29. Spinazzola A, Marti R, Nishino I, *et al.* Altered thymidine metabolism due to defects of thymidine phosphorylase. *J Biol Chem* 2002; **277**: 4128–4133.

30. Rahman S, Poulton J. Diagnosis of mitochondrial DNA depletion syndromes. *Arch Dis Child* 2009; **94**: 3–5.

31. Alpers BJ. Diffuse progressive degeneration of gray matter of cerebrum. *Arch Neurol Psychiatry* 1931; **25**: 469–505.

32. Huttenlocher PR, Solitare GB, Adams G. Infantile diffuse cerebral degeneration with hepatic cirrhosis. *Arch Neurol* 1976; **33**: 186–192.

33. McFarland R, Hudson G, Taylor RW, *et al.* Reversible valproate hepatotoxicity due to mutations in mitochondrial DNA polymerase gamma (POLG1). *Arch Dis Child* 2008; **93**: 151–153.

34. Wolf NI, Rahman S, Schmitt B, *et al.* Status epilepticus in children with Alpers' disease caused by POLG1 mutations: EEG and MRI features. *Epilepsia* 2009; **50**: 1596–1607.

35. Chan SS, Copeland WC. DNA polymerase gamma and mitochondrial disease: understanding the consequence of POLG mutations. *Biochim Biophys Acta* 2009; **1787**: 312–319.

36. Mandel H, Szargel R, Labay V, *et al.* The deoxyguanosine kinase gene is mutated in individuals with depleted hepatocerebral mitochondrial DNA. *Nat Genet* 2001; **29**: 337–341.

37. Bourdon A, Minai L, Serre V, *et al.* Mutation of RRM2B, encoding p53-controlled ribonucleotide reductase (p53R2), causes severe mitochondrial DNA depletion. *Nat Genet* 2007; **39**: 776–780.

38. Spinazzola A, Viscomi C, Fernandez-Vizarra E, *et al.*

MPV17 encodes an inner mitochondrial membrane protein and is mutated in infantile hepatic mitochondrial DNA depletion. *Nat Genet* 2006; **38**: 570–575.

39. Saada A, Shaag A, Mandel H, *et al.* Mutant mitochondrial thymidine kinase in mitochondrial DNA depletion myopathy. *Nat Genet* 2001; **29**: 342–344.

40. Elpeleg O, Miller C, Hershkovitz E, *et al.* Deficiency of the ADP-forming succinyl-CoA synthase activity is associated with encephalomyopathy and mitochondrial DNA depletion. *Am J Hum Genet* 2005; **76**: 1081–1086.

41. Ostergaard E, Christensen E, Kristensen E, *et al.* Deficiency of the alpha subunit of succinate-coenzyme A ligase causes fatal infantile lactic acidosis with mitochondrial DNA depletion. *Am J Hum Genet* 2007; **81**: 383–387.

42. Goto Y, Nonaka I, Horai S. A mutation in the tRNA(Leu) (UUR) gene associated with the MELAS subgroup of mitochondrial encephalomyopathies. *Nature* 1990; **348**: 651–653.

43. Santorelli FM, Tanji K, Kulikova R, *et al.* Identification of a novel mutation in the mtDNA ND5 gene associated with MELAS. *Biochem Biophys Res Commun* 1997; **238**: 326–328.

44. van den Ouweland JWM, Lemkes HHPJ, Ruitenbeek K. Mutation in mitochondrial tRNA$^{Leu(UUR)}$ gene in a large pedigree with maternally transmitted type II diabetes mellitus and deafness. *Nat Genet* 1992; **1**: 368–371.

45. Moraes CT, Ciacci F, Silvestri G, *et al.* Atypical clinical presentations associated with the MELAS mutation at position 3243 of human mitochondrial DNA. *Neuromuscul Disord* 1993; **3**: 43–50.

46. Ciafaloni E, Ricci E, Shanske S, *et al.* MELAS: clinical features,

biochemistry, and molecular genetics. *Ann Neurol* 1992; **31**: 391–398.

47. Shoffner JM, Lott MT, Lezza AM, *et al*. Myoclonic epilepsy and ragged-red fiber disease (MERRF) is associated with a mitochondrial DNA tRNA(Lys) mutation. *Cell* 1990; **61**: 931–937.

48. Silvestri G, Moraes CT, Shanske S. A new mtDNA mutation in the tRNA(Lys) gene associated with myoclonic epilepsy and ragged-red fibers (MERRF). *Am J Hum Genet* 1992; **51**: 1213–1217.

49. Larsson NG, Tulinius MH, Holme E, Oldfors A. Pathogenetic aspects of the A8344G mutation of mitochondrial DNA associated with MERRF syndrome and multiple symmetric lipomas. *Muscle Nerve* 1995; **3**: S102–S106.

50. Traff J, Holme E, Ekbom K, Nilsson BY. Ekbom's syndrome of photomyoclonus, cerebellar ataxia and cervical lipoma is associated with the tRNA(Lys) A8344G mutation in mitochondrial DNA. *Acta Neurol Scand* 1995; **92**: 394–397.

51. Leigh D. Subacute necrotizing encephalomyelopathy in an infant. *J Neurol Neurosurg Psychiatry* 1951; **1951**: 216–221.

52. Zhu Z, Yao J, Johns T, *et al*. SURF1, encoding a factor involved in the biogenesis of cytochrome c oxidase, is mutated in Leigh syndrome. *Nat Genet* 1998; **20**: 337–343.

53. Rahman S, Blok RB, Dahl HH, *et al*. Leigh syndrome: clinical features and biochemical and DNA abnormalities. *Ann Neurol* 1996; **39**: 343–351.

54. Holt IJ, Harding AE, Petty RK, Morgan-Hughes JA. A new mitochondrial disease associated with mitochondrial DNA heteroplasmy. *Am J Hum Genet* 1990; **46**: 428–433.

55. Wallace DC, Singh G, Lott MT, *et al*. Mitochondrial DNA mutation associated with Leber's hereditary optic neuropathy. *Science* 1988; **242**: 1427–1430.

56. Taylor RW, Jobling MS, Turnbull DM, Chinnery PF. Frequency of rare mitochondrial DNA mutations in patients with suspected Leber's hereditary optic neuropathy. *J Med Genet* 2003; **40**: e85.

57. Newman NJ, Lott MT, Wallace DC. The clinical characteristics of pedigrees of Leber's hereditary optic neuropathy with the 11778 mutation. *Am J Ophthalmol* 1991; **111**: 750–762.

58. Johns DR, Heher KL, Miller NR, Smith KH. Leber's hereditary optic neuropathy. Clinical manifestations of the 14484 mutation. *Arch Ophthalmol* 1993; **111**: 495–498.

59. Harding AE, Sweeney MG, Miller DH, *et al*. Occurrence of a multiple sclerosis-like illness in women who have a Leber's hereditary optic neuropathy mitochondrial DNA mutation. *Brain* 1992; **115**: 979–989.

60. Hanna MG, Nelson I, Sweeney MG, *et al*. Congenital encephalomyopathy and adult-onset myopathy and diabetes mellitus: different phenotypic associations of a new heteroplasmic mtDNA tRNA glutamic acid mutation. *Am J Hum Genet* 1995; **56**: 1026–1033.

61. Hao H, Bonilla E, Manfredi G, DiMauro S, Moraes CT. Segregation patterns of a novel mutation in the mitochondrial tRNA glutamic acid gene associated with myopathy and diabetes mellitus. *Am J Hum Genet* 1995; **56**: 1017–1025.

62. Ballinger SW, Shoffner JM, Hedaya EV, *et al*. Maternally transmitted diabetes and deafness associated with a 10.4 kb mitochondrial DNA deletion. *Nat Genet* 1992; **1**: 11–15.

63. Harvey JN, Barnett D. Endocrine dysfunction in Kearns–Sayre syndrome. *Clin Endocrinol (Oxf)* 1992; **37**: 97–103.

64. Morten KJ, Cooper JM, Brown GK, *et al*. A new point mutation associated with mitochondrial encephalomyopathy. *Hum Mol Genet* 1993; **2**: 2081–2087.

65. de Lonlay P, Valnot I, Barrientos A, *et al*. A mutant mitochondrial respiratory chain assembly protein causes complex III deficiency in patients with tubulopathy, encephalopathy and liver failure. *Nat Genet* 2001; **29**: 57–60.

66. Cheong HI, Chae JH, Kim JS, *et al*. Hereditary glomerulopathy associated with a mitochondrial tRNA(Leu) gene mutation. *Pediatr Nephrol* 1999; **13**: 477–480.

67. Richardson C, Smith T, Schaefer A, Turnbull D, Griffiths P. Ocular motility findings in chronic progressive external ophthalmoplegia. *Eye (London)* 2004; **19**: 258–263.

68. Jackson MJ, Schaefer JA, Johnson MA, *et al*. Presentation and clinical investigation of mitochondrial respiratory chain disease. *Brain* 1995; **118**: 339–357.

69. McDonnell MT, Schaefer AM, Blakely EL, *et al*. Noninvasive diagnosis of the 3243A>G mitochondrial DNA mutation using urinary epithelial cells. *Eur J Hum Genet* 2004; **12**: 778–781.

70. Sciacco M, Bonilla E, Schon EA, *et al*. Distribution of wild-type and common deletion forms of mtDNA in normal and respiration-deficient muscle fibers from patients with mitochondrial myopathy. *Hum Mol Genet* 1994; **3**: 13–19.

71. Gempel K, Topaloglu H, Talim B, *et al*. The myopathic form of coenzyme Q10 deficiency is caused by mutations in the electron-transferring-flavoprotein

dehydrogenase (ETFDH) gene. *Brain* 2007; **130**: 2037–2044.

72. Montini G, Malaventura C, Salviati L. Early coenzyme Q10 supplementation in primary coenzyme Q10 deficiency. *N Engl J Med* 2008; **358**: 2849–2850.

73. Rotig A, Appelkvist EL, Geromel V, *et al.* Quinone-responsive multiple respiratory-chain dysfunction due to widespread coenzyme Q10 deficiency. *Lancet* 2000; **356**: 391–395.

74. Quinzii CM, Lopez LC, Naini A, DiMauro S, Hirano M. Human CoQ10 deficiencies. *Biofactors* 2008; **32**: 113–118.

75. Shoubridge EA. Nuclear genetic defects of oxidative phosphorylation. *Hum Mol Genet* 2001; **10**: 2277–2284.

76. Loeffen J, Smeitink J, Treipels R, *et al.* The first nuclear-encoded complex I mutation in a patient with Leigh syndrome. *Am J Hum Genet* 1998; **63**: 1598–1608.

77. Benit P, Chretien D, Kadhom N, *et al.* Large-scale deletion and point mutations of the nuclear NDUFV1 and NDUFS1 genes in mitochondrial complex I deficiency. *Am J Hum Genet* 2001; **68**: 1344–1352.

78. Loeffen J, Elpeleg O, Smeitink J, *et al.* Mutations in the complex I *NDUFS2* gene of patients with cardiomyopathy and encephalomyopathy. *Ann Neurol* 2001; **49**: 195–201.

79. Benit P, Beugnot R, Chretien D, *et al.* Mutant NDUFV2 subunit of mitochondrial complex I causes early onset hypertrophic cardiomyopathy and encephalopathy. *Hum Mutat* 2003; **21**: 582–586.

80. Van den Heuvel L, Ruitenbeek W, Smeets R, *et al.* Demonstration of a new pathogenic mutation in human complex I deficiency: a 5-bp duplication in the nuclear gene encoding the 18kD (AQDQ)

subunit. *Am J Hum Genet* 1998; **62**: 262–268.

81. Procaccio V, Wallace DC. Late-onset Leigh syndrome in a patient with mitochondrial complex I NDUFS8 mutations. *Neurology* 2004; **62**: 1899–1901.

82. Benit P, Slama A, Cartault F, *et al.* Mutant NDUFS3 subunit of mitochondrial complex I causes Leigh syndrome. *J Med Genet* 2004; **41**: 14–17.

83. Bougeron T, Rustin P, Birch-Machin M, *et al.* A mutation of nuclear succinate dehydrogenase gene results in mitochondrial respiratory chain deficiency. *Nat Genet* 1995; **11**: 144–149.

84. Astuti D, Douglas F, Lennard TW, *et al.* Germline SDHD mutation in familial phaeochromocytoma. *Lancet* 2001; **357**: 1181–1182.

85. Niemann S, Muller U. Mutations in SDHC cause autosomal dominant paraganglioma, type 3. *Nat Genet* 2000; **26**: 268–270.

86. Haut S, Brivet M, Touati G, *et al.* A deletion in the human QP-C gene causes a complex III deficiency resulting in hypoglycaemia and lactic acidosis. *Hum Genet* 2003; **113**: 118–122.

87. Massa V, Fernandez-Vizarra E, Alshahwan S, *et al.* Severe infantile encephalomyopathy caused by a mutation in COX6B1, a nucleus-encoded subunit of cytochrome c oxidase. *Am J Hum Genet* 2008; **82**: 1281–1289.

88. Ogilvie I, Kennaway NG, Shoubridge EA. A molecular chaperone for mitochondrial complex I assembly is mutated in a progressive encephalopathy. *J Clin Invest* 2005; **115**: 2784–2792.

89. Dunning CJ, McKenzie M, Sugiana C, *et al.* Human CIA30 is involved in the early assembly of mitochondrial complex I and mutations in its gene cause

disease. *EMBO J* 2007; **26**: 3227–3237.

90. Sugiana C, Pagliarini DJ, McKenzie M, *et al.* Mutation of C20orf7 disrupts complex I assembly and causes lethal neonatal mitochondrial disease. *Am J Hum Genet* 2008; **83**: 468–478.

91. Saada A, Vogel RO, Hoefs SJ, *et al.* Mutations in NDUFAF3 (C3ORF60), encoding an NDUFAF4 (C6ORF66)-interacting complex I assembly protein, cause fatal neonatal mitochondrial disease. *Am J Hum Genet* 2009; **84**: 718–727.

92. Saada A, Edvardson S, Rapoport M, *et al.* C6ORF66 is an assembly factor of mitochondrial complex I. *Am J Hum Genet* 2008; **82**: 32–38.

93. Ghezzi D, Goffrini P, Uziel G, *et al.* SDHAF1, encoding a LYR complex-II specific assembly factor, is mutated in SDH-defective infantile leukoencephalopathy. *Nat Genet* 2009; **41**: 654–656.

94. de Lonlay P, Valnot I, Barrientos A, *et al.* A mutant mitochondrial respiratory chain assembly protein causes complex III deficiency in patients with tubulopathy, encephalopathy and liver failure. *Nat Genet* 2001; **29**: 57–60.

95. Visapaa I, Fellman V, Vesa J, *et al.* GRACILE syndrome, a lethal metabolic disorder with iron overload, is caused by a point mutation in BCS1L. *Am J Hum Genet* 2002; **71**: 863–876.

96. Ramos-Arroyo MA, Hualde J, Ayechu A, *et al.* Clinical and biochemical spectrum of mitochondrial complex III deficiency caused by mutations in the BCS1L gene. *Clin Genet* 2009; **75**: 585–587.

97. Zhu Z, Yao J, Johns T, *et al.* SURF1, encoding a factor involved in the biogenesis of cytochrome c oxidase, is mutated

in Leigh syndrome. *Nat Genet* 1998; **20**: 337–343.

98. Tiranti V, Hoertnagel K, Carrozzo R, *et al*. Mutations of SURF-1 in Leigh disease associated with cytochrome c oxidase deficiency. *Am J Hum Genet* 1998; **63**: 1609–1621.

99. Valnot I, Ormond S, Gigarel N. Mutations of the SCO 1 gene in mitochondrial cytochrome c oxidase (COX) deficiency with neonatal-onset hepatic failure and encephalopathy. *Am J Hum Genet* 2000; **67**: 1104–1109.

100. Papadopoulou LC, Sue CM, Davidson M. Fatal infantile cardioencephalomyopathy with cytochrome c oxidase (COX) deficiency due to mutations in SCO2, a human COX assembly gene. *Nat Genet* 1999; **23**: 333–337.

101. Mootha VK, Lepage P, Miller K, *et al*. Identification of a gene causing human cytochrome c oxidase deficiency by integrative genomics. *Proc Natl Acad Sci USA* 2003; **100**: 605–610.

102. De Meirleir L, Seneca S, Lissens W, *et al*. Respiratory chain complex V deficiency due to a mutation in the assembly gene ATP12. *J Med Genet* 2004; **41**: 120–124.

103. Ghezzi D, Saada A, D'Adamo P, *et al*. FASTKD2 nonsense mutation in an infantile mitochondrial encephalomyopathy associated with cytochrome c oxidase deficiency. *Am J Hum Genet* 2008; **83**: 415–423.

104. van der Knaap MS, van der Voorn P, Barkhof F, *et al*. A new leukoencephalopathy with brainstem and spinal cord involvement and high lactate. *Ann Neurol* 2003; **53**: 252–258.

105. Jin H, May M, Tranebjaerg L, *et al*. A novel X-linked gene, DDP, shows mutations in families with deafness (DFN-1), dystonia, mental deficiency and blindness. *Nat Genet* 1996; **14**: 177–180.

106. Horvath R, Hudson G, Ferrari G, *et al*. Phenotypic spectrum associated with mutations of the mitochondrial polymerase gamma gene. *Brain* 2006; **129**: 1674–1684.

107. Moraes CT, Ciacci F, Bonilla E, *et al*. Two novel pathogenic mitochondrial DNA mutations affecting organelle number and protein synthesis. Is the tRNA(Leu (UUR)) gene an etiologic hot spot? *J Clin Invest* 1993; **92**: 2906–2915.

108. Goto Y-I, Nonaka I, Horai S. A new mtDNA mutation associated with mitochondrial myopathy, encephalomyopathy, lactic acidosis and stroke-like episodes (MELAS). *Biochem Biophys Acta* 1991; **1097**: 238–240.

109. Goto Y, Tsugane K, Tanabe Y, *et al*. A new point mutation at nucleotide pair 3291 of the mitochondrial tRNA(Leu(UUR)) gene in a patient with mitochondrial myopathy, encephalopathy, lactic acidosis, and stroke-like episodes (MELAS). *Biochem Biophys Res Commun* 1994; **202**: 1624–1630.

110. Hanna MG, Nelson IP, Morgan-Hughes JA, Wood NW. MELAS: a new disease associated mitochondrial DNA mutation and evidence for further genetic heterogeneity. *J Neurol Neurosurg Psychiatry* 1998; **65**: 512–517.

111. Manfredi G, Schon EA, Moraes CT, *et al*. A new mutation associated with MELAS is located in a mitochondrial DNA polypeptide-coding gene. *Neuromuscul Disord* 1995; **5**: 391–398.

112. Corona P, Antozzi C, Carrara F, *et al*. A novel mtDNA mutation in the ND5 subunit of complex I in two MELAS patients. *Ann Neurol* 2001; **49**: 106–110.

113. Taylor RW, Taylor GA, Durham SE, Turnbull DM. The determination of complete human mitochondrial DNA sequences in single cells: implications for the study of somatic mitochondrial DNA point mutations. *Nucleic Acids Res* 2001; **29**: E74–4.

114. Ingman M, Kaessmann H, Paabo S, Gyllensten U. Mitochondrial genome variation and the origin of modern humans. *Nature* 2000; **408**: 708–713.

115. Herrnstadt C, Elson JL, Fahy E, *et al*. Reduced-median-network analysis of complete mitochondrial DNA coding-region sequences for the major African, Asian, and European haplogroups. *Am J Hum Genet* 2002; **70**: 1152–1171.

116. DiMauro S, Schon EA. Mitochondrial DNA mutations in human disease. *Am J Med Genet* 2001; **106**: 18–26.

117. McFarland R, Elson JL, Taylor RW, Howell N, Turnbukk DM. Assigning pathogenicity to mitochondrial tRNA mutations: when "definitely maybe" is not good enough. *Trends Genet* 2004; **20**: 591–596.

118. Sacconi S, Salviati L, Nishigaki Y, *et al*. A functionally dominant mitochondrial DNA mutation. *Hum Mol Genet* 2008; **17**: 1814–1820.

119. McFarland R, Clark KM, Morris AA, *et al*. Multiple neonatal deaths due to a homoplasmic mitochondrial DNA mutation. *Nat Genet* 2002; **30**: 145–146.

120. Chinnery PF, Brown DT, Andrews RM, *et al*. The mitochondrial ND6 gene is a hot spot for mutations that cause Leber's hereditary optic neuropathy. *Brain* 2001; **124**: 209–218.

121. Liolitsa D, Rahman S, Benton S, *et al*. Is the mitochondrial complex I ND5 gene a hot-spot for MELAS causing mutations? *Ann Neurol* 2003; **53**: 128–132.

122. McFarland R, Kirby DM, Fowler KJ, *et al*. De novo mutations in the mitochondrial ND3 gene as a cause of infantile mitochondrial

encephalopathy and complex I deficiency. *Ann Neurol* 2004; **55**: 58–64.

123. Kirby DM, McFarland R, Ohtake A, *et al.* Mutations of the mitochondrial ND1 gene as a cause of MELAS. *J Med Genet* 2004; **41**: 784–789.

124. Chinnery PF, DiMauro S, Shanske S, *et al.* Risk of developing a mitochondrial DNA deletion disorder. *Lancet* 2004; **364**: 592–596.

125. Cree LM, Samuels DC, de Sousa Lopes SC, *et al.* A reduction of mitochondrial DNA molecules during embryogenesis explains the rapid segregation of genotypes. *Nat Genet* 2008; **40**: 249–254.

126. Wai T, Teoli D, Shoubridge EA. The mitochondrial DNA genetic bottleneck results from replication of a subpopulation of genomes. *Nat Genet* 2008; **40**: 1484–1488.

127. Brown DT, Samuels DC, Michael EM, *et al.* Random genetic drift determines the level of mutant mtDNA in human primary oocytes. *Am J Hum Genet* 2000; **68**: 533–536.

128. Poulton J, Turnbull DM. 74th ENMC International Workshop. Mitochondrial diseases. *Neuromuscul Disord* 2000; **10**: 460–462.

129. Man PY, Griffiths PG, Brown DT, *et al.* The epidemiology of Leber hereditary optic neuropathy in the North East of England. *Am J Hum Genet* 2003; **72**: 333–339.

130. Harding A, Holt I, Sweeney M, *et al.* Prenatal diagnosis of mitochondrial DNA$^{8993\ T>G}$ disease. *Am J Hum Genet* 1992; **50**: 629–633.

131. Leshinsky–Silver E, Perach M, Basilevsky E, *et al.* Prenatal exclusion of Leigh syndrome due to T8993C mutation in the mitochondrial DNA. *Prenat Diagn* 2003; **23**: 31–33.

132. Weber K, Wilson JN, Taylor L, *et al.* A new mtDNA mutation showing accumulation with time and restriction to skeletal muscle. *Am J Hum Genet* 1997; **60**: 373–380.

133. Jenuth JP, Peterson AC, Shoubridge EA. Tissue-specific selection for different mtDNA genotypes in heteroplasmic mice. *Nat Genet* 1997; **16**: 93–95.

134. White SL, Shanske S, Biros I, *et al.* Two cases of prenatal analysis for the pathogenic T to G substitution at nucleotide 8993 in mitochondrial DNA. *Prenat Diagn* 1999; **19**: 1165–1168.

135. Steffann J, Frydman N, Gigarel N, *et al.* Analysis of mtDNA variant segregation during early human embryonic development: a tool for successful NARP preimplantation diagnosis. *J Med Genet* 2006; **43**: 244–247.

136. Dean NL, Battersby BJ, Ao A, *et al.* Prospect of preimplantation genetic diagnosis for heritable mitochondrial DNA diseases. *Mol Hum Reprod* 2003; **9**: 631–638.

137. Thorburn DR, Dahl HHM. Mitochondrial disorders: genetics, counseling, prenatal diagnosis and reproductive options. *Am J Med Genet* 2001; **106**: 102–114.

138. Brown DT, Herbert M, Lamb VK, *et al.* Transmission of mitochondrial DNA disorders: possibilities for the future. *Lancet* 2006; **368**: 87–89.

139. Tachibana M, Sparman M, Sritanaudomchai H, *et al.* Mitochondrial gene replacement in primate offspring and embryonic stem cells. *Nature* 2009; **461**: 367–372.

140. Chinnery P, Majamaa K, Turnbull D, Thorburn D. Treatment for mitochondrial disorders. *Cochrane Database Syst Rev* 2006; **1**: CD004426.

141. Jacobs HT. Mitochondrial deafness. *Ann Med* 1997; **29**: 483–491.

142. Ponchaut S, van Hoof F, Veitch K. Cytochrome aa3 depletion is the cause of the deficient mitochondrial respiration induced by chronic valproate administration. *Biochem Pharmacol* 1992; **43**: 644–647.

143. Lamperti C, Naini A, Hirano M, *et al.* Cerebellar ataxia and coenzyme Q10 deficiency. *Neurology* 2003; **60**: 1206–1208.

144. Van Maldergem L, Trijbels F, DiMauro S, *et al.* Coenzyme Q-responsive Leigh's encephalopathy in two sisters. *Ann Neurol* 2002; **52**: 750–754.

145. Naini A, Lewis VJ, Hirano M, DiMauro S. Primary coenzyme Q10 deficiency and the brain. *Biofactors* 2003; **18**: 145–152.

146. Cooper JM, Schapira AH. Friedreich's ataxia: disease mechanisms, antioxidant and coenzyme Q10 therapy. *Biofactors* 2003; **18**: 163–171.

147. Geromel V, Darin N, Chretien D, *et al.* Coenzyme Q(10) and idebenone in the therapy of respiratory chain diseases: rationale and comparative benefits. *Mol Genet Metab* 2002; **77**: 21–30.

148. De Stefano N, Matthews PM, Ford B, *et al.* Short-term dichloroacetate treatment improves indices of cerebral metabolism in patients with mitochondrial disorders. *Neurology* 1995; **45**: 1193–1198.

149. Kaufmann P, Engelstad K, Wei Y, *et al.* Dichloroacetate causes toxic neuropathy in MELAS: a randomized, controlled clinical trial. *Neurology* 2006; **66**: 324–330.

150. Hirano M, Marti R, Casali C, *et al.* Allogeneic stem cell transplantation corrects biochemical derangements in MNGIE. *Neurology* 2006; **67**: 1458–1460.

151. Koga Y, Akita Y, Nishioka J, *et al.* L-arginine improves the symptoms of strokelike episodes

in MELAS. *Neurology* 2005; **64**: 710–712.

152. Taivassalo T, Shoubridge EA, Chen J, *et al.* Aerobic conditioning in patients with mitochondrial myopathies: physiological, biochemical, and genetic effects. *Ann Neurol* 2001; **50**: 133–141.

153. Taivassalo T, Fu K, Johns T, *et al.* Gene shifting: a novel therapy for mitochondrial myopathy. *Hum Mol Genet* 1999; **8**: 1047–1052.

154. Murphy JL, Blakely EL, Schaefer AM, *et al.* Resistance training in patients with single, large-scale deletions of mitochondrial

DNA. *Brain* 2008; **131**: 2832–2840.

155. Taivassalo T, Gardner JL, Taylor RW, *et al.* Endurance training and detraining in mitochondrial myopathies due to single large-scale mtDNA deletions. *Brain* 2006; **129**: 3391–3401.

The neurofibromatoses and related disorders

Rosalie E. Ferner

Neurofibromatosis 1 and 2

Advances in molecular biology and the development of sophisticated imaging techniques have permitted the clinical and genetic characterization of two distinct neurocutaneous conditions: neurofibromatosis 1 (NF1) and neurofibromatosis 2 (NF2). NF1 and NF2 are tumor suppressor disorders in which affected individuals are predisposed to develop benign and malignant tumors. This chapter discusses the clinical and genetic features of NF1 and NF2 and evaluates the current diagnosis and management of these conditions.

Neurofibromatosis 1

Historical introduction and definition

Cases suggestive of neurofibromatosis are thought to have been depicted in manuscripts dating from 1000 AD. The Cistercian monastery in Rein in southern Austria houses a thirteenth century illustration of a man with swellings emanating from his face and trunk. The drawing is purported to be an early portrayal of neurofibromatosis 1 [1]. More convincingly, Tilesius reported "A case of extraordinarily unsightly skin." He requested alms for the patient, Johann Gottfried Rheinhard, who emitted an unpleasant odor. He had limb pigmentation, countless skin tumors, a large head, short stature, and a curved spine [2]. Subsequently, von Recklinghausen established that the tumors arose from the connective tissue of nerve sheaths, especially the endoneurium, and he coined the term "neurofibroma" [3]. Furthermore, he reported innumerable brown spots on the skin of Marie Kientz, a manual worker with 11 children from different husbands, who died aged 55 years from a ruptured pulmonary artery aneurysm. However, it was not until a century later that the National Institutes of Health consensus development conference proposed the current diagnostic criteria for neurofibromatosis 1 (Table 14.1) [4].

Table 14.1. Diagnostic criteria for neurofibromatosis 1*

Two or more criteria are needed for diagnosis
- Six or more *cafe au lait* patches >15 mm in adults and >5 mm in children
- Two or more neurofibromas or one plexiform neurofibroma
- Axillary or groin freckling
- Lisch nodules (iris hamartomas)
- Optic pathway glioma
- A first-degree relative with NF1
- A distinctive osseous lesion such as sphenoid wing dysplasia or thinning of the long bone cortex with or without pseudoarthrosis

* NIH Consensus Development Conference (1988) [4], with permission.

Neurofibromatosis 1 is a common autosomal dominant disease with an estimated birth incidence of 1 in 2500 and a prevalence of 1 in 4000 [5]. The *NF1* gene is on chromosome 17q11.2 and the protein product is called neurofibromin, which acts as a tumor suppressor [6–8]. NF1 arises as a new mutation in 50% of patients and there is almost complete penetrance by the age of three years. The major and defining manifestations are *café au lait* patches, neurofibromas, skin-fold freckling, iris Lisch nodules, and characteristic osseous dysplasia [9]. There is a wide phenotypic variation in NF1, even within families, and the complications affect many of the body systems.

Genetics and molecular biology

The *NF1* gene was identified on chromosome 17q11.2 and the coding region comprises 60 exons spanning 350 kb of genomic DNA [6,7]. Three embedded genes *EVI2A*, *EVI2B*, and *OMGP* (oligodendrocyte myelin glycoprotein) are transcribed off the opposite strand of intron 27b of the *NF1* gene. The function of these genes is uncertain, but there is no evidence to date that altered expression in patients with NF1 results in clinical heterogeneity [10].

The *NF1* gene encodes neurofibromin, a protein that is found predominantly in the cytoplasm and has multiple isoforms, which may be expressed at different times during fetal development [11]. Neurofibromin is ubiquitously expressed, but the greatest levels of expression are in the brain, Schwann cells, oligodendrocytes, and peripheral nerves [12]. Neurofibromin is structurally and functionally related to the guanosine triphosphatase-activating proteins (GAP), which negatively regulate a cellular protooncogene, $p21^{RAS}$ [13]. One of the functions of neurofibromin is to reduce cell proliferation by promoting the inactivation of $p21^{RAS}$, which has a key role in mitogenic intracellular signaling pathways.

Pathogenesis of neurofibromas

Neurofibromas contain a mixture of Schwann cells, fibroblasts, perineurial cells, mast cells, and axons lying within a collagen-rich extracellular matrix [14]. Schwann cells exhibit loss of NF1 expression, and recent research has shown that the Schwann cell initiates neurofibroma growth and increased numbers of mast cells may contribute to neurofibroma formation [15,16]. RAS-GTP levels are increased in some neurofibroma Schwann cells but not in fibroblasts [17]. Expression of epidermal and vascular endothelial growth factors and their receptors and matrix metalloproteinases may also play a role in neurofibroma development [18,19].

Clinical manifestations

The skin

Café au lait macules contain melanin macroglobules, often appear at birth, and are usually present by the age of three years [9]. Skin-fold freckling develops in most NF1 children [9].

Cutaneous neurofibromas usually appear in adulthood and the growth rate is unpredictable. Some tumors are visible, initially with a purplish hue, and may become pedunculated, while others are only evident on palpation [9]. Neurofibromas increase in size and number during puberty and pregnancy, implying that hormones influence their development. About 75% of neurofibromas express progesterone receptors but only 5% express estrogen receptors, suggesting a

potential role for anti-progesterone therapy [20]. Patients experience itching and stinging, but the overriding psychological burden arises from disfigurement [21]. Surgery and carbon dioxide laser are used to remove the lesions, albeit with hypertrophic scarring in some individuals [22]. Subcutaneous neurofibromas are firmer, deeper, discrete benign tumors, which cause pain, neurological symptoms, and deficit owing to pressure on peripheral nerves [9].

Plexiform neurofibromas contain the same cell types as cutaneous neurofibromas, but may involve multiple nerves or fascicles, and have an expanded extracellular matrix and a rich vascular supply [14]. Superficial lesions are characterized by skin thickening and hyperpigmentation, and diffuse pigmentation may betray the presence of a deep-seated plexiform neurofibroma. The tumors are found in about 50% of NF1 individuals and many are congenital [23,24].

The natural history of plexiform neurofibromas has not been established and the growth rate is variable. The diffuse nature of the tumors often precludes accurate measurement and total removal. Radiotherapy is contraindicated because of the risk of malignant transformation. Several chemotherapy trials have been conducted to develop treatments for plexiform neurofibromas, including antihistamines, maturation agents, and anti-angiogenesis drugs [24]. A randomized, placebo-controlled trial is in progress to assess an oral farnesyltransferase inhibitor, and the antifibrotic agent pirfenidone is being evaluated in adults with progressive plexiform and spinal neurofibromas [24,25].

NF individuals have about a 10% lifetime risk of developing a malignant peripheral nerve sheath tumor (MPNST) [26,27]. Extensive and centrally located plexiform neurofibromas, neurofibromatous neuropathy, previous personal or family history of malignancy, and radiotherapy treatment increase the likelihood of developing MPNST [27,28]. Individuals with a microdeletion of the NF1 locus also need careful surveillance [29]. Malignant peripheral nerve sheath tumors are difficult to diagnose and often herald a poor outcome. The clinical features of malignancy are persistent pain, change in texture, rapid increase in size of a neurofibroma, and the onset of neurological deficit. However, the symptoms and magnetic resonance imaging (MRI) manifestations of malignancy overlap with benign neurofibromas, and a biopsy may miss the site of malignant change because the tumors are heterogeneous [27,30].

A retrospective study suggested that ^{18}FDG PET (fluorodeoxyglucose positron emission tomography) may be useful in evaluating malignant change in plexiform neurofibromas [31].

Malignant peripheral nerve sheath tumors from NF1 individuals exhibit loss of NF1 expression and high levels of RAS [32]. However, malignant change depends on additional genetic events that inactivate key cell cycle regulators including p53, p16, and p27-kip1 [33,34]. Moreover, mice with targeted mutations of the *NF1* and *p53* genes develop MPNSTs when these genes are inactivated [35].

The mainstay of treatment for MPNST is surgical excision with tumor-free margins [27]. Radiotherapy improves local control and chemotherapy with ifosfamide and doxorubicin is palliative in metastatic disease [27]. Farnesyl transferase inhibitors targeting the RAS pathway may be useful, novel therapeutic agents [24].

The eye

Lisch nodules are visualized on slit-lamp examination as dome-shaped hamartomas of the iris in over 90% of postpubertal NF1 individuals [36,37]. Cutaneous and plexiform neurofibromas may involve the eyelid and orbit. Idiopathic congenital ptosis, congenital and acquired glaucoma, choroidal hamartomas, and diffuse or nodular enlargement of the corneal nerves have also been described. Sphenoid wing dysplasia affects the greater sphenoid wing in about 1% of NF1 patients and disrupts the posterior, superior wall of the orbit [9].

Cardiovascular problems

Cardiovascular disease is a major cause of early death in NF1 individuals and the manifestations range from hypertension, vasculopathy, and congenital heart defects to rare complications caused by neurofibromas obstructing, compressing, or invading the heart or major vessels [38]. Small and large caliber vessels may be involved and stenosis, occlusion, aneurysm, rupture, and fistulas have been reported. Coarctation of the aorta has also been reported. Vasculopathy is not always symptomatic, but the renal arteries are the most common source of clinical problems.

Essential hypertension occurs frequently, and 1% of patients present with hypertension from renal artery stenosis in childhood, young adulthood, or pregnancy. Pheochromocytomas are detected in 0.1%–1.5% of NF1 individuals, causing severe sustained or paroxysmal hypertension and life-threatening cardiovascular compromise, particularly during anesthesia and pregnancy [9]. Biochemical diagnosis of pheochromocytoma is determined by measuring 24-hour urinary catecholamines, preferably when the patient is symptomatic. Alternative techniques include abdominal CT or MRI, arteriography, and adrenal scintigraphy with metaiodobenzylguanidine.

There is a higher than expected frequency of congenital heart disease in NF1 individuals, particularly of valvular pulmonary stenosis. The latter is also associated with clinical subtypes of NF1, including Watson syndrome, NF1-Noonan syndrome, and patients with large NF1 deletions [39].

Respiratory complications

Asymptomatic intrapulmonary neurofibromas, pectus excavatum, and carinatum are observed in NF1 individuals. Significant scoliosis may lead to restrictive lung disease and the chest is the most common site of metastases from MPNSTs [9,27].

Gastrointestinal complications

Gastrointestinal neurofibromas cause abdominal distension, pain, dyspepsia, hemorrhage, and constipation in 2% of patients [9]. Carcinoid tumors are located predominantly in the duodenum and produce facial flushing, diarrhea, right-sided cardiac lesions, facial telangiectasiae, and bronchoconstriction [40]. Increased urinary levels of the serotonin metabolite 5-hydroxyindolacetic acid confirm the diagnosis and clinicians should be alert to the possibility of coexisting pheochromocytoma. Gangliocytic paraganglioma and ganglioneuromatosis are rare complications, the latter representing dysplastic proliferation of the myenteric plexuses and ganglion cells of the gastrointestinal system [41,42].

Orthopedic complications

Orthopedic complications result from intrinsic defects of the skeletal system [43]. Pseudoarthrosis, a false joint in a long bone, affects 2% of NF1 patients, and the tibia is the most common bone involved [9]. Bowing of the affected long bone is apparent at birth or in the first few months of life, and a fracture develops after trivial injury, with delayed healing. Most patients require surgery and amputation is necessary in severe cases [44].

Scoliosis affects 10% of NF1 patients, most commonly involves the cervical and thoracic spine, and may be either idiopathic or dystrophic. A dystrophic curve entails four to six segments, causes distortion of the vertebral bodies and ribs, and is rapidly progressive, needing early spinal fusion [45].

Neurological complications
Tumors and malformations

Gliomas arise in all parts of the central nervous system (CNS), including the spinal cord, optic pathways, brainstem, and cerebellum [46]. Ependymomas have been reported in NF1 individuals, but vestibular schwannomas and meningiomas do not occur with increased frequency. Brainstem gliomas appear to have a more indolent course in NF1 children than in the general population and some tumors show spontaneous remission [47]. However, a recent study observed that gliomas located outside the optic pathway were more aggressive [48].

NF1 inactivation has been detected in late-onset astrocytomas and some tumors harbor deletions of the *NF1* gene. Mutation of TP53 and deletion of CDKN2A/p16 have been detected in NF1 associated high-grade astrocytomas as well as in their sporadic counterparts [49].

A population-based study reported optic pathway gliomas (OPG) in 1.5% of NF1 individuals, but a clinic-based investigation observed OPG in 15% of patients [9,50]. These low-grade pilocytic astrocytomas are often asymptomatic but may cause visual impairment, pupillary abnormalities, strabismus, proptosis, and hypothalamic dysfunction. Optic pathway gliomas usually arise in the first six years of life and the development of symptomatic tumors in older children and adults is unusual. Nonetheless, progression of known OPG requiring therapy has been reported in patients in their third decade [51]. Screening for asymptomatic OPG is not advocated, as it does not influence the need for treatment or the outcome. Chemotherapy with vincristine and cisplatinum is the optimum treatment for progressive symptomatic OPG, but radiotherapy is not recommended for young children because of the neuropsychiatric, endocrinological, and vascular sequelae [52,53].

Cerebrovascular disease

Cerebrovascular disease occurs with increased frequency in NF1 and results from stenosis or occlusion of the internal carotid, middle cerebral, and anterior cerebral arteries [54,55]. Intracranial and cervical aneurysms and cervical arteriovenous fistulae have also been reported in older patients [38].

Multiple sclerosis

Primary progressive multiple sclerosis has been reported in association with NF1 [56], but the etiology is uncertain. No mutations have been detected in the *OMGP* gene, which is involved in CNS myelination [57]. However, it is conceivable that a mutation within the *NF1* gene may lead to altered function of the *OMGP* gene and predispose to both NF1 and demyelination.

Epilepsy

About 7% of NF1 patients have epilepsy, which cannot be explained by underlying tumors, malformations, or cerebrovascular disease. An underlying cortical dysgenesis might account for this phenotype in NF1 individuals [58,59].

Cognitive impairment

Cognitive impairment is the most common complication of NF1 and patients present with low IQ, specific learning problems, and behavioral difficulties. Abnormal executive function and language deficits have also been observed [60,61]. The majority of patients have an IQ in the low average range, about 90, but mental retardation (IQ <70) is uncommon, occurring in 4%–8% of NF1 individuals [61]. There is no evidence that cognitive ability improves with age [60,62].

Learning difficulties have been reported in 30%–60% of NF1 children and include visual spatial deficits, poor coordination, and difficulty with reading, handwriting, and spelling [61,63]. Disruptive behavior, misinterpretation of social cues, and hyperactivity attention deficit disorder are evident [60]. Investigators have demonstrated that NF1 children and adolescents are less conscientious and more emotionally unstable and irritable than their peers in the general population [64]. NF1 individuals demonstrate poor organizational skills, inflexibility, and an inability to select appropriate strategies to cope with unfamiliar and complex tasks, consistent with impaired executive function [60].

The etiology of cognitive impairment has not been determined. A neuropathological study hypothesized that cognitive problems are related to underlying migrational abnormalities in the developing brain [58]. Unidentified bright objects (UBOs) have been identified as focal areas of high signal intensity of T2-weighted MRI, predominantly in the basal ganglia, brainstem, and cerebellum [61,65,66]. The lesions do not cause overt neurological deficits and develop in the majority of children with NF1, but tend to disappear in adulthood. Their nature and significance are unclear, but they may represent aberrant myelination or gliosis [67]. There have been reports that the presence of UBOs is associated with cognitive dysfunction, and in some cases, this was related to the site and volume of the UBOs [68]. UBOs may represent a marker for impaired fine motor performance in individuals with NF1 [69]. However, other studies have not found any relationship between the number, size, and sites of T2-weighted hyperintensities and cognitive problems in NF1 [66,70]. The presence of UBOs in childhood is purported to be the best predictor of cognitive impairment in adulthood [62]. Mouse models suggest that cognitive impairment in NF1 is a result of excessive RAS activity and that farnesyltransferase inhibitors may reverse the deficit, implying that increased RAS activity might play a significant role in the etiology of cognitive impairment in NF1 [71].

Neurofibromatous neuropathy

Neurofibromatous neuropathy affects about 1% of NF1 individuals and is characterized by a mild distal sensorimotor neuropathy associated with diffuse neurofibromatous change in thickened peripheral nerves [28,72].

Molecular diagnosis

The clinical diagnosis of NF1 is evident by the age of three years in the majority of NF1 patients (see NIH consensus development conference diagnostic criteria, Table 14.1). Current mutation testing permits the identification of pathogenic mutations in over 95% of NF1 patients and the majority of mutations result in truncation of the gene product [73]. Prenatal testing of fetal DNA extracted from chorionic villous sampling or from aminiocentesis is possible. However, requests for prenatal testing are limited because of the inability to predict disease severity.

Mosaic neurofibromatosis 1

Somatic mutations arising early in embryogenesis result in generalized disease clinically indistinguishable from non-mosaic NF1. There have been few reported cases of somatic mosaicism for the *NF1* gene in individuals with sporadic generalized NF1. Somatic mutations occurring later produce localized disease restricted to the affected area and the estimated prevalence of mosaic localized NF1 is between 1 in 36 000 and 1 in 40 000 [74]. The risk of an individual passing on generalized disease to an offspring is unquantifiable, as it depends on the percentage of the body that is affected [74].

Phenotype–genotype correlations

There is marked clinical heterogeneity between individuals with NF1, even within families. Recent research suggests that individuals with *NF1* microdeletions are at higher risk of developing MPNST, but a larger cohort needs to be assessed to verify this premise [29]. It has been hypothesized that the variation in clinical expression in NF1 is a result of the nature, timing, or location of second-hit mutations at the *NF1* gene locus, to somatic mosaicism, or to the presence of modifying genes [75,76]. The presence of modifying genes is supported by frequent observations that identical *NF1* gene mutations give rise to different clinical phenotypes.

Screening

Annual assessment of children and adults with NF1 should be undertaken by a clinician who is conversant with the management of the disease. Children require developmental and educational monitoring, examination of the spine and skin, and blood pressure measurement. Formal visual examination with color vision, fundoscopy, and visual fields is recommended from the developmental age of eight years. Adults need annual blood pressure monitoring and assessment of the skin, and patients and clinicians should be alert to the symptoms suggesting the development of MPNST.

Neurofibromatosis 2
Definition and historical introduction

Neurofibromatosis 2 (NF2) is a rare autosomal dominant neurocutaneous disorder caused by inactivating mutations of the tumor suppressor gene *NF2* on chromosome 22 [77,78]. The hallmark of NF2 is bilateral vestibular schwannomas, but affected individuals may develop schwannomas on other cranial nerves, or on the spinal, peripheral, or cutaneous nerves [79,80]. Central nervous system tumors including meningioma, astrocytoma, and ependymoma occur, ophthalmological abnormalities are prominent, and skin manifestations may be visible. Schwannomatosis is characterized by the development of multiple schwannomas without vestibular schwannomas and the annual incidence of newly identified cases has been estimated to be 1 in 1 700 000 [81,82]. Schwannomatosis and NF2 are clinically and molecularly distinct, although there is some clinical overlap between the two conditions.

James Wishart reported the first case of NF2, formerly known as bilateral acoustic or central neurofibromatosis [83,84]. Wishart described a young baker with progressive hearing loss who died following surgery and who had multiple tumors of the dura mater and brain in addition to bilateral eighth nerve tumors.

Clinical diagnosis

The diagnostic criteria for NF2 proposed by the National Institutes of Health (1998) [4] state the necessity for bilateral vestibular schwannomas or a family history of the disease in combination with two or more other manifestations – meningioma, glioma, schwannoma, neurofibroma, and juvenile posterior subcapsular lenticular opacity. However, 50% of patients have no family history of NF2, and skin and ocular problems may develop before a vestibular schwannoma [85,86]. This was reflected in the modified NF2 diagnostic criteria [87] (Table 14.2). In 1992, the birth incidence of NF2 was 1 in 33 000 and the symptomatic prevalence was 1 in 210 000 in the United Kingdom [88].

Clinical manifestations

Cranial nerve, cerebral, and spinal tumors

Schwannomas are benign encapsulated tumors that rarely undergo malignant change [79]. Bilateral vestibular schwannomas are pathognomonic for NF2 and occur in 95% of adult patients [85]. They arise from the vestibular branch of the eighth cranial nerve and usually cause sensorineural hearing loss,

Table 14.2. Revised diagnostic criteria for neurofibromatosis 2

A. Bilateral vestibular schwannomas

B. First-degree relative with NF2, plus:
Unilateral vestibular schwannoma, or 2 of:
Meningioma, schwannoma, glioma,
neurofibroma, posterior subcapsular lens opacity

C. Unilateral vestibular schwannoma, plus 2 of:
Meningioma, schwannoma, glioma,
neurofibroma, posterior subcapsular lens opacity

D. Multiple meningiomas, plus:
Unilateral schwannoma, or 2 of:
Schwannoma, glioma,
neurofibroma, posterior subcapsular lens opacity

From Baser *et al.* (2002) [87], with permission from Lippincott, Williams, and Wilkins.

which is unilateral initially and associated with tinnitus and ataxia [85].

The mean age at diagnosis is 27 years (range 5–66 years) for individuals with NF2-associated vestibular schwannomas, in contrast to patients with unilateral sporadic tumors who usually present in the fourth decade [85]. The growth rate of vestibular schwannomas varies greatly even within the same family and is not related to overall disease severity or the number of peripheral nerve or CNS tumors [89]. The growth rate of vestibular schwannomas declines in older patients and does not depend on the type of constitutional *NF2* gene mutation [89,90]. The inference is that the rate of growth of vestibular schwannomas is determined by unknown environmental or molecular mechanisms distinct from those that control schwannoma formation. Hence, the management of vestibular schwannomas should be tailored to the individual and not based on the growth pattern observed in other family members. Early operative intervention does not necessarily preserve hearing, and suitability for cochlear or brainstem auditory implants varies between individuals.

Gadolinium-enhanced MRI permits the early detection of tumors, and the current options for treatment range from observation for individuals with a tumor in the hearing ear to microsurgery and stereotactic radiosurgery [91–93]. The possible advantages of stereotactic radiosurgery need to be evaluated against the possible long-term risk of malignancy following radiotherapy [94].

Schwannomas are observed on other cranial nerves in 38% of patients; the trigeminal nerve is most commonly affected [95]. Mautner *et al.* (1996) [95] identified spinal tumors in 90% of patients on whole spine MRI, predominantly in the thoracic and lumbar regions, and only 30% of spinal extramedullary tumors were symptomatic.

Cranial meningiomas affect 45%–58% of NF2 individuals, are usually supratentorial, and are multiple in 38% of patients [85,95]. The tumors do not differ pathologically from sporadic meningiomas, but are a major cause of morbidity and mortality in NF2. Cerebral pilocytic astrocytomas and intramedullary ependymomas are found mostly in the brainstem and upper cervical region [85,95].

Peripheral neuropathy and mononeuropathy

Axonal peripheral neuropathy is common in NF2 individuals with severe disease and may be progressive [96]. Mononeuropathy causing foot drop or facial nerve weakness may be the presenting symptom in children with NF2 [85].

The skin

The cutaneous manifestations of NF2 are less pronounced than in NF1 but may be the presenting features of the disease. *Café au lait* patches are observed in 40% of patients but are found in smaller numbers than in NF1 [85]. Skin tumors occur in 68% of patients and comprise three types [85]. The most common are discrete, slightly raised, roughened areas of skin that may be associated with pigmentation or excess hair growth. Well-circumscribed, subcutaneous peripheral nerve tumors accompanied by peripheral nerve thickening are observed in 33% of individuals, and intra-dermal tumors similar in appearance to those in NF1 are found in 20% of NF2 patients.

The eye

The most frequent ophthalmological abnormalities are presenile posterior subcapsular lens opacities, which may be the presenting symptom of NF2 [85,86]. Juvenile-onset cortical cataracts, retinal hamartomas, and optic nerve sheath meningiomas have also been described [97].

Mosaic neurofibromatosis 2

A significant number of individuals with sporadic generalized NF2 (approximately 20%) have somatic mosaicism, and the risk of passing on the condition to children may be less than 50%. In one study, only one out of nine children of three patients with mosaic NF2 inherited the condition [98]. Mildly affected individuals with mosaic NF2 should be counseled about the possibility of more severe disease in offspring, as all the cells will harbor the constitutional *NF2* gene mutation [74]. The frequency of mosaic localized NF2 has not been determined, but individuals present with NF2-related tumors in one part of the nervous system [74].

Screening

Screening, including ophthalmological examination for lens opacities and inspection of the skin for cutaneous schwannomas, is recommended from infancy. Children require annual neurological examination and audiometry; brain and spine MRI should be performed every three years in asymptomatic at-risk individuals over the age of 10 years. Imaging of the brain and spine is undertaken at yearly intervals in patients with known brain and spinal tumors. Individuals with a family history of NF2, those who develop unilateral vestibular schwannomas or meningiomas before the age of 30 years, and patients with multiple spinal schwannomas or meningiomas require further evaluation as they are at risk for development of NF2.

Genetic diagnosis

About 35%–66% of pathogenic *NF2* gene mutations are detected by employing standard mutation techniques and most are truncating mutations, resulting in smaller and probably nonfunctional protein products [99]. About 25% of cases are a result of somatic mosaicism and large deletions and rearrangements at the NF2 locus may not be detected by standard mutation testing [100]. The constitutional mutation should be sought in peripheral blood and the somatic mutation sought in tumor tissue from individuals with new mutations. Prenatal diagnosis is also available by analysis of DNA extracted from fetal cells.

Phenotype–genotype correlations

Patients with more severe disease usually have constitutional frameshift or nonsense mutations resulting in a truncated, unstable protein [101]. Conversely, missense mutations, inframe deletions, or large deletions are detected in families with milder clinical manifestations of NF2 [102]. Patients with splice-site mutations have variable disease severity [103]. Although disease severity is comparable within NF2 families, specific disease manifestations and progression of the condition vary even between monozygotic twins with NF2, presumably as a result of stochastic inactivation of the second NF2 allele [104]. A greater number of patients with nonsense and frameshift mutations have intramedullary spinal tumors than patients with other constitutional *NF2* gene mutations [105]. New evidence suggests that the relative risk of cataracts is less than one in patients with somatic mosaicism, large deletions, or new unfound mutations compared with individuals with classic NF2 and nonsense and frameshift mutations [106].

Baser *et al.* (2002) [107] reported a decrease in the mortality risk in NF2 commensurate with increasing age, the absence of intracranial meningiomas, treatment at a specialist center, and the presence of a constitutional NF2 missense mutation.

Genetics and molecular biology

The *NF2* gene was cloned on chromosome 22q11.2 and encodes a protein known as merlin (or schwannomin) [77,78]. Merlin is structurally related to the esrin moesin radixin proteins from the protein 4.1 family, which link the actin cytoskeleton to cell surface glycoproteins and involve cellular remodeling [108]. During embryonic development, many tissues show abundant merlin expression. In adults, merlin is expressed in Schwann cells, meningeal cells, nerve, and the lens, reflecting the clinical manifestations in NF2 [92,109]. Merlin's role as a growth regulator may be related to its capacity to exist in an open inactive form and a closed growth suppressor form [110]. Merlin phosphorylation, association with interacting proteins, or specific *NF2* gene mutations may influence the conformation [110]. In vitro studies have demonstrated that merlin interacts with a number of molecules, including the cell surface glycoprotein CD44 and paxillin, which is involved in cell–cytoskeleton dynamics [111,112]. These molecules may have a pivotal function in merlin growth regulation.

NF2-associated tumors and many sporadic nervous system tumors have inactivation of both alleles of the *NF2* gene and loss of merlin expression [81]. Conditional inactivation of *NF2* in mouse Schwann

cells results in Schwann cell hyperplasia and schwannomas [113]. Similarly, conditional inactivation of *NF2* in leptomeningeal cells leads to leptomeningeal hyperplasia and meningioma formation [114], emphasizing that loss of *NF2* in the relevant tissue is sufficient for tumor development. These recent insights are of particular interest because NF2 tumors are usually benign and grow slowly. The mechanisms of growth control are different from those operating in other syndromes where malignant tumors are more common.

Conclusion

Ideally, patients with NF1 and NF2 should be managed by a multidisciplinary team with input from neurology, genetics, neurosurgery, plastic surgery, sarcoma, orthopedics, ophthalmology, and otolaryngology specialists. Uncomplicated NF1 can be monitored in the local community by an experienced clinician with expertise in the disorder. Links should be fostered between the community and a tertiary specialist center, and a dedicated specialist nurse would be in an ideal position to fulfill this role. Advances in molecular genetics and the development of mouse disease models offer the tantalizing hope of targeted therapies for these distressing neurocutaneous disorders.

Von Hippel–Lindau disease

Many authors have considered von Hippel–Lindau (VHL) disease in the same category as the neurofibromatoses and tuberous sclerosis. Undoubtedly, VHL is a tumor suppressor syndrome; however, there are no skin manifestations in VHL and it cannot be regarded as a neurocutaneous disorder. The clinical and genetic manifestations of this disease are considered here as a discrete entity.

Definition and historical description

Since the 1930s, the term von Hippel–Lindau disease has been applied to describe an autosomal dominant condition in which individuals are at risk of developing benign and malignant tumors of the CNS, eye, endolymphatic sac, kidneys, pancreas, adrenal glands, and reproductive adnexal organs [115,116].

Eugen von Hippel (1867–1939) observed the evolving clinical and histological features affecting the right eye of Otto Mayer, a 23-year-old man with visual

Table 14.3. Diagnostic criteria for VHL

1. Family history of VHL and one of: clear cell renal carcinoma, pheochromocytoma, brain, retinal or spinal hemangioblastoma

2. Two or more central nervous system hemangioblastomas or:

3. One central nervous system hemangioblastoma and one visceral tumour*

* excluding renal cysts, which are common in the general population.
Melman and Rose (1964) [125]; Maher et al. (1991) [131].

Table 14.4. Mean age of presentation and frequency of clinical manifestations in VHL

Clinical features of VHL	Age of presentation in years (range)	Disease frequency (%)
Renal cell carcinoma/cysts	40 (16–67)	24–60
Pheochromocytoma	30 (5–58)	10–20
Pancreatic cysts/ tumors	37 (5–70)	17–56
Pancreatic neuroendocrine tumors	35	8–17
Epididymal tumors	adolescence	25–60
Retinal hemangioblastomas	25 (1–67)	25–60
Endolymphatic sac tumors	22 (12–50)	11–16
CNS hemangioblastomas	33 (9–78)	10–72
Spinal cord hemangioblastomas	33 (12–66)	13–50

Maher et al. (1990) [121]; Kaelin and Maher (1998) [142]; Lonser et al. (2003, 2004) [116,128].

impairment. Von Hippel concluded that his patient's retinal lesions arose from a congenital cystic capillary angiomatosis or angiomatosis retinae [117,118]. Otto Mayer developed headaches, nausea, unsteadiness, and facial weakness before his death in 1917 at the age of 47 years. Brandt reported Otto Mayer's postmortem findings and attributed the multiple vascular tumors and cysts in the cerebellum, medulla, pancreas, kidneys, and epididymis to developmental malformations [119]. Arvid Lindau (1892–1958) recognized that the tumors in multiple organs were part of a single disease entity and that the condition was familial [120]. Von Hippel and Lindau's meticulous observations and pathological descriptions, combined with clinical acumen, have facilitated the categorization of an important cancer predisposition syndrome.

Clinical features

In a study of 152 patients with VHL, the mean age at presentation was 26.3 years and penetrance was 95% by the age of 65 years [121]. Renal cell carcinoma was the principal cause of death and the median actuarial survival in patients with VHL was 49 years. The diagnostic criteria for VHL are described in Table 14.3. The frequency of the major clinical manifestations and the mean age of presentation are delineated in Table 14.4.

Renal carcinomas and cysts

Renal cell carcinoma is the first manifestation of VHL in 13% of individuals [121]. The tumor is often asymptomatic for protracted periods and hematuria, flank pain, or a mass are features of advanced disease. Renal cysts are asymptomatic and do not require treatment, but complex cysts often contain areas of

renal cell carcinoma. Presymptomatic screening with contrast abdominal CT or MRI allows early detection of tumors. Nephron-sparing surgery for lesions smaller than 3 cm permits preservation of renal function and reduces the risk of metastases [122]. Partial or total nephrectomy is necessary for large renal tumors and renal transplantation has been successful in individuals requiring bilateral nephrectomy.

Pheochromocytoma

Pheochromocytomas may be bilateral and extra-adrenal, and 5% undergo malignant change. Patients are often asymptomatic, but may present with episodic or sustained hypertension, palpitations, sweating, nausea, headache, or tachycardia [123]. Screening for pheochromocytoma before surgery and labor is recommended to avert hypertensive crises. Diagnosis is confirmed by measurement of 24-hour urinary catecholamines, plasma-free metanephrines, abdominal CT, or MRI. Metaiodobenzylguanidine (MIBG) scintigraphy identifies extra-adrenal tumors. Alpha and beta blockade is a prerequisite before surgery, which is undertaken for large lesions or those with abnormal function or cancerous change [116].

Pancreatic lesions

Pancreatic cysts are often multiple and rarely symptomatic [124]. Similarly, neuroendocrine tumors of the pancreas are usually indolent, although hepatic metastases have been reported [116]. These tumors are identified on CT scan and large lesions require resection.

Epididymal tumors

Benign epididymal papillary cystadenomas are encountered in adolescence; they are detected on ultrasound scanning, are often multiple and bilateral, and are treated conservatively [116]. There are infrequent reports of asymptomatic, broad ligament cystadenomas occurring in females with VHL between the ages of 22 and 46 years [116].

Retinal hemangioblastomas

Retinal lesions, formerly termed angiomas, are indistinguishable histologically from hemangioblastomas. Hemangioblastomas are encapsulated tumors with a rich vascular plexus and surrounded by polygonal stromal cells. The lesions may be bilateral and multiple and have a predilection for the temporal periphery of the retina, but also form on or near the optic disk. Patients may be asymptomatic, but retinal detachment, exudation, or hemorrhage are heralded by visual field defects or impaired visual acuity [125,126]. Dilated ophthalmoscopy allows early detection of retinal hemangioblastomas and laser photocoagulation or cryotherapy preserves vision in many cases. Extensive retinal detachment may require vitrectomy and enucleation is the only option for severe glaucoma. Recovery of visual function following therapy with a vascular endothelial growth factor (VEGF) receptor inhibitor has been reported [127].

Endolymphatic sac tumors

Endolymphatic sac tumors are locally invasive lesions arising in the temporal bone and are frequently bilateral in individuals with VHL. Symptoms include acute hearing loss that may be progressive, tinnitus, dizziness, aural fullness, and facial nerve weakness [128]. The tumors are imaged by MRI and CT scan,

the latter demonstrating bony erosion; complete surgical resection is curative [128].

Brain and spine hemangioblastomas

Central nervous system hemangioblastomas are most commonly located in the cerebellum (9%–78%) and spinal cord (13%–25%), but also involve the brainstem and, infrequently, the lumbosacral nerve roots and supratentorium. Peripheral nerve hemangioblastomas are rare. Symptomatic tumors grow ten times faster than quiescent lesions and the symptoms are related to the site of the tumor, associated cysts, and surrounding edema [116,129]. Gadolinium-enhanced MRI is the imaging method of choice and treatment is surgical removal. Radiotherapy has been advocated for tumors less than 3 cm, but the long-term sequelae of this treatment have not been evaluated.

Screening

The optimum care for patients is within a multidisciplinary service comprising a geneticist, neurologist, neurosurgeon, renal physician, ophthalmologist, and specialist nurse. Ophthalmology assessment with dilated fundoscopy should be undertaken annually from infancy; blood pressure and urinary catecholamines are measured yearly from the age of two years; and abdominal ultrasound is undertaken yearly from eight years of age. Annual abdominal CT after the age of 18 years is recommended by some centers and imaging of the neuroaxis is performed at one- to three-year intervals from the age of 11 years [116,130].

Genetics and molecular biology

VHL disease affects one in 36000 individuals [121,131]; about 20% of individuals do not have an affected parent and parental mosaicism has been reported, although the incidence has not been determined [132]. VHL is caused by germline mutations in the tumor suppressor gene *VHL* on chromosome 3p25–26 [133], and mutation detection is virtually 100% in patients fulfilling the clinical criteria for VHL [134]. Although germline mutations are present in all cells of patients with VHL, tumors occur only in susceptible organs, when a deletion or mutation occurs in the remaining wild-type allele. Somatic inactivation of the *VHL* gene has been demonstrated in sporadic CNS hemangioblastomas and renal cell carcinomas [135–138].

The *VHL* gene product, VHL, is a tumor suppressor protein that is widely expressed and its localization in the nucleus or cytoplasm is determined by cell density [139]. VHL has a putative role in transcriptional regulation, by its interaction with B and C subunits of the elongin C transcription factor [140]. It is hypothesized that mutations of the *VHL* gene facilitate transcription of specific mRNA and thereby promote tumor growth [141]. However, the VHL protein does not inhibit transcription in vivo, implying that the VHL–elongin B and C complex may have other functions [142]. The VHL–elongin B and C complex also binds with the cullin family of proteins (CUL2), and is thought to be involved in the ubiquitin-mediated degradation of cell cycle regulatory proteins [143,144]. Recent evidence suggests that the VHL tumor suppressor protein regulates hypoxia inducible transcripts such as VEGF by altering mRNA stability [145,146]. Impaired or absent VHL leads to increased expression of VEGF and proliferation of endothelial cells and pericytes, and accounts for the vascular nature of the tumors that occur in VHL disease [116]. VHL interacts with fibronectin, which is required for assembly of the extracellular matrix. Cells derived from *VHL* knockout mouse embryo fibroblasts fail to form a fibronectin matrix, suggesting a mechanism of tumor formation [147].

Phenotype–genotype correlations

Germline mutations that produce distinct cancer phenotypes have been detected and will be helpful in presymptomatic testing. Four phenotypic groups related to the risk of developing renal cell carcinoma or pheochromocytoma have been identified [148,149]. Type 1 families develop all types of tumors, but have a lower risk of pheochromocytoma. Type 2A VHL is characterized by a reduced risk of renal cell carcinoma, while Type 2B families have a high risk of developing these tumors. The hallmark of type C VHL is pheochromocytomas, in the absence of other tumor manifestations. The majority of type 1 families have either premature termination mutations or deletions, while most type 2 families have missense mutations [148,149].

Conclusions

The diagnosis and clinical care of patients with VHL have been enhanced by the identification of the *VHL* gene, and functional studies of the *VHL* gene product have provided an insight into the role of hypoxia response pathways in tumor formation. The preliminary use of VEGF inhibitors to stabilize retinal and CNS disease heralds exciting prospects for the development of targeted therapy for this rare condition.

References

1. Zanca A, Zanca A. Antique illustrations of neurofibromatosis. *Int J Dermatol* 1980; **19**: 55–58.

2. Von Tilesius WG. *Historia pathologica singularis cutis turpitudinis Jo. Godfredi Rheinhardi viri 50 annorum.* Leipzig: SL Crusius, 1793.

3. Von Recklinghausen FD. *Uber die multiplen fibrome der haut und ihre Beziehung zu den multiplen neuromen.* Berlin: A Hirschwald, 1882.

4. National Institutes of Health Consensus Development Conference Statement. Neurofibromatosis. *Arch Neurol* 1988; **45**: 575–578.

5. Huson SM, Compston DAS, Clark P, Harper PS. A genetic study of von Recklinghausen neurofibromatosis in south east Wales. 1. Prevalence, fitness, mutation rate, and effect of parental transmission on severity. *J Med Genet* 1989; **26**: 704–711.

6. Viskochil D, Buchberg AN, Xu G, *et al.* Deletions and a translocation interrupt a cloned gene at the neurofibromatosis type 1 locus. *Cell* 1990; **62**: 1887–1892.

7. Wallace MR, Marchuk DA, Anderson LB, *et al.* Type 1 neurofibromatosis gene: indentification of a larger transcript disrupted in three NG1 patients. *Science* 1990; **249**: 181–186.

8. Gutmann DH, Wood DL, Collins FS. Identification of the neurofibromatosis 1 gene product. *Proc Natl Acad Sci USA* 1991; **88**: 9658–9662.

9. Huson SM, Harper PS, Compston DAS. Von Recklinghausen neurofibromatosis: clinical and population study in South East Wales. *Brain* 1988; **111**: 155–181.

10. Johnson MR, Ferner RE, Bobrow M, Hughes RAC. Detailed analysis of the oligodendrocyte myelin glycoprotein gene in four patients with neurofibromatosis 1 and primary progressive multiple sclerosis. *J Neurol Neurosurg Psychiatry* 2000; **8**: 643–646.

11. DeClue J, Cohen BD, Lowy DR. Identification and characterisation of the neurofibromatosis type 1 gene

product. *Proc Natl Acad Sci USA* 1991; **88**: 9914–9918.

12. Daston MM, Scrable H, Nordlund M, *et al.* The protein product of the neurofibromatosis type 1 gene is expressed at highest abundance in neurons, Schwann cells and oligodendrocytes. *Neuron* 1992; **8**: 415–428.

13. Xu GF, O'Connell P, Viskochil D, *et al.* The neurofibromatosis type 1 gene encodes a protein related to GAP. *Cell* 1990; **62**: 599–608.

14. Kimura M, Kamata Y, Matsumoto K, Takaya H. Electron microscopical study on the tumour of von Recklinghausen's neurofibromatosis. *Acta Pathol Jpn* 1974; **24**: 79–91.

15. Rutkowski JL, Wum K, Gutmannn DH, *et al.* Genetic and cellular defects contributing to benign tumour formation in neurofibromatosis type 1. *Hum Mol Genet* 2000; **9**: 1059–1066.

16. Zhu Y, Ghosh P, Charnay P, *et al.* Neurofibromas in NF1: Schwann cell origin and role of tumour environment. *Science* 2002; **296**: 920–922.

17. Sherman LS, Atit R, Rosenbaum T, Cox AD, Ratner N. Single cell RAS-GTP analysis reveals altered RAS activity in a subpopulation of neurofibroma Schwann cells but not fibroblasts. *J Biol Chem* 2000; **275**: 30740–30745.

18. Muir D. Differences in proliferation and invasion by normal, transformed and NF1 Schwann cell cultures are influenced by matrix metalloproteinase expression. *Clin Exp Metastasis* 1995; **13**: 303–314.

19. DeClue JE, Heffelfinger S, Benvenuto G, *et al.* Epidermal growth factor receptor expression in neurofibromatosis type 1-related tumors and NF1

animal models. *J Clin Invest* 2000; **105**: 1233–1241.

20. McLaughlin ME, Jacks T. Progesterone receptor expression in neurofibromas. *Cancer Res* 2003; **63**: 752–755.

21. Wolkenstein P, Zeller J, Revuz J, *et al.* Quality-of-life impairment in neurofibromatosis type 1: a cross-sectional study of 128 cases. *Arch Dermatol* 2001; **137**: 1421–1425.

22. Moreno JC, Mathoret C, Lantieri L, *et al.* Carbon dioxide laser for removal of multiple cutaneous neurofibromas. *Br J Dermatol* 2001; **144**: 1096–1098.

23. Tonsgard JH, Kwak SM, Short MP, Dachman AH. CT imaging in adults with neurofibromatosis-1: frequent asymptomatic plexiform lesions. *Neurology* 1998; **50**: 1755–1760.

24. Packer RJ, Gutmann DH, Rubenstein A, *et al.* Plexiform neurofibromas in NF1: toward biologic-based therapy. *Neurology* 2002; **58**: 1461–1470.

25. Gurujeyalakshmi G, Hollinger MA, Giri SN. Pirfenidone inhibits PDGF isoforms in bleomycin hamster model of lung fibrosis at the translational level. *Am J Physiol* 1999; **276**: L311–L318.

26. Evans DG, Baser ME, McGaughran J, *et al.* Malignant peripheral nerve sheath tumours in neurofibromatosis 1. *J Med Genet* 2002; **39**: 311–314.

27. Ferner RE, Gutmann DH. International consensus statement on malignant peripheral nerve sheath tumours in neurofibromatosis 1. *Canc Res* 2002; **62**: 1573–1577.

28. Ferner RE, Hall SM, Hughes RAC, *et al.* Neurofibromatous neuropathy in neurofibromatosis 1. *J Med Genet* 2004; **41**: 837–841.

29. De Raedt T, Brems H, Wolkenstein P, *et al.* Elevated

risk for MPNST in NF1 microdeletion patients. *Am J Hum Genet* 2003; **72**: 1288–1292.

30. Ducatman B, Scheithauer B, Piepgras D, *et al.* Malignant peripheral nerve sheath tumours: a clinicopathological study of 120 cases. *Cancer* 1986; **57**: 2006–2021.

31. Ferner R, Lucas JD, O'Doherty MJ, *et al.* Evaluation of 18-fluorodeoxyglucose positron emission tomography (18FDGPET) in the detection of malignant peripheral nerve sheath tumours arising from within plexiform neurofibromas in neurofibromatosis 1. *J Neurol Neurosur Psychiatry* 2000; **68**: 353–357.

32. Guha A, Lau N, Huvar I, *et al.* RAS-GTP levels are elevated in human peripheral nerve tumours. *Oncogene* 1996; **12**: 507–513.

33. Kourea HP, Cordon-Cardo C, Dudas M, *et al.* The emerging role of p27kip in malignant transformation of neurofibromas. *Am J Pathol* 1999; **155**: 1885–1891.

34. Nielsen GP, Stemmer-Rachamimov AO, Ino Y, *et al.* Malignant transformation of neurofibromas in neurofibromatosis 1 is associated with CDKNA/p16 inactivation. *Am J Pathol* 1999; **155**: 1879–1884.

35. Cichowski K, Shih TS, Schmitt E, *et al.* Mouse models of tumour development in neurofibromatosis type 1. *Science* 1999; **286**: 2172–2176.

36. Lisch K. Ueber beteilgung der augen, inbesondere das Vorkommen von irisknotchen bei der neurofibromatose (Recklinghausen). *Z Augenheilkd* 1936; **93**: 137–143.

37. Nichols JC, Amato JE, Chung SM. Characteristics of Lisch nodules in patients with

neurofibromatosis type 1. *J Paediatr Ophthalmol Strabismus* 2003; **40**: 293–296.

38. Friedman JM, Arbiser J, Epstein JA, *et al.* Cardiovascular disease in neurofibromatosis 1: report of the NF1 cardiovascular task force. *Genet Med* 2002; **4**: 105–111.

39. Lin AE, Birch PH, Korf B, *et al.* Cardiovascular malformations and other cardiac abnormalities in neurofibromatosis 1. *Am J Med Genet* 2000; **95**: 108–117.

40. Hough DR, Usar MC, Chan A, Davidson H. Von Recklinghausen's disease associated with gastrointestinal carcinoid tumours. *Cancer* 1983; **51**: 2206–2208.

41. Phat VN, Sezzzeur A, Danne M. Primary myenteric plexus alterations as a cause of megacolon in von Recklinghausen's disease. *Pathol Biol* 1980; **28**: 585–588.

42. Stephens M, Williams GT, Jasani B, Williams ED. Synchronous duodenal neuroendocrine tumours in von Recklinghausen disease. A case report of co-existing paraganglioma and somatostatin-rich glandular carcinoid. *Histopathology* 1987; **11**: 1331–1340.

43. Kuorilehto T, Poyhonen M, Bloigu R, *et al.* Decreased bone mineral density and content in neurofibromatosis type 1: lowest local values are located in the load-carrying parts of the body. *Osteoporosis Int* 2005; **16**: 928–936.

44. Jacobsen ST, Crawford AH, Millar EA, Steel HH. The Syme amputation in patients with congenital pseudoarthrosis of the tibia. *J Bone Joint Surg* 1983; **65**: 533–537.

45. Crawford AH Jr, Bagamery N. Osseous manifestations of neurofibromatosis in childhood. *J Pediatr Orthop* 1986; **6**: 72–88.

46. Guillamo JS, Créange A, Kalifa C, *et al.* Prognostic factors of CNS tumours in neurofibromatosis 1 (NF1): a retrospective study of 104 patients. *Brain* 2003; **126**: 152–160.

47. Pollack IF, Shultz B, Mulvihill JJ. The management of brainstem gliomas in patients with neurofibromatosis 1. *Neurology* 1996; **46**: 1652–1660.

48. Créange A, Zeller J, Rostaing-Rigattieri S, *et al.* Neurological complications of neurofibromatosis type 1 in adulthood. *Brain* 1999; **122**: 473–481.

49. Gutmann DH, James CD, Poyhonen M, *et al.* Molecular analysis of astrocytomas presenting after age 10 in individuals with NF1. *Neurology* 2003; **61**: 1397–1400.

50. Lewis RA, Gerson LP, Axelson KA, *et al.* Von Recklinghausen neurofibromatosis. II. Incidence of optic gliomata. *Ophthalmology* 1984; **91**: 929–935.

51. Listernick R, Ferner RE, Piersall L, *et al.* Late-onset optic pathway tumors in children with neurofibromatosis 1. *Neurology* 2004; **63**: 1944–1946.

52. Packer RJ, Alter J, Allen J, *et al.* Carboplatin and vincristine chemotherapy for children with newly diagnosed progressive low-grade gliomas. *J Neurosurg* 1997; **86**: 747–754.

53. Listernick R, Charrow J, Tomita T, Goldman S. Carboplatin therapy for optic pathway tumors in children with neurofibromatosis type-1. *J Neurooncol* 1999; **45**: 185–190.

54. Zochodne D. Von Recklinghausen's vasculopathy. *Am J Med Sci* 1984; **287**: 64–65.

55. Sasaki J, Miura S, Kikuchi K. Neurofibromatosis associated with multiple intracranial vascular lesions, stenosis of the internal carotid artery and peripheral aneurysm of the Heubner's artery: report of a case. *Neurol Surg* 1995; **23**: 813–817.

56. Ferner RE, Hughes RAC, Johnson MR. Neurofibromatosis 1 and multiple sclerosis. *J Neurol Neurosurg Psychiatry* 1995; **56**: 492–495.

57. Johnson MR, Ferner RE, Bobrow M, Hughes RA. Detailed analysis of the oligodendrocyte myelin glycoprotein gene in four patients with neurofibromatosis 1 and primary progressive multiple sclerosis. *J Neurol Neurosurg Psychiatry* 2000; **68**: 643–646.

58. Rosman NP, Pearce J. The brain in multiple neurofibromatosis (von Recklinghausen's disease): a suggested neuropathological basis for the associated mental defect. *Brain* 1967; **90**: 829–838.

59. Vivarelli R, Grosso S, Calabrese F, *et al.* Epilepsy in neurofibromatosis 1. *J Child Neurol* 2003; **18**: 338–342.

60. Ferner RE, Hughes RAC, Weinman J. Intellectual impairment in neurofibromatosis 1. *J Neurol Sci* 1996; **138**: 125–133.

61. North KN, Riccardi V, Samango-Sprouse C, *et al.* Cognitive function and academic performance in neurofibromatosis. 1: consensus statement from the NF1 Cognitive Disorders Task Force. *Neurology* 1997; **48**: 1121–1127.

62. Hyman SL, Gill DS, Shores EA, *et al.* Natural history of cognitive deficits and their relationship to MRI T2-hyperintensities in NF1. *Neurology* 2003; **60**: 1139–1145.

63. Lorch M, Ferner R, Golding J, Whurr R. The nature of speech and language impairment in adults with neurofibromatosis 1. *J Neurolinguistics* 1999; **12**: 167–165.

64. Prinzie P, Descheemaeker MJ, Vogels A, *et al.* Personality profiles of children and adolescents with neurofibromatosis type 1. *Am J Med Genet* 2003; **118A**: 1–7.

65. Bognanno JR, Edwards MK, Lee TA, *et al.* Cranial MR imaging in neurofibromatosis. *Am J Radiol* 1988; **151**: 381–388.

66. Ferner RE, Chaudhuri Bingham J, Cox T, Hughes RAC. MRI in neurofibromatosis 1. The nature and evolution of increased intensity T2 weighted lesions and their relationship to intellectual impairment. *J Neurol Neurosurg Psychiatry* 1993; **56**: 492–495.

67. DiPaolo DP, Zimmerman RA, Rorke LB, *et al.* Neurofibromatosis type 1: pathologic substrate of high-signal-intensity foci in the brain. *Radiology* 1995; **195**: 721–724.

68. Denckla MB, Hofman K, Mazzocco MM, *et al.* Relationship between T2 weighted hyperintensities (unidentified bright objects) and lower IQs in children with neurofibromatosis type 1. *Am J Med Genet* 1996; **67**: 98–102.

69. Feldmann R, Denecke J, Grenzebachm M, *et al.* Neurofibromatosis 1: motor and cognitive function and T2-weighted MRI hyperintensities. *Neurology* 2003; **61**: 1725–1728.

70. Legius E, Descheemaeker MJ, Steyaert J, *et al.* Neurofibromatosis type 1 in childhood: correlation of MRI findings with intelligence. *J Neurol Neurosurg Pschyiatry* 1995; **59**: 638–640.

71. Costa RM, Federov NB, Kogan JH, *et al.* Mechanisms for the learning deficits in a mouse model of neurofibromatosis 1. *Nature* 2002; **415**: 526–530.

72. Thomas PK, King RH, Chiang TR, *et al.* Neurofibromatous neuropathy. *Muscle Nerve* 1990; **13**: 93–101.

73. Messiaen LM, Callens T, Mortier G, *et al.* Exhaustive mutation analysis of the NF1 gene allows identification of 95% of mutations and reveals a high frequency of unusual splicing defects. *Hum Mutat* 2000; **15**: 541–555.

74. Ruggieri M, Huson SM. The clinical and diagnostic implications of mosaicism in the neurofibromatoses. *J Neurol* 2001; **56**: 1433–1443.

75. Easton DF, Ponder MA, Huson SM, Ponder BA. An analysis of variation in expression of neurofibromatosis type 1 (NF1): evidence for modifying genes. *Am J Hum Genet* 1993; **53**: 305–313.

76. Castle B, Baser ME, Huson SM, *et al.* Evaluation of genotype-phenotype correlations in neurofibromatosis type 1. *J Med Genet* 2003; **40**: e109.

77. Rouleau G, Merel P, Lutchman M, *et al.* Alteration in a new gene encoding a putative membrane – organising protein causes neurofibromatosis type 2. *Nature* 1993; **363**: 515–521.

78. Trofatter J, Maccollin MM, Rutter JL, *et al.* A novel moesin-, esrin-, radixin-like gene is a candidate for the neurofibromatosis 2 tumour suppressor. *Cell* 1993; **72**: 791–800.

79. Wiestler OD, Radner H. Pathology of neurofibromatosis 1 and 2. In Huson SM, Hughes RAC, eds. *The Neurofibromatoses: A Pathogenetic and Clinical Overview.* Cambridge, UK: Chapman and Hall, 1994; 135–160.

80. Ferner RE, O'Doherty MJ. Neurofibroma and schwannoma. *Curr Opin Neurol* 2002; **15**: 679–684.

81. Antinheimo J, Sankila R, Carpen O, *et al.* Population-based analysis of sporadic and type 2 neurofibromatosis-associated meningiomas and schwannomas. *Neurology* 2000; **54**: 71–76.

82. MacCollin M, Chiocca EA, Evans DG, *et al.* Diagnostic criteria for schwannomatosis. *Neurology* 2005; **64**: 1838–1845.

83. Wishart JH. Case of tumours in the skull, dura mater, and brain. *Edinburgh Med Surg J* 1822; **18**: 393–397.

84. National Institutes of Health Consensus Development Conference Statement. Acoustic Neuroma. *Neurofibromatosis Res Newsletter* 1992; **8**: 1–17.

85. Evans DGR, Huson SM, Donnai D, *et al.* A clinical study of type 2 neurofibromatosis. *Q J Med* 1992; **84**: 603–618.

86. Nunes F, MacCollin M. Neurofibromatosis 2 in the pediatric population. *J Child Neurol* 2003; **18**: 718–724.

87. Baser ME, Friedman JM, Wallace AJ, *et al.* Evaluation of clinical diagnostic criteria for neurofibromatosis 2. *Neurology* 2002; **59**: 1759–1765.

88. Evans DGR, Huson SM, Donnai D, *et al.* A genetic study of type 2 neurofibromatosis in the United Kingdom. 1. Prevalence, mutation rate, fitness, and confirmation of maternal transmission effect on severity. *J Med Genet* 1992; **29**: 841–846.

89. Baser ME, Erini V, Makariou MD, *et al.* Predictors of vestibular schwannoma growth in patients with neurofibromatosis type 2. *J Neurosurg* 2002; **96**: 217–222.

90. Mautner FM, Baser ME, Sarang D, *et al.* Vestibular schwannoma growth in patients with neurofibromatosis type 2: a longitudinal study. *J Neurosurg* 2002; **96**: 223–228.

91. Brackmann DE, Fayad JN, Slattery WH, *et al.* Early proactive management of vestibular schwannomas in

225

neurofibormatosis type 2. *Neurosurgery* 2001; **49**: 274–280.

92. Baser ME, Evans DGR, Gutmann DH. Neurofibromatosis 2. *Curr Opin Neurol* 2003; **16**: 27–33.

93. Rowe JG, Radatz MW, Walton L, *et al.* Clinical experience with gamma knife stereotactic radiosurgery in the management of vestibular schwannomas secondary to type 2 neurofibromatosis. *J Neurol Neurosurg Psychiatry* 2003; **9**: 1288–1293.

94. Thomsen J, Mirz F, Wetke R, *et al.* Intracranial sarcoma in a patient with neurofibromatosis type 2 treated with gamma knife radiosurgery for vestibular schwannoma. *Am J Otol* 2000; **21**: 364–370.

95. Mautner VF, Lindenau M, Baser ME, *et al.* The neuroimaging and clinical spectrum of neurofibromatosis 2. *Neurosurgery* 1996; **38**: 880–885.

96. Sperfeld AD, Hein C, Schroder JM, *et al.* Occurrence and characterisation of peripheral nerve involvement in neurofibromatosis type 2. *Brain* 2002; **125**: 996–1004.

97. Ragge NK, Baser ME, Klein J, *et al.* Ocular abnormalities in neurofibromatosis 2. *Am J Ophthalmol* 1995; **120**: 634–641.

98. Evans DG, Wallace AJ, Wu CL, *et al.* Somatic mosaicism: a common cause of classic disease in tumour-prone syndromes? Lessons from type 2 neurofibromatosis. *Am J Hum Genet* 1998; **63**: 727–736.

99. MacCollin M, Ramesh V, Jacoby LB, *et al.* Mutational analysis of patients with neurofibromatosis 2. *Am J Hum Genet* 1994; **55**: 314–320.

100. Kluwe L, Mautner V, Heinrich B, *et al.* Molecular study of frequency of mosaicism in neurofibromatosis 2 patients with bilateral vestibular schwannomas. *J Med Genet* 2003; **40**: 109–114.

101. Evans DG, Trueman L, Wallace A, *et al.* Genotype/phenotype correlations in type 2 neurofibromatosis (NF2): evidence for more severe disease associated with truncating mutations [published erratum in *J Med Genet* 1999; **36**: 87]. *J Med Genet* 1998; **35**: 450–455.

102. Ruttledge MH, Andermann AA, Phelan CM, *et al.* Type of mutation in the neurofibromatosis type 2 gene (NF2) frequently determines severity of disease. *Am J Hum Genet* 1996; **59**: 331–342.

103. Kluwe L, MacCollin M, Tatagiba M, *et al.* Phenotypic variability associated with 14 splice-site mutations in the NF2 gene. *Am J Med Genet* 1998; **77**: 228–233.

104. Baser ME, Ragge NK, Riccardi VM, *et al.* Phenotypic variability in monozygotic twins with neurofibromatosis 2. *Am J Med Genet* 1996; **64**: 563–567.

105. Patronas NJ, Courcoutsakis N, Bromley CM, *et al.* Intramedullary and spinal canal tumors in patients with neurofibromatosis 2: MR imaging findings and correlation with genotype. *Radiology* 2001; **218**: 434–442.

106. Baser ME, Kuramoto L, Joe H, *et al.* Genotype-phenotype correlations for cataracts in neurofibromatosis 2. *J Med Genet* 2003; **40**: 758–760.

107. Baser ME, Friedmanm JM, Aeschliman D, *et al.* Predictors of the risk of mortality in neurofibromatosis 2. *Am J Hum Genet* 2002; **71**: 715–723.

108. Tsukita S, Yonemura S, Tsukita S. ERM family: from cytoskeleton to signal transduction. *Curr Opin Cell Biol* 1997; **9**: 70–75.

109. Claudio JO, Veneziale RW, Menko AS, Rouleau GA. Expression of schwannomin in lens and Schwann cells. *Neuroreport* 1997; **8**: 2025–2030.

110. Sherman L, Xu H-M, Geist RT, *et al.* Interdomain binding mediates tumour growth suppression by the NF2 gene product. *Oncogene* 1997; **15**: 2505–2509.

111. Xu H-M, Gutmann DH. Merlin differentially associates with microtubule and actin cytoskeleton. *J Neurosci Res* 1998; **51**: 403–415.

112. Morrison H, Sherman L/S, Legg J, *et al.* The NF2 tumour suppressor gene product, merlin, mediates contact inhibition of growth through interactions with CD44. *Genes Dev* 2001; **15**: 968–980.

113. Giovannini M, Robanus-Maandag E, Niwa-Kawakita M, *et al.* Schwann cell hyperplasia and tumours in transgenic mice expressing a naturally occurring mutant NF2 protein. *Genes Dev* 1999; **13**: 978–986.

114. Kalamarides M, Niwa-Kawakita M, Leblois H, *et al.* NF2 gene inactivation in arachnoidal cells is rate-limiting for meningioma development in the mouse. *Genes Dev* 2002; **16**: 1060–1065.

115. Davison C, Brock S, Dyke CG. Retinal and central nervous hemangioblastomatosis with visceral changes (von Hippel–Lindau's disease). *Bull Neurol Instit New York* 1936; **5**: 72–93.

116. Lonser RR, Glenn GM, McClellan W, *et al.* Von Hippel Lindau disease. *Lancet* 2003; **361**: 2059–2067.

117. Von Hippel E. Uber eine sehr seltene Erkrankung der Netzhaut. Klinische Beobachtungen. *A von Graefes Arch Ophthalmol* 1904; **59**: 83–106.

118. Von Hippel E. Die anatomische Grundlage der von mir beschriebenen "sehr seltene Erkrankung der Netzhaut." *A von Graefes Arch Ophthalmol* 1911; **79**: 350–377.

119. Brandt R. Zur frage der angioatosis retinae. *A von Graefes Arch Ophthalmol* 1921; **106**: 127–165.

120. Lindau A. Studien uber Kleinhirnzystern. Bau, Pathogenese und Beziehungen zur Angiomatosis retinae. *Acta Pathol Microbiol Scand* 1926; **S1**: 1–28.

121. Maher ER, Yates JR, Harries R, *et al.* Clinical features and natural history of von Hippel–Lindau disease. *Q J Med* 1990; 77: 1151–1163.

122. Walther MM, Lubensky IA, Venzon D, *et al.* Prevalence of microscopic lesions in grossly normal renal parenchyma from patients with von Hippel–Lindau disease, sporadic renal cell carcinoma and no renal disease: clinical implicatons. *J Urol* 1995; **154**: 2010–2014.

123. Walther MM, Reiter R, Keiser HR, *et al.* Clinical and genetic characterisation of phaeochromocytoma in von Hippel–Lindau families: comparison with sporadic phaeochromocytoma gives insight into natural history of phaeochromocytoma. *J Urol* 1999; **162**: 659–664.

124. Neumann HP, Dinkel E, Brambs H, *et al.* Pancreatic lesions in the von Hippel–Lindau syndrome. *Gastroenterology* 1991; **101**: 465–471.

125. Melman KL, Rose SW. Lindau's disease. *Am J Med* 1964; **36**: 595–617.

126. Dollfus H, Massin P, Taupin P, *et al.* Retinal hemangioblastoma in von Hippel–Lindau disease: a clinical and molecular study. *Invest Ophthalmol Vis Sci* 2002; **43**: 3067–3074.

127. Aiello DJ, George DJ, Cahill MT, *et al.* Rapid and durable recovery of visual function in a patient with von Hippel–Lindau syndrome after systemic therapy with vascular endothelial growth factor receptor inhibitor su5416. *Ophthalmology* 2002; **109**: 1745–1751.

128. Lonser RR, Kim HJ, Butman JA, *et al.* Tumours of the endolymphatic sac in von Hippel–Lindau disease. *N Engl J Med* 2004; **350**: 2481–2486.

129. Wanebo JE, Lonser RR, Glenn GM, Oldfield EH. The natural history of central nervous system haemangioblastomas in patients with von Hippel–Lindau disease. *J Neurosurg* 2003; **98**: 82–94.

130. Choyke PL, Glenn GM, Walther MM, *et al.* Von Hippel–Lindau disease: genetic, clinical, and imaging features. *Radiology* 1995; **194**: 629–642.

131. Maher ER, Iselius L, Yates JR, *et al.* Von Hippel–Lindau disease: a genetic study. *J Med Genet* 1991; **28**: 443–447.

132. Sgambati MT, Stolle C, Choyke PL, *et al.* Mosaicism in von Hippel–Lindau disease: lessons from kindreds with germline mutations identified in offspring with mosaic parents. *Am J Med Genet* 2000; **66**: 84–91.

133. Latif K, Tory J, Gnarra J, *et al.* Identification of the von Hippel–Lindau disease tumour suppressor gene. *Science* 1993; **260**: 1317–1320.

134. Stolle C, Glenn G, Zbar B, *et al.* Improved detection of germline mutations in the von Hippel–Lindau disease tumor suppressor gene. *Hum Mutat* 1998; **12**: 417–423.

135. Gnarra R, Tory K, Weng Y, *et al.* Mutations of the VHL tumour suppressor gene in renal carcinoma. *Nat Genet* 1994; 7: 85–90.

136. Kanno H, Kondo K, Ito S, *et al.* Somatic mutations of the von Hippel–Lindau tumour suppressor gene in sporadic central nervous system hemangioblastomas. *Cancer Res* 1994; **54**: 4845–4847.

137. Lee JY, Dong SM, Park WS, *et al.* Loss of heterozygosity and somatic mutations of the VHL tumour suppressor gene in sporadic cerebellar hemangioblastomas. *Cancer Res* 1998; **58**: 504–508.

138. Kondo K, Yao M, Yoshida M, *et al.* Comprehensive mutational analysis of the VHL gene in sporadic renal cell carcinoma: relationship to clinicopathological parameters. *Genes Chromosomes Cancer* 2002; **34**: 58–68.

139. Lee DY, Chen JS, Humphrey JR, *et al.* Nuclear/cytoplasmic localization of the von Hippel–Lindau tumour suppressor gene product is determined by cell density. *Proc Natl Acad Sci USA* 1996; **93**: 1770–1775.

140. Ohh M, Kaelin GW Jr. The von Hippel–Lindau tumour suppressor protein: new perspectives. *Mol Med Today* 1999; **5**: 257–263.

141. Duan DR, Pause A, Burgess WH, *et al.* Inhibition of transcription elongation by the VHL tumor suppressor protein. *Science* 1995; **269**: 1402–1406.

142. Kaelin WG Jr, Maher ER. The VHL tumour-suppressor gene paradigm. *Trends Genet* 1998; **14**: 423–426.

143. Pause A, Lee S, Worrell RA, *et al.* The von Hippel–Lindau tumor-suppressor gene product forms a stable complex with human CUL-2, a member of the Cdc53 family of proteins. *Proc Natl Acad Sci USA* 1997; **94**: 2156–2161.

144. Patton EE, Willems AR, Tyers M. Combinatorial control in ubiquitin-dependent proteolysis:

don't Skp the F-box hypothesis. *Trends Genet* 1998; **14**: 236–243.

145. Gnarra JR, Zhou S, Merrill MJ, *et al.* Post-transcriptional regulation of vascular endothelial growth factor mRNA by the product of the VHL tumor suppressor gene. *Proc Nat Acad of Sci USA* 1996; **93**: 10589–10594.

146. Mukhopadhyay D, Knebelmann B, Cohen HT, *et al.* The von Hippel–Lindau tumor suppressor gene product interacts with Sp1 to repress vascular endothelial growth factor promoter activity. *Mol Cell Biol* 1997; **17**: 5629–5639.

147. Ohh M, Yauch RL, Lonergan KM, *et al.* The von Hippel-Lindau tumour suppressor protein is required for proper assembly of an extracellular fibronectin matrix. *Mol Cell* 1998; **1**: 959–968.

148. Chen F, Kishida T, Yao M, *et al.* Germline mutations in the von Hippel-Lindau disease tumour suppressor gene: correlations with phenotype. *Hum Mutat* 1995; **5**: 66–75.

149. Zbar B, Kishida F, Chen F, *et al.* Germline mutations in the Von Hippel-Lindau disease gene in families from North America, Europe and Japan. *Hum Mutat* 1996; **8**: 348–357.

Chapter 15

The future of neurogenetics

Thomas D. Bird

Predicting the future can be viewed as both foolish and dangerous, but we all like to do it from time to time. In 1865, Jules Verne wrote a fantasy predicting travel to the moon and it became reality little more than 100 years later. To predict where we are going, it should be helpful to review where we have been. I have chosen to look back over the past 50-plus years of neurogenetics and then guess where those accomplishments might lead in the next 50 years.

Table 15.1 lists a personal and idiosyncratic view of important accomplishments in neurogenetics between 1953 and 2009. The year 1953 is an auspicious date because it coincides with the publication of the Watson and Crick model of the DNA double helix. That same year saw the identification of the biochemical defect in phenylketonuria (PKU). Research related to neurogenetic disorders in the 1950s and 1960s focused on understanding the chemical basis of metabolic disorders such as PKU and lipid storage diseases and the identification of chromosomal aberrations such as trisomy 21 in Down syndrome. The 1970s saw the advent of a few successful genetic linkage studies related to neurogenetic disorders such as myotonic dystrophy, hereditary ataxia, and Charcot–Marie–Tooth neuropathy, but these studies were severely limited by the small number of available blood markers known to have chromosomal assignments. The advent of DNA-based markers, such as restriction fragment length polymorphisms (RFLP), in the early 1980s led to a flurry of positive genetic linkage studies epitomized by the assignment of the Huntington's disease (HD) gene to chromosome 4p in 1983. The identification of regional chromosomal assignments of multiple disease genes then led naturally to the discovery and cloning of the relevant genes in the 1980s and 1990s. This included the unexpected discovery of the fascinating phenomenon of nucleotide repeat expansion disorders and diseases of the peripheral and central nervous system associated with duplication or even triplication of the underlying gene. Genome-wide association (GWA) studies looking for genetic risk-factors for complex and polygenic neurogenetic disorders have proven to be a more difficult task, but the association of Apo E4 with Alzheimer's disease (AD) remains a model for future studies. Recent positive GWA studies of stroke, amyotropic lateral sclerosis (ALS), multiple sclerosis (MS), autism, Parkinson's disease (PD) and AD have begun to provide an extensive new list of genes potentially involved in the pathogenesis of these common disorders.

An obvious result of all of this work has been the dramatic realization of the magnitude of genetic heterogeneity underlying all diseases including those of the nervous system. The continuing multiplication of subtypes of hereditary neuropathy and ataxia are prominent examples of this phenomenon. Another consistent and related theme is the discovery that single-gene Mendelian causes of common disorders such as AD and PD have been found to represent only a small fraction of the larger disease population, but provide critical information for understanding the underlying biology and biochemistry (e.g. the central roles of amyloid, tau, and α-synuclein).

It should be pointed out that the advances in neurogenetics over the past 50 years have been intimately tied to the advances in both laboratory technology and basic molecular science. This includes the discovery of the DNA double helix and breaking of the genetic code followed by the use of improved DNA-based markers for linkage studies, the polymerase chain reaction (PCR) technology, the development of highly efficient and time-saving laboratory robotic machines, and new computer technology all culminating in the completion of the human genome project in 2000. Transgenic animal research, especially with mice and drosophila, has also contributed a great deal.

Looking back on the past 50 years, it is clear that we have been highly successful in locating and

Table 15.1. The past 50+ years of neurogenetics

(1953–2009)	
1950s and 1960s	
1953	Identification of the biochemical defect in phenylketonuria (PKU)
1958	Identification of sulfatide excess in metachromatic leukodystrophy (MLD)
1959	Identification of trisomy 21 as the cause of Down syndrome
1962	Identification of GM_2 storage in Tay–Sachs disease
1963	Identification of arylsulfatase A deficiency in MLD
1970s	
1971	Myotonic dystrophy linked to Lutheran and ABH secretor markers
1976	Treatment of dopa-responsive dystonia
1977	SCA1 linked to HLA on 6p
1980s	
1980	CMT1B linked to Fy on 1q
1983	Huntington's disease (HD) linked to RFLP markers on 4p
1985	Duchenne muscular dystrophy and NFI genes identified
1988	Mitochondrial mutations in neurological disease
1989	Prion gene mutations in familial Creutzfeldt–Jakob disease (CJD)
1990s	
1990	Channelopathy gene identified: hyper-K periodic paralysis
1991	Mutations in APP found in early onset familial Alzheimer's disease (AD)
	Duplication of PMP22 found in CMT1A
	Trinucleotide repeat diseases discovered: XLSBMA, FRAX
1993	Discovery of HD gene
	Identification of SOD1 mutation in familial amyotropic lateral sclerosis (ALS)
1995	Apo E4 association with AD
	PS1/PS2 mutations found in early onset AD
	CHRNA4 mutations in nocturnal frontal lobe epilepsy
1997	α-synuclein mutations found in familial Parkinson's disease (PD)
1998	tau mutations found in frontotemporal dementia (FTD); parkin mutations found in familial PD
1999	Identification of genetic defect in Rett syndrome
1999–2006	Enzyme replacement therapy for Pompe's glycogen storage disease
2000s	
2000	Completion of the Human Genome Project
2001	Aberrant regulation of splicing described in DM1 GFAP mutations in Alexander disease
2002	Attempt to treat AD with β-amyloid vaccination
2003	α-synuclein triplication found in familial PD
2006	Progranulin (GRN) mutations in FTD
2008	TARDBP (TDP43) mutations in ALS
2007–2009	Successful genome-wide association (GWA) of stroke, multiple sclerosis, autism, ALS, PD, AD

identifying disease causing genes and in discovering the chemicals and proteins involved in disease pathogenesis. However, we are still left with many genes the protein products of which are unclear and many proteins the normal and abnormal functions of which are largely unknown. A major thrust of future research obviously will be a better understanding of the normal function of these proteins, how they interact with one another, how their aberrations lead to cell dysfunction, and finally and most importantly, how this knowledge will lead to treatment, reversal, and prevention of these diseases.

Table 15.2 reveals personal insights from viewing a neurogenetic crystal ball and gazing 50 years into the future of neurogenetic research. The table is divided into six major sections. The first section relates to gene discovery, which has been so elegantly begun in the past two decades. There are many more genes to be discovered, which are related to diseases of the nervous system, and the identification of more than 2000 such genes and their related diseases is certainly feasible.

The second section relates to an improved understanding of the basic genetic mechanisms underlying neurogenetic diseases. A critical issue is the selective neuronal vulnerability that is apparent in so many neurogenetic disorders. For example, why does the huntingtin gene primarily select medium spiny neurons in the striatum for destruction, whereas ataxin 1 is focused on Purkinje cells in the cerebellum? We will gain a better understanding of how chromatin and other epigenetic factors influence the regulation of gene expression. There will be clarification of the genetic control of early development of the nervous system including factors determining cell fate and migration of cells to their appropriate positions in the brain, spinal cord, and nerves. Complex neurogenetic diseases such as AD, PD, MS, epilepsy, and stroke are widely regarded as resulting from the interaction of multiple genes (polygenic) with many environmental factors (multifactoral). For example, in AD there will be a better understanding of the interplay between aggregation of amyloid and tau proteins, aging of the nervous system, and environmental factors such as head trauma and cognitive stimulation. A common theme in several neurogenetic disorders of the brain has proven to be protein aggregation in such diseases as AD, PD, HD, the spinocerebellar ataxias (SCA), and familial Creutzfeldt–Jakob disease (CJD). The relationship of these aggregates to neuronal dysfunction and death will be clarified.

The third section deals with clinical diagnostic genetic testing. In the past decade, neurology has been in the forefront of studying diseases for which genetic testing has become commercially available. These tests represent powerful tools for diagnosis, classification, and identification of asymptomatic gene mutation carriers. The future will see the development of hundreds of additional DNA-based genetic tests. Most important, this testing will become less expensive, faster, and more readily available to practicing neurologists. These techniques will also be used to expand the field of preimplantation diagnosis of neurogenetic diseases, which is proving to be a highly attractive alternative to parents whose children are at risk for these disorders. To be more readily utilized, this technology will acquire improved efficiency and lower cost.

This identification of neurogenetic diseases by mutations in the relevant genes will result in new systems of classification or nosology. New ways of thinking about how we name diseases will be forced upon us by the knowledge that mutations in the same gene can produce several different phenotypes, and the same phenotype can be caused by mutations in different genes. New classifications will also be needed simply because of the shear unattractiveness of assigning endless numbers to different diseases (e.g. SCA1, 2, 3, 4, 5, 6, 7, etc.).

The fourth section deals with the treatment of neurogenetic diseases. The genetic revolution of the past 20 years has raised the expectations of the public for the successful treatment and prevention of hereditary diseases. These expectations have led to an unfortunate degree of urgency and impatience. However, although slow to emerge, such treatments are bound to come. It should be noted that discovery of effective treatment does not require complete understanding of pathogenesis (e.g. anticonvulsants for epilepsy, L-DOPA for PD and dopa-responsive dystonia). However, new therapies are likely to be tied to a better understanding of basic molecular mechanisms in the pathogenesis of these diseases, as mentioned previously. The treatments may be drugs targeted at the dysfunctional proteins, or dietary manipulations such as those already used effectively for diseases such as PKU, and vitamin E and pyridoxine deficiencies. It is also likely that drugs will be tailored to the individual patient's genotype. Slow and rapid metabolizers of various drugs will be identified and specific drugs will be used to treat specific genetic subtypes of diseases. In addition, this should lead to the early intervention and prevention of neurogenetic disorders by identifying gene mutation carriers in the presymptomatic stages of their diseases. There is now evidence that neurodegenerative disorders that once were thought of as irreversible may be capable of being reversed to a healthier state. The reversal of amyloid pathology in the transgenic mouse model of AD by β-amyloid vaccination is a model of this therapeutic approach, although it has not yet been proven to be safe in

Table 15.2. The next 50 years of human neurogenetics

(2010–2060)

1. Gene discovery
   - More than 2000 genes associated with common and rare diseases of the central and peripheral nervous system will be identified

2. Basic disease mechanisms: better understanding of
   - Selective neuronal vulnerability
   - Protein aggregation diseases
   - Influence of chromatin and epigenetic phenomena
   - Genetic factors in embryological development of the brain and nerves
   - Polygenic factors resulting in complex diseases
   - Gene/environment interactions
   - Role of glial cells in genetic diseases

3. Diagnostic genetic testing
   - More tests
   - Better availability
   - Less expensive
   - Greater use of preimplantation diagnosis
   - New systems of disease classification

4. Treatments
   - Effective treatment for neurogenetic disease
     - drugs
     - diets
     - stem cells
     - altered genes
   - Treatments tailored to genotype
   - Reversal of neurodegenerative diseases
   - Treatment delivery to affected cells
     - neurons
     - glia
     - nerves
     - muscles
   - Prevention and early intervention in mutation carriers

5. Neurogenetic healthcare providers
   - Education of the public
   - Education of physicians and other providers
   - Neurogenetics as a subspecialty
   - Need for genetic counselors

6. Neurogenetics and behavior
   - Better understanding of the genetic control of
     - Language
     - Mood (e.g. depression, bipolar)
     - Schizophrenia
     - Cognition/intellect
     - Addiction
     - Violence

humans. The removal of other intraneuronal protein aggregates (such as ataxins, Lewy bodies, and huntingtin) may also be feasible by manipulation of chaperons, heat shock proteins, or the proteosome complex. Stem cells may be used to alter disease progression, as has been demonstrated in mouse models of leukodystrophy. Altered genes may be introduced directly into the nuclei of diseased cells to redirect metabolism into more normal pathways. Abnormal genetic programs within the cell may be corrected by the use of RNA interference technology.

The fifth section relates to healthcare providers and the field of neurogenetic diseases. Because genetic diseases of the nervous system are of such major social importance, it is critical that the general public be educated about these diseases and appreciates the critical role of the scientific method in understanding and eventually treating these disorders. General physicians and related healthcare providers should be trained in the basic principals of medical genetics, which must include neurogenetics. This is especially important with regard to genetic factors in common neurological diseases such as AD, PD, stroke, migraine, peripheral neuropathy, and MS. Neurogenetic training will be especially important for tomorrow's clinical neurologists. Particularly, they must become competent in neurogenetic diagnosis, testing, and test interpretation. However, the field of neurogenetics is too complex to be mastered by general physicians or even neurologists. Therefore, there is likely to be a role for neurologists who have had detailed and focused training in neurogenetics and will call themselves clinical neurogeneticists. Medicine has become so super-subspecialized that many clinical neurogeneticists will probably specialize further in specific groups of diseases such as genetic myopathies or movement disorders. In addition, there should be an expanding role for genetic counselors, persons specifically trained to educate patients and families about genetic diseases. Neurogenetics is such a large and complex field that it would make sense for a subgroup of genetic counselors to focus on neuro-genetic diseases.

The sixth section predicts a better understanding of the genetic control of human behavior. This is a highly controversial topic that includes identifying genetic factors underlying language, mood, cognition/intellect, addictive behavior, and violence. This category also includes psychiatric diseases of the brain such as schizophrenia, depression, and bipolar disease. That such genetic factors exist is undeniable. Their pursuit must be accomplished in a thoughtful and ethical manner that preserves human dignity and privacy. Recognizing that our genetic background plays an important role in these human behaviors should not ignore the recognition that environmental and social factors are also clearly involved. The nature versus nurture argument is simplistic and unproductive. Identifying both kinds of influences and understanding their interactions will pave the way for improvement in some of the most basic activities of human life. An optimist can look back on the past 50 years of neuro-genetic research and eagerly anticipate an equally pro-ductive future filled with impressive advances and delightful surprises.

Index

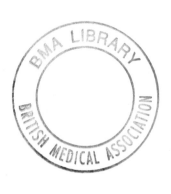

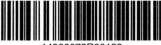
Printed in Great Britain
by Amazon.co.uk, Ltd.,
Marston Gate.